D1514968

DUE DATE	RETURN DATE	DUE DATE	RETURN DATE

Current Topics in Microbiology

110 and Immunology

The Molecular Biology of Adenoviruses 2

30 Years of Adenovirus Research 1953–1983

Edited by Walter Doerfler

With 49 Figures

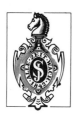

Springer-Verlag
Berlin Heidelberg New York Tokyo 1984

Professor Dr. Walter Doerfler
Institut für Genetik
der Universität zu Köln
Weyertal 121
D-5000 Köln 41

ISBN 3-540-13127-2 Springer-Verlag Berlin Heidelberg New York Tokyo
ISBN 0-387-13127-2 Springer-Verlag New York Heidelberg Berlin Tokyo

© by Springer-Verlag Berlin Heidelberg 1984
Library of Congress Catalog Card Number 15-12910
Printed in Germany.

Typesetting, printing and bookbinding:
Universitätsdruckerei H. Stürtz AG, Würzburg
2123/3130-543210

Table of Contents

Indexed in Current Contents

List of Contributors

BERNARDS, R., Department of Medical Chemistry, Sylvius Laboratories, Wassenaarseweg 72, NL-2333 AL Leiden

COOK, J.L., Department of Medicine, National Jewish Hospital and Research Center, Denver, CD 80206, USA

FIELD, J., Departments of Developmental Biology and Cancer, Albert Einstein College of Medicine, Bronx, NY 10461, USA

FRIEFELD, B.R., Departments of Cell Biology, Albert Einstein College of Medicine, Bronx, NY 10461, USA

FUJINAGA, K., Department of Molecular Biology, Cancer Research Institute, Sapporo Medical College, S-1, W-17, Chuo-ku, Sapporo 060, Japan

GALIBERT, F., Laboratory of Experimental Hematology, Centre Hayem, Hôpital St-Louis, F-Paris

GRONOSTAJSKI, R.M., Departments of Developmental Biology and Cancer, Albert Einstein, College of Medicine, Bronx, NY 10461, USA

GUGGENHEIMER, R.A., Departments of Developmental Biology and Cancer, Albert Einstein College of Medicine, Bronx, NY 10461, USA

HORWITZ, M.S., Departments of Cell Biology, Microbiology and Immunology, Pediatrics, Albert Einstein College of Medicine, Bronx, NY 10461, USA

HURWITZ, J., Departments of Developmental Biology and Cancer, Albert Einstein College of Medicine, Bronx, NY 10461, USA

KREVOLIN, M.D., Departments of Microbiology and Immunology, Albert Einstein College of Medicine, Bronx, NY 10461, USA

LEVINE, A.J., State University of New York at Stony Brook, School of Medicine, Department of Microbiology, Stony Brook, NY 11794, USA

LEWIS, A.M., Jr., Laboratory of Molecular Microbiology, National Institute of Allergy and Infectious Diseases, National Institutes of Health, Bethesda, MD 20205, USA

LICHY, J.H., Departments of Developmental Biology and Cancer, Albert Einstein College of Medicine, Bronx, NY 10461, USA

NAGATA, K., Departments of Developmental Biology and Cancer, Albert Einstein College of Medicine, Bronx, NY 10461, USA

SHIMIZU, Y., Department of Molecular Biology, Cancer Research Institute, Sapporo Medical College S-1, W-17, Chuo-ku, Sapporo 060, Japan

TIKCHONENKO, T.I., D.I. Ivanovsky, Institute of Virology, 16, Gamaleya Street, 123098 Moscow, USSR

VAN DER EB, A.J., Department of Medical Biochemistry, Sylvius Laboratories, Wassenaarseweg 72, NL-2333 AL Leiden

VAN ORMONDT, H., Department of Medical Biochemistry, University of Leiden, NL-2333 AL Leiden

WADELL, G., Department of Virology, University of Umeå, S-901 85 Umeå

YAMASHITA, T., Department of Molecular Biology, Cancer Research Institute, Sapporo Medical College S-1, W-17, Sapporo 060, Japan

YOSHIDA, K., Department of Molecular Biology, Cancer Research Institute, Sapporo Medical College S-1, W-17, Sapporo 060, Japan

The Interface Between Adenovirus-Transformed Cells and Cellular Immune Response in the Challenged Host

A.M. Lewis, Jr.[1] and J.L. Cook[2]

1 Introduction

The discovery by TRENTIN et al. (1962) that human adenoviruses were capable of producing tumors when inoculated into hamsters created a major role for these agents in the field of viral oncology. As participants in this field, several of the adenovirus (Ad) serotypes are among the most thoroughly studied animal viruses. One of the primary objectives of the study of these agents as tumor viruses has been to elucidate the mechanisms that are associated with their capacity to convert normal cells to neoplastic cells that produce tumors in animals. In approaching this objective, theoretical and technical developments have focused current research on the structure, organization, and expression of the Ad genome, and much has been accomplished. The functional arrangement of the Ad2 genome has been determined and the DNA sequence structure of several Ad serotypes is far advanced. The processing of Ad RNA into cytoplasmic mRNA that is translated into viral proteins has provided new insights into the mechanisms of RNA transcription in eukaryotic organisms. The mode of replication of the Ad genomes is under intensive investigation. The regions of the viral genome that are associated with the conversion of normal cells to neoplastic cells have been located, and many of the proteins encoded by these genes have been identified and in some cases purified. For detailed discussions of these developments, we refer the reader to other chapters in this volume and to recent reviews by FLINT (1980a, b), PERSSON and PHILIPSON (1982),

---

1 Laboratory of Molecular Microbiology, National Institute of Allergy and Infectious Diseases, National Institutes of Health, Bethesda, MD 20205, USA
2 Department of Medicine, National Jewish Hospital and Research Center, Denver, CO 80206, USA

Current Topics in Microbiology and Immunology, Vol. 110
© Springer-Verlag Berlin·Heidelberg 1984

CHALLBERG and KELLY (1982), and DOERFLER (1982). In spite of these impressive accomplishments, the goal of defining the mechanism of Ad-induced carcinogenesis has remained elusive, and it is becoming increasingly apparent that the question of how viruses and neoplastic cells produce tumors in animals will most likely remain after understanding of the molecular mechanisms of cell transformation (as defined by the induction of immortality) in vitro has been reached. The complexities of the interactions between cells rendered neoplastic by adenoviruses and the cellular immune defenses of the potential animal host suggest that new concepts and approaches to the possible mechanism of viral carcinogenesis are needed.

As tumors develop only in intact animal hosts, the cumulative studies of tumor-host relationships lead us to believe that the interactions at the interface between the incipient tumor and the cellular immune system of the potential host are the critical elements in the success or failure in the events leading to tumor development. To define these interactions and to develop the conceptual framework and the biological assays that will be essential for the success of a more refined molecular approach to the problems of tumor induction, the systematic study of the potential for tumor development in a number of animal models by oncogenic and nononcogenic Ad serotypes and the cells they transform will be necessary. In this chapter we will consider those phenomena that appear to be associated with the capacity of adenoviruses and Ad-transformed cells to induce the formation of tumors in animal hosts. To accomplish this objective, we will direct our remarks to the studies of Ad2, the most thoroughly studied nononcogenic Ad serotype, and Ad12, the most thoroughly studied oncogenic Ad serotype.

2 Patterns of Ad2- and Ad12-Induced Neoplasia In Vivo and In Vitro

Neoplasia as a biological entity is poorly understood. Basic concepts of the process have been derived from clinical and pathological studies of patients with neoplastic diseases. During the past half century, these clinicopathological observations, coupled with studies of tumor development in animals inoculated with oncogenic viruses or treated with chemical carcinogens, have provided a plausible sequence of events that appears to outline the conversion of normal cells to tumor cells in vivo (FOULDS 1969). The steps in this neoplastic conversion comprise an initiating event followed by a series of progressions from a more organized abnormal or atypical growth through a less organized hyperplastic or premalignant type of growth to invasive, metastasizing tumors. However, foci of tumor cells can appear within these lesions at any of the stages of development. To unravel the components of this process as it occurs in vivo, models are needed that mimic the various events in the conversion of normal cells to tumor cells.

Particularly relevant to the study of the sequential conversion of normal cells to tumor cells is the range of neoplastic capacities represented among the various subgroups of human adenoviruses. Based upon the differences in their ability to induce tumors when inoculated into newborn Syrian hamsters (*Mesocricetus auratus*), adenoviruses have been classified into the highly onco-genic human subgroup A (serotypes 12, 18, 31); the weakly oncogenic subgroup B (serotypes 3, 7, 11, 14, 16, 21, 34, 35); and the nononcogenic subgroups C (serotypes 1, 2, 5, 6) and D (serotypes 8–10, 13, 15, 17, 19, 20, 22–30, 32, 33). HUEBNER et al. (1962, 1963b) found that hamsters carrying tumors induced by Ad12 and Ad18 developed antibodies that reacted by complement fixation to early nonvirion T (tumor) antigens. These antibodies were subsequently found to be subgroup specific, and their reactivity by the complement fixation test was used to further characterize the highly oncogenic, weakly oncogenic, and nononcogenic subgroups (HUEBNER 1967; GILDEN et al. 1968; MCALLISTER et al. 1969). The classification of human adenoviruses according to their oncogeni-city for rodents and the subgroup specificity of their T antigens by complement fixation assays has been extended by studies of the degree of homology among Ad genomes (GREEN et al. 1979), restriction endonuclease analysis of viral DNA, and the characterization of virion polypeptides (WADELL et al. 1980). Based upon these studies, the subgroup similarities of these viruses have been substan-tiated. Ad4 has been classified as the only member of subgroup E (WADELL 1979), and the enteric adenoviruses have been classified as subgroup F (WADELL et al. 1980). The nonviron early virus T antigens in Ad-induced tumors and the presence of virus-specific antibodies in animals carrying virus-free tumor cells implied the continued presence of specific regions of the Ad genome in tumor cells that were free of infectious virions. The pursuit of this implication led to much of the current understanding of the molecular structure and func-tional organization of the Ad genome. Many of the proteins expressed by specific Ad genes that are present in these tumor cells have been characterized, and their functions are currently being investigated (FLINT 1980a, b; PERSSON and PHILIPSON 1982).

The tumor-inducing capacity of Ad12 for Syrian hamsters and other rodents has been well documented. Sixty-one percent (314/519) of hamsters in four independent studies that used both laboratory and field strains of Ad12 devel-oped tumors described as undifferentiated sarcomas (Table 1). Other studies have shown that Ad12 can induce tumors when inoculated into Sprague-Dawley rats, mastomys, and C3H and CBA mice (Table 1). The data used to substantiate the lack of oncogenicity of Ad2 in rodents have been less well publicized. Of the four studies of which we are aware, only two tumors have been observed in 159 hamsters inoculated with infectious Ad2 or Ad2 inactivated by exposure to ultraviolet (UV) light (Table 1). No tumors were observed in 16 Fisher or Sprague-Dawley rats or in 35 BALB or NIH Swiss mice. We are not aware of studies in which the oncogenicity of Ad2 has been tested in C3H or CBA mice. The Ad2 inoculum used to inject the hamster that developed one of the tumors listed in Table 1 (GIRARDI et al. 1964) was subsequently found to be contaminated with SV40. Cells from this tumor were not reported to have been examined for the presence of Ad2 or SV40 genetic information. The second tumor in Table 1 developed in a hamster inoculated with Ad2 inactivated with UV light (LEWIS and COOK 1979). Histopathologically, this

Table 1. Oncogenicity of Ad2 and Ad12 in rodents less than 24 h old inoculated with varying doses of virus by several routes of injection

Virus	Tumor incidence (no. with tumors/no. surviving)				References
	Hamsters	Rats	Mastomys	Mice	
Ad2	0/105	0/16	–	0/35	GILDEN and HUEBNER (unpublished)
	0/8	–	–	–	TRENTIN et al. (1962)
	1/5	–	–	–	GIRARDI et al. (1964)
	1/41	–	–	–	LEWIS and COOK (1979)
Ad12	100/183	–	–	–	TRENTIN et al. (1962, 1968)
	83/144	–	–	–	YABE et al. (1962, 1963)
	89/135	–	–	–	HUEBNER et al. (1962, 1963a)
	42/57	–	–	–	GIRARDI et al. (1964)
		3/10	–	–	HUEBNER et al. (1963b)
	–	2/32	7/29		RABSON et al. (1964)
	–	–	3/13		YABE et al. (1964)
	–	–	21/24		ALLISON et al. (1967)
	–	–	5/14		SJÖGREN et al. (1967)

tumor was an adenocarcinoma of a skin appendage, probably of the mammary gland. Cells from this tumor did not contain Ad2 T antigens or Ad2 DNA, and hamsters carrying transplants of this tumor did not develop antibodies to Ad2 antigens. Thus this tumor would appear to be a spontaneous neoplasm. Based upon these findings, Ad2 is considered to be nononcogenic for rodents while Ad12 is considered to be oncogenic for rats and mice and highly oncogenic for hamsters.

Several explanations have been advanced for the differences in tumor-inducing capacity between Ad2 and Ad12. Since both these viruses are capable of inducing neoplastic changes (i.e., transforming) in hamster and rat cells in tissue culture, differences in their efficiencies of transformation could explain the differences in their oncogenicity. Several studies have addressed this possibility (Table 2). McALLISTER and MacPHERSON (1968) and McALLISTER et al. (1969) noted that nononcogenic Ad19 (subgroup D) was approximately 50 times more efficient in transforming rat embryo cells in tissue culture than was the highly oncogenic Ad12 ($10^{4.5}$ PFU/FFU for Ad19; $10^{6.2}$ PFU/FFU for Ad12). GALLI-MORE and PARASKEVA (1980) found no difference in the efficiency with which Ad2 and Ad12 transformed identical batches of rat embryo brain cells (both $10^{5.9}$ PFU/FFU); and one of us (A.M. LEWIS JR., unpublished) found that these two viruses are approximately equally efficient ($10^{7.8}$ PFU/FFU for Ad2; $10^{8.0}$ PFU/FFU for Ad12) in transforming identical batches of LSH hamster embryo cells. Thus there appear to be no inherent differences in the capacity of Ad2 and Ad12 to induce neoplastic changes in cells removed from the intact animal host that can satisfactorily explain the differences in the oncogenicity of these two viruses.

The ability of nononcogenic Ad2 and oncogenic Ad12 to transform normal rodent cells to neoplastic cells in vitro with essentially the same efficiency implies

Table 2. Evidence for the lack of correlation between tumor induction in rodents and the efficiency of transforming rodent cells in vitro by human adenoviruses

Ad serotype	Tumor-inducing capacity in vivo	Efficiency of cell transformation in vitro ($\log_{10}$ PFU/FFU)	
		Rat cells	Hamster cells
1	Nononcogenic	5.8[a]	–
2	Nononcogenic	7.6 5.9[b]	7.8[c]
19	Nononcogenic	4.5	–
12	Oncogenic	6.2 5.9	8.0

[a] Data from MCALLISTER and MACPHERSON (1968) and MCALLISTER et al. (1969)
[b] Estimated from the data of GALLIMORE and PARASKEVA (1980)
[c] Unpublished data from A.M. LEWIS, Jr

that the factors determining the tumor-inducing capacity of these viruses are related to the interactions between cells transformed by these viruses in vivo and the prospective rodent host being used to evaluate viral oncogenicity. A number of observations support this conclusion. Ad2 produced tumors when inoculated into newborn rats that were immunosuppressed with antithymocyte serum (HARWOOD and GALLIMORE 1975). Ad12 is oncogenic only when inoculated into newborn rodents or adults that have been immunosuppressed by thymectomy or treatment with antithymocyte serum or steroids (YABE et al. 1962; KIRSCHSTEIN et al. 1964; YOHN et al. 1965, 1968; ALLISON et al. 1967). As the virus produces tumors more efficiently in immunoimmature or immunosuppressed rodents, the degree of maturation of the immune system of the prospective host appears to play a critical role in the outcome of the oncogenic process. Several studies have considered a possible role in the tumor-producing process for those properties of cells transformed in vitro that differentiate them from normal cells. These studies have been unable to consistently associate any of these properties (i.e., cell morphology, immortality, doubling times, saturation densities, serum growth requirements, anchorage independence, proteolytic enzyme activity, and the presence of surface glycoproteins) with the differences in the tumor-inducing capacities between hamster and rat cells transformed by Ad2 and Ad12 (GALLIMORE et al. 1977; GALLIMORE and PARASKEVA 1980; COOK and LEWIS 1979). In spite of our inability to differentiate between cells transformed in vitro by these two viruses, syngeneic rats and hamsters readily perceive the differences that have eluded us (Table 3). All the lines of Ad12-transformed rat and hamster cells that have been tested produce tumors in syngeneic newborn animals. Furthermore, Ad12-transformed inbred hamster cells are highly tumorigenic when transplanted into fully immunocompetent adult syngeneic hamsters (LEWIS and COOK 1982). In contrast, only 23% of the lines of Ad2-transformed rat cells developed by HARWOOD and GALLIMORE (1975) and GALLIMORE and PARASKEVA (1980) produced tumors in immunoimmature newborn rats further immunosuppressed by treatment with antirat thymocyte serum. The majority (87%) of the lines of Ad2-transformed inbred hamster cells that we have tested are highly tumorigenic in immunoimmature

Table 3. Tumor-inducing capacity of Ad2- and Ad12-transformed inbred rat and hamster cells in syngeneic rats and hamsters

Transforming virus	No. cell lines oncogenic/no. cell lines tested (%)			
	ATS newborn rats[a]	Normal newborn rats	Newborn hamsters[b]	Adult hamsters
Ad2	16/70 (23)	1/70 (1)	13/15 (87)	0/15 (0)
Ad12	NT	25/25 (100)	5/5 (100)	5/5 (100)

ATS, treated with antirat thymocyte serum; NT, not tested
[a] Rat data from GALLIMORE and PARASKEVA (1980). Animals were challenged with 2×10^6 cells
[b] Hamster data from COOK and LEWIS (1979) and LEWIS and COOK (1980, 1982). Hamsters were challenged with 10^7 cells

newborn hamsters but nontumorigenic when 10^7 cells are inoculated into immunocompetent syngeneic adult hamsters (COOK and LEWIS 1979). These results strongly support the conclusion that it is the interactions between the host and Ad2- or Ad12-transformed cells that ultimately determine the outcome of the neoplastic processes which lead to tumor development.

3 Virus-Specific Immunogenicity of Ad2- and Ad12-Transformed Rodent Cells

Tumor-specific transplantation antigens (TSTAs) have been discovered on cells from tumors induced by a number of chemical carcinogens and oncogenic viruses. These antigens are detected by their ability to induce cellular immune reactions in a host immunized with tumor viruses or tumor cells, resulting in the destruction of viable antigen-containing tumor cells. The discovery of TSTAs on neoplastic cells was of major theoretical significance, as it offered an immunological approach to tumor therapy and suggested the importance of host immune mechanisms in determining the outcome of virus-induced neoplastic disease. The presence of TSTAs on the surface of tumor cells also offered an explanation for the observed differences in the tumor-inducing capacities among oncogenic viruses and the cells they transformed in vitro. This explanation suggested that the different levels of immunogenicity expressed by cells transformed in tissue cultures should evoke different degrees of immune recognition and rejection in the potential host. By this reasoning, weakly immunogenic neoplastic cells should be highly tumorigenic and highly immunogenic neoplastic cells should be weakly tumorigenic. Conversely, immunoincompetent animals should be more susceptible to tumor induction by transformed cells that express transplantation antigens than fully immunocompetent animals.

One of the first indications that the immune system of the host plays a role in tumor induction by adenoviruses was provided by KIRSCHSTEIN et al. (1964), who found that Ad12 could produce tumors only in thymectomized BALB/c or C3H mice. Shortly after this initial observation, YOHN et al. (1965)

found that thymectomy increased the incidence of tumor induction by Ad12 in male syrian hamsters, and ALLISON et al. (1967) reported that thymectomized CBA mice and CBA mice treated with antilymphocyte serum and inoculated with doses of Ad12 that were marginally tumorigenic developed a higher percentage of tumors than did untreated normal animals.

EDDY et al. (1964) and TRENTIN and BRYAN (1966) described the induction of immunity to Ad12 TSTAs in virus-immunized hamsters and mice. BERMAN (1967) demonstrated the presence of Ad12 TSTAs on cells from tumors induced by Ad12 in CBA mice and found that protection against tumor challenge was mediated by immune lymphoid cells and not by serum containing antibodies to Ad12 T antigens. SJÖGREN et al. (1967) demonstrated the presence of TSTAs on tumor cells induced in C3H mice by Ad12, and also found that immunization with Ad7 and Ad18 but not Ad5 could protect mice against a challenge with Ad12 tumor cells. ANKERST and SJÖGREN (1969, 1970) extended this observation; they found that Ad serotypes 3, 7, 12, and 14 seemed to share a common TSTA and that TSTAs on cells from tumors induced in mice and hamsters by Ad12 shared immunological specificities. These results suggested that the Ad12 genome codes for common TSTA specificities that are independent of the species of animal cell undergoing neoplastic transformation.

Thus far, the role of the viral genome in inducing TSTAs in cells transformed in vitro and in vivo by human adenoviruses has not been precisely defined. SHIROKI et al. (1979) have shown that rat cells transformed by subgenomic fragments of Ad12 (*Eco*RI C fragment map position 0–16 and *Hind*III G fragment map position 0–7.2) protected immunized rats inoculated as newborns with Ad12 against subsequent tumor development. Cells transformed by the *Acc*I/*Bpa*I H fragment (map position 0–4.5) did not protect immune rats against Ad12 tumor development. RASKA et al. (1980) found that rats carrying tumors induced by cells transformed by the same Ad12 *Eco*RI C fragment developed lymphoid cells in their spleens that were specifically cytotoxic for syngeneic but not allogeneic Ad12-transformed rat cells in vitro. The tumor-bearing animals also developed complement-dependent antibodies that were cytotoxic for Ad12-transformed cells in vitro. Ad2-transformed rat embryo cells containing only the left-hand 14% of Ad genome produced similar complement-dependent cytotoxic antibodies and cytolytic T lymphocytes in the sera and spleens of immune rats (RASKA et al. 1982). These data imply that the early region 1 (E1) of the Ad12 and Ad2 genomes encode proteins that specify TSTAs in virus-transformed cells. The E1 region of the viral genome is located between map position 1.0 and map position 11.5. Proteins encoded by this region apparently interact with cell surface histocompatibility antigens to produce a specific complex that can be recognized by cytotoxic T lymphocytes from virus-immune syngeneic animals in a manner similar to those described for the papovavirus SV40 TSTA system (TEVETHIA 1980). The E1 region of the Ad genome has been divided into two transcription units (E1A and E1B) by the presence of two distinct promoters (SEHGAL et al. 1979; WILSON et al. 1979). The E1A region extends from about map position 1.0 to map position 4.4, while the E1B region extends from about map position 4.5 to map position 11.5. Thus the data of SHIROKI et al. (1979) and RASKA et al. (1980) indicate that polypeptides from the E1B region of the Ad genome are responsible for the Ad-specific TSTAs present on Ad2-transformed rodent cells. PERSSON et al. (1982) have purified a 15 000-dalton protein encoded by the E1B region of the Ad2 genome. Monospecific antiserum prepared with this protein immunoprecipitated a 15 000-dalton protein from human and rodent cells transformed by Ad2 and Ad5. Since this protein was found to be tightly associated with cell membranes, it may be an Ad2 gene product that conveys virus-specific immunogenicity to transformed cells.

KVIST et al. (1978) found that antiserum prepared against Ad2-transformed rat A2T2C4 cells and antiserum against the rat major histocompatibility antigens immunoprecipitate the same 19 000-dalton glycosylated cell surface antigen from A2T2C4 cells. Antiserum that was specific for β_2-microglobulin [a subunit of cell surface histocompatibility antigens: RASK et al. (1974); SILVER and HOOD (1974); VITETTA et al. (1975)] also precipitated the 19 000-dalton polypeptide. Their data suggest that the 19 000-dalton polypeptide is a virus-coded protein that forms a ternary complex with the subunits of the rat histocompatibility antigens on the surface of the A2T2C4 cells. Subsequent studies (PERSSON et al. 1980; SIGNAS et al. 1982) identified the 19 000-dalton Ad glycoprotein as a product of early region 3 (E3, map position 76.0 to map position 86.0) of the Ad2 genome and showed that it binds specifically to the heavy chain of class 1 antigens of the major histocompatibility complex present on the surface of Ad2-infected human cells. These studies also demonstrated that the complex formed between this Ad glycoprotein and class 1 histocompatibility antigens are recognized by cytotoxic T lymphocytes. Thus both the E1 and E3 regions of the adenovirus genome appear to encode proteins that may be associated with the virus-specific immunogenicity of infected and transformed cells.

MCALLISTER et al. (1969) suggested that the induction of highly immunogenic transplantation antigens on rodent cells transformed in vivo and in vitro might determine the oncogenicity of the Ad serotype and the tumor-inducing capacity of the virus-transformed cell. Subsequent studies demonstrated that rat cells transformed by nononcogenic Ad2 were capable of inducing tumors only in immunosuppressed newborn rats (GALLIMORE 1972; HARWOOD and GALLIMORE 1975). Since rat cells transformed by oncogenic Ad12 produced tumors quite readily in newborn rats, these findings supported the concept that differences in the immunogenicity of rodent cells transformed by the highly oncogenic, weakly oncogenic, and nonocogenic adenoviruses could explain the differences in their tumor-inducing capacities.

The evidence obtained by successfully grafting nontumorigenic transformed cells into immunosuppressed hosts implies that some type of immunological mechanism is at work in determining the success or failure of the transformed cells in establishing themselves as a neoplasm. Such studies provide only indirect evidence that the immunogenicity of the transformed cell is the determining factor. In a direct attempt to correlate tumorigenicity and immunogenicity, AKAGI and OGAWA (1972) found no correlation between the expression of TSTAs and the "intensity of tumorigenicity" among three cell lines derived from hamster cells transformed in vitro by Ad12 and one cell line established from a tumor induced in hamsters by Ad12. In more recent studies, GALLIMORE

Table 4. Evidence for the lack of correlation between the immunogenicity and tumorigenicity of Ad2- and Ad12-transformed rat and hamster cells

Cell line	Tumor-inducing capacity								Resistance index
	Nude mice	Rats			Hamsters				
		ATS newborns	Normal newborns	Adults	ALS newborns	Normal newborns	Adults		
Ad2F4[a]	+(4.8)	+	0	−	−	−	−		>400
Ad2F17	+(7.3)	0	0	−	−	−	−		>400
Ad2F19	+(6.0)	0	0	−	−	−	−		>635
Ad250A	+(2.3)	+	+	+	−	−	−		>635
Ad2HE7[b]	+(5.5)[f]	−	−	−	+(5.5)	0(>8.5)	0(>8.5)		107
Ad2HE1	+(3.9)	−	−	−	NT	+(5.3)	0(>8.5)		1,961
Ad2HE3	+(4.9)	−	−	−	NT	+(3.6)	0(>8.5)		2,511
Ad2HE3-ATCL-1	NT	−	−	−	NT	NT	+(4.1)		1,149
Ad12HE1	+(4.1)	−	−	−	NT	+(3.4)	+(4.5)		10,000

Resistance index, no. of cells per TPD_{50} in immune animals/no. cells per TPD_{50} in nonimmune controls; ATS, treated with antirat thymocyte serum; ALS, treated with antihamster lymphocyte serum; +, tumorigenic when animals were challenged with single doses (10^{6-3}) of transformed cells in parentheses, no. of cells per TPD at the 100% end point [top half of table) or no. of cells per TPD_{50} (bottom half of toble]; NT, not tested

[a] Ad2-transformed rat embryo brain cells (Ad2F4, Ad2F17, Ad2F19) or Ad2-transformed rat embryo fibroblasts (Ad250A). From the data of *Gallimore* and *Paraskeva* (1980)

[b] Ad2- or Ad12-transformed inbred LSH hamster embryo cells (Ad2HE7, Ad2HE3, Ad12HE1). To establish the Ad2HE3-ATCL-1 cell line, tumors were induced in newborn hamsters with Ad2HE3 cells. These tumors were adapted to grow in adult hamsters by serial passage in newborns. After multiple passages in adult hamsters, cells from a single tumor were established in vitro

and PARASKEVA (1980) and LEWIS and COOK (1982) have attempted to correlate the expression of virus-specific immunogenicity of Ad2-transformed rat and hamster cells with their tumor-inducing capacities (Table 4). Ad2-transformed rat embryo brain cells and Ad2-transformed rat embryo fibroblasts that exhibited a variety of tumor-inducing capacities for nude mice, normal syngeneic newborn rats, and antirat-thymocyte-serum-treated syngeneic newborn rats were all highly immunogenic (resistance indices > 400) in bioassays for the expression of Ad2-specific transplantation antigen. Three lines of Ad2-transformed LSH hamster embryo cells and one line of Ad12-transformed LSH hamster embryo cells that exhibited three distinct tumorigenic phenotypes – tumorigenic in nude mice and nontumorigenic in hamsters (Ad2HE7); tumorigenic in nude mice and syngeneic newborn hamsters but nontumorigenic in adult hamsters (Ad2HE1 and Ad2HE3); tumorigenic in nude mice and in syngeneic newborn hamsters and adult hamsters (Ad2HE3-ATCL-1 and Ad12HE1) – were widely divergent in their ability to convey protection to immune hamsters challenged with graded tumor-producing doses of viable transformed cells. Indeed, the least tumorigenic of the cell lines (Ad2HE7), which produced tumors only in nude mice, was the least immunogenic in repetitive assays (average resistance index of 107) in which immune animals were challenged with Ad2HE3-ATCL-1 cells. Ad12HE1 cells that produced tumors quite efficiently [$10^{4.5}$ cells/tumor-producing dose at the 50% end point (TPD$_{50}$)] in syngeneic adult hamsters were highly immunogenic in that no tumors developed in immune hamsters challenged with more than 10000 TPD$_{50}$ of Ad12HE3 cells. These results imply that the differences in the immunogenicity of Ad-transformed cells as reflected by their expression of TSTAs which can be detected by bioassay are not related to the differences in their tumor-inducing capacity. Furthermore, the minor differences in the immunogenicities of the Ad2HE3 cells (resistance index 2511) and the cells selected during in vivo tumor passage that become the more highly oncogenic Ad2HE3-ATCL-1 cell line (resistance index 1149) imply that the cell selection process involved in tumor induction in animals that possess a greater degree of immunocompetence does not result in the overgrowth of cells that are markedly deficient in Ad2 TSTAs.

4 Adenovirus-Transformed Cell Tumorigenic Phenotypes Defined in the Context of the Host Cellular Immune Response

By definition, bioassays evaluating virus-specific immunogenicities of adenovirus-transformed cells reveal the ability of the immunized host to respond to a repeated exposure to TSTAs. It is apparent from the above data that the elicitation of such secondary host responses does not discriminate among adenovirus-transformed rodent cells that differ in their tumor-inducing capacities. Rather, the key factor differentiating highly oncogenic Ad12-transformed cells from weakly oncogenic Ad2-transformed rodent cells appears to be the outcome of the interactions between the transformed cells and the primary host defenses mounted by the naive host. The nature of these host defenses has been examined in several studies evaluating the ontogeny of host cellular immune responses related to tumor susceptibility, the effects of suppression of host cellular immune defenses on tumor susceptibility, and the characteristics of in situ host inflammatory cell responses to incipient neoplasms.

As documented in Table 3, there is a distinct age-related difference in susceptibility of Syrian hamsters to challenge with most Ad2-transformed cell lines. Conversely, Ad12-transformed cells efficiently induce tumors in hamsters irrespective of the age of the host at the time of challenge (COOK and LEWIS 1979; LEWIS and COOK 1982). Thirteen of 15 different tissue culture cell lines of Ad2-transformed inbred LSH hamster cells induced progressive tumors when 10^7 cells were inoculated into syngeneic newborn (<4-day-old) hamsters (range of tumor incidence 20–100%), while none of six of these Ad2-transformed cell lines induced tumors in similarly challenged syngeneic weanling (>28-day-old) hamsters. Conversely, five different Ad12-transformed LSH hamster cell lines induced tumors in 100% of both syngeneic newborn and weanling hosts. Tumor induction studies using syngeneic hamsters challenged at various ages between these two extremes revealed that resistance to Ad2 tumor challenge had matured by the beginning of the 2nd week of life, a time at which functional hamster-cell-mediated immune responses are first detected (BILLINGHAM et al. 1960; COOK and LEWIS 1979; COOK et al. 1979a). Hence, the age-related resistance of syngeneic hamsters to challenge with Ad2-transformed-cell-induced tumors is temporally associated with the early maturation of host-cell-mediated immune responses. The results of tumor induction studies in weanling hamsters rendered immunodeficient by neonatal thymectomy further supported the role of host cellular defenses in Ad2 tumor rejection (COOK et al. 1979b). Thymectomy did not prevent the production of antibody specific for nonvirion Ad2 T antigen, but did result in increased host susceptibility to Ad2 tumor challenge unless the cellular defenses of the recipient had been reconstituted by adoptive transfer of syngeneic lymphoid cells. Thus it appears that the maturation of host cellular defenses during the early stages of hamster immune ontogeny are responsible for efficient rejection of syngeneic neoplastic cells transformed by Ad2, while hamster cells transformed by Ad12 escape such rejection and cause fatal malignancies in this host.

In spite of their apparently meager immunological defenses, newborn hamsters and rats may also exhibit remarkable resistance to challenge with certain syngeneic Ad2-transformed cells (HARWOOD and GALLIMORE 1975; GALLIMORE and PARASKEVA 1980; LEWIS and COOK 1982). Two of 15 Ad2-transformed LSH hamster cell lines that have been repeatedly evaluated have consistently failed to induce tumors in syngeneic newborn hamsters challenged with 10^7–10^8 cells. In the Ad2 rat system described by GALLIMORE and his co-workers, only one of 70 Ad2-transformed syngeneic cell lines induced tumors in syngeneic newborn rats challenged with 2×10^6 cells. That the rejection of such Ad2-tranformed cell lines in newborns of both species is mediated by host cells sharing antigenic determinants with components of the adult cellular defense system is suggested by the increased susceptibility of neonates in Ad2-transformed-cell challenges when the recipients are treated with antilymphocyte serum produced by rabbits following immunization with isologous adult hamster or rat lymphoid cells.

Table 5. Histopathological observations during tumor evolution in inbred LSH Syrian hamsters challenged with Ad2 tumor cells[a]

Parameter	Recipient of tumor challenge	
	Syngeneic newborn	Syngeneic adult
Early vascularization	+ + +	+ +
Polymorphonuclear leukocyte infiltration	+ (Early, transient)	+ (Early, transient)
Lymphohistiocytic cell cell infiltration (<3 days post challenge)	+ (*Peripheral*)	+ + + + (*Invasive*)
Status 7 days post challenge	Tumor nodules with peripheral mononuclear cells	Granulomatous inflammation, multi- nucleated giant cells, rare tumor cells
Status 15 days post challenge	Enlarging tumor nodules, some with peripheral mono- nuclear cells, some with no surrounding inflammation. Some areas of granulomatous inflammation and multi- nucleated giant cells	Granulomatous re- action with focal calcification. No tumor cells
Outcome	Progressive tumor causing death of the host in 4–6 weeks	Tumor rejection

[a] Animals were challenged subcutaneously with 0.2 ml of a standard suspension of Ad2HTL3 or Ad2HTL6 tumor cells. An 0.2 ml suspension of tumor cells contained between $10^{3.0}$ and $10^{5.0}$ TPD_{50} in newborn syngeneic hamsters. At 1- to 3-day intervals through the 15th day postinoculation, two to five animals from each group were killed and biopsies of the tumor nodules and adjacent tissues were fixed in formalin and embedded in paraffin. Sections taken at 100–200 µm intervals through each tissue specimen were stained with hematoxylin and eosin. Adapted from Cook et al. (1979a)

To begin to directly evaluate the interface between Ad-transformed cells and the cellular defenses of the host, serial histopathological studies of neo-plasms have been performed during the course of tumor evolution in syngeneic newborn, weanling, and neonatally thymectomized weanling Syrian hamsters (Table 5; Cook et al. 1979a). Light-microscopic examination of serial step sec-tions taken at 100–200 µm intervals from evolving Ad2 tumor masses revealed early formation of new capillaries and a transient polymorphonuclear leukocyte infiltration of approximately the same intensity in animals from each of the three groups. Conversely, the migration of lymphocytic and histiocytic (macro-phage-like) cells into the tumor site occurred earlier (within the first 3 days) and with much greater intensity in normal weanling hamsters than in newborns or in the immunocompromised weanlings that had been thymectomized at birth. The mononuclear cells that did appear in tumor sites in newborn or thymectomized weanling hamsters tended to remain at the periphery of growing tumor nodules, whereas in normal weanling hamsters the inflammatory cells often infiltrated the tumor masses, apparently leading to tumor rejection within 1 week of challenge. Interestingly, some sections of tumors removed after 15 days from animals inoculated as newborns also revealed fairly intensive mononuclear cell responses. However, these late inflammatory reactions were obviously insufficient to prevent the progression of the Ad2 tumors that had become established under the cover of inadequate host cellular responses. The results of recent histopathological studies of evolving Ad12 tumors in normal weanling hamsters indicate that the immunocompetent host may mount an early, invasive mononuclear cell response to Ad12-transformed cells similar to the response seen in Ad2 tumor studies (COOK et al. 1982). However, in contrast to the rapid destruction of Ad2 tumor cells that is associated with such a response, Ad12 tumors appear to progress in spite of the presence of these host inflammatory cells.

The results of these in vivo studies of tumor induction by Ad2- and Ad12-transformed hamster and rat cells demonstrate the importance of qualifying the tumorigenicity of an Ad-transformed cell line in terms of the cellular immune responsiveness of the host. The histopathological correlations obtained from the hamster tumor model emphasize the importance of host cellular defenses in determining the course of tumor evolution and also suggest the existence of differences in the susceptibilities of Ad2- and Ad12-transformed cells to destruction by the inflammatory cells that comprise the early host response to tumor cell challenge.

5 Adenovirus-Transformed Cell-Host Effector Cell Interactions

There is increasing evidence from studies in several different species and tumor models of a role for immunologically nonspecific host effector cells as a first line of defense against neoplastic cells (HALLER et al. 1980; HERBERMAN and ORTALDO 1981). The importance of this type of host effector cell activity, termed spontaneous or natural cell-mediated cytotoxicity, is that such host cells can destroy tumor cells without prior specific sensitization to tumor antigens and that augmentation of such effector cell cytolytic activity appears to occur rapidly. The in vivo experimental data summarized in Sect. 3 indicates that the immunogenicity (induction of immunity to TSTAs) of Ad-transformed rodent cell lines, as determined in bioassays, does not correlate with the tumor-inducing capacities of those cell lines. TSTA-specific tumor rejection in sensitized hosts is mediated largely by cytolytic thymus-derived lymphocytes (CTLs). However, there is very little experimental evidence that such CTLs play a decisive role in the early host response to syngeneic tumor cells grafted to normal, unsensitized recipients (KIESSLING and WIGZELL 1979; HERBERMAN 1981). Studies by RASKA and GALLIMORE (1982) and RASKA et al. (1982), in which Ad2- and Ad12-transformed inbred rat cell lines exhibiting several different tumorigenic phenotypes were tested for susceptibility to lysis by specifically sensitized, syngeneic CTLs, suggest that such secondary host responses are also of little importance in determining tumor cell rejection by native hosts in the Ad-transformed rodent cell system. All cell lines tested, whether of high or low tumorigenic potential in unsensitized syngeneic rats, were found to be approximately equally susceptible to lysis by virus-specific CTLs. The histopathological studies of evolving Ad hamster tumors discussed in Sect. 4 suggested that early host mononuclear cell responses (those occurring within the first few days following tumor challenge) play a decisive role in Ad2-transformed cell rejection and also that such early host effector cells may be the host factor that discriminates between weakly oncogenic Ad2-transformed and highly oncogenic Ad12-transformed cells. The different tumorigenic phenotypes in Ad2- and Ad12-transformed hamster and rat cells and the suggested importance of early nonspecific effector cells in the host response provided a framework within which the results of spontaneous cell-mediated cytotoxicity assays using Ad-transformed cells could be interpreted.

We had previously observed that a weakly oncogenic Ad2-transformed Syrian hamster cell line, Ad2HE7 (see Table 4), was highly sensitive to lysis by activated hamster macrophages when compared to highly oncogenic SV40-transformed hamster cell lines that were resistant to macrophage-mediated cytolysis (COOK et al. 1980). Therefore, since lymphocytes and macrophages were the predominant early host inflammatory cell types present in Ad tumor sites (see Sect. 4), we were interested in comparing Ad2-, Ad12-, and SV40-transformed cells for susceptibility to lysis by spontaneously cytolytic hamster lymphoid cells (unsensitized spleen cells) and activated hamster macrophages. The results of these studies (Table 6) revealed that Ad2-transformed hamster cell lines that induce tumors only in immunologically compromised hosts were significantly

Table 6. Correlations between host-defined tumorigenic phenotypes and susceptibilities of Ad2-, Ad12-, and SV40-transformed LSH Syrian hamster cells to lysis by unsensitized hamster spleen cells and activated hamster peritoneal macrophages

Tumorigenic phenotype[a]	Representative cell line	Tumor-inducing capacity[b]				Susceptibility to lysis by[c]	
		Nude mice	Syngeneic newborn hamsters	Syngeneic adult hamsters	Allogeneic adult hamsters	Normal spleen cells	Activated macrophages
I	Ad2HE7	5.5	>8.5	>8.5	>8.5	62.1±2.4	92.1±1.4
II	Ad2HE1	3.9	5.3	>8.5	>8.5	74.4±4.1	96.2±1.8
III	Ad12HE1	4.1	3.4	4.5	>8.5	29.0±6.0	90.2±4.1
IV	SV40HE1	2.7	3.5	4.2	5.0	16.6±2.4	19.5±1.3

[a] Classification of transformed cell lines according to tumor-inducing capacity. Type I, lowest capacity; Type IV, highest capacity
[b] No. of cells ($\log_{10}$) required to induce tumors in 50% of animals (>8.5=no tumors observed within 10–12 weeks following challenge with 10^8 cells)
[c] Effector-cell-induced release of nuclear label ([^{3}H-]thymidine) in 48-h cytolysis assays. Each value represents the mean ±SEM result of all published assays for each cell line. The number of experiments represented is as follows (spleen cell, macrophage): Ad2HE7 55, 29; Ad2HE1 5, 6; Ad12HE1 20, 7; SV40HE1 39, 64. Macrophages were activated by intraperitoneal infection with BCG. Adapted from COOK et al. (1980, 1982)

more susceptible to the lytic effects of unsensitized hamster spleen cells than were Ad12- or SV40-transformed hamster cells (COOK et al. 1982). Ad12-transformed cell lines were consistently more resistant to spleen-cell-induced lysis than Ad2-transformed cells, but were not as resistant as SV40-transformed cells. Furthermore, Ad2- and Ad12-transformed cell lines were both highly susceptible to the cytolytic effects of activated macrophages compared to resistant SV40-transformed cells. Analogous in vitro cytolysis assays performed by RASKA and GALLIMORE (1982), using Ad2- and Ad12-transformed rat cells as targets for unsensitized rat spleen cells or specifically sensitized rat CTLs, produced similar results. The least tumorigenic Ad2-transformed rat cell line, which induced tumors only in immunosuppressed newborn rats, was the most sensitive to lysis by naturally cytolytic lymphoid cells, while highly oncogenic Ad12-transformed rat cell lines were resistant to lysis by the same effector cell populations. As previously mentioned, the Ad2- and Ad12-transformed rat cell lines were equally susceptible to lysis by specifically sensitized CTLs. Comparisons between these two in vitro assay systems for measurement of cytolytic susceptibility among Ad-transformed cells from different species are instructive. In both systems, weakly oncogenic Ad2-transformed cells were more susceptible to destruction by spontaneously cytolytic host lymphoid cells than were highly oncogenic Ad12-transformed cells. The reproducibility of this correlation in different species using Ad-transformed cells from different laboratories suggests the importance of these observations to the understanding of adenovirus tumor biology. When viewed in the context of the previously described tumor induction studies and the histological studies of adenovirus tumor evolution, these results suggest that one of the key differences in highly oncogenic (e.g., Ad12) and nononcogenic (e.g., Ad2) Ad serotypes may be the differences in cytolytic susceptibility that may be induced during host cell transformation. While differences in susceptibility to destruction by spontaneously cytolytic host lymphoid cells were observed between Ad2 (sensitive)-transformed and Ad12 (resistant)-transformed cells in both experimental models, cells transformed by both Ad serotypes were equally susceptible to lysis by immunologically nonspecific activated macrophages (hamster model) and by Ad-specific CTLs (rat model). These results indicate that the transformed cell properties responsible for the resistance of Ad12 transformed cells observed with spontaneously cytolytic lymphoid cells are inadequate to prevent destruction by host effector cells with greater cytolytic potential. The relative resistance of Ad12-transformed rodent cells to spontaneous, but not to nonspecifically or specifically activated, host cytolytic effector cells offers an interesting in vitro correlate for the previously reported in vivo observation that treatment of Ad12-inoculated animals with nonspecific or specific immunostimuli during the latent period of tumor induction can cause a marked reduction in the incidence of primary Ad12-induced tumors (SJÖGREN and ANKERST 1969).

It is generally accepted that many of the properties of adenovirus-transformed cells are the phenotoypic expressions of early adenovirus-encoded gene products, some of which are detected as Ad-specific T antigens. It is therefore possible that the degree of Ad-transformed cell susceptibility to effector cell lysis may also be under control of the integrated adenoviral genome. Initial studies evaluating the role of Ad2 early gene products in determining the level of susceptibility of transformed hamster cells to cytolysis by effector cells have been performed using somatic cell hybrids formed between a highly susceptible Ad2-transformed (Ad2HE1) and a highly resistant SV40-transformed (SV40HE1) hamster cell line (PATCH et al. 1983; COOK et al. 1983). One of the characteristics of such intraspecific rodent cell hybrids is that a proportion of the chromosomes present following cell fusion will be lost during subsequent cell divisions. While this instability is usually viewed as a disadvantage in the genetic study of cell hybrids, it proved to be useful in analyzing the relative effects of Ad2 and SV40 early gene products on transformed-cell cytolytic susceptibility. As an indicator of the presence of virus-specific early gene products, cell hybrids were tested for the presence of Ad2- and SV40-specific T antigens by indirect immunofluorescence assays using specific antisera. All nine Ad2HE1 × SV40HE1 hybrid cell lines tested continued to express SV40 T antigen throughout the hybrid cell selection process and the evaluation of cytolytic susceptibility. However, three of these lines lost the ability to express Ad2 T antigen. The results of reassociation kinetics studies suggest that the lack of expression of Ad2 T antigen by these immunofluorescence-negative hybrid cell lines is due to their loss of the cellular chromosome(s) bearing integrated Ad2 DNA. The availability of these Ad2 T-antigen-positive and -negative hybrid cell lines allowed an examination of the effect of Ad2 T antigens on the cytolytic resistant phenotype of this SV40-transformed hamster cell line (Table 7; COOK et al. 1983). When evaluated for sensitivity to lysis by unsensitized spleen cells and activated macrophages, the three Ad2 T-antigen-negative hybrid cell lines were as resistant to lysis as was the nonhybrid SV40HE1 parental cell line. Conversely, all six Ad2 T-antigen-positive hybrid cell lines (two of which are shown in Table 7) were significantly more susceptible than SV40HE1 to lysis by both types of effector cells. Thus in each case in which Ad2 T antigen could be detected serologically in weekly oncogenic Ad2 × SV40-transformed cell hybrids, susceptibility to destruction by nonspecific host effector cells was significantly greater than in the cytolytic resistant parental cell (SV40HE1) or in Ad2 T-antigen-negative hybrid cells both of which were highly oncogenic. These results suggest the existence of a novel function for early Ad2-genome-encoded polypeptides (T antigens) expressed in transformed hamster cells – the induction of susceptibility to immunologically nonspecific effector-cell-mediated destruction.

In summary, these in vitro data suggest that the differential susceptibilities of Ad-transformed rodent cells to destruction by the putative early host effector cells that appear to invade adenoviral malignancies provides one explanation for the differences in the tumor-inducing capacities of highly oncogenic Ad12 and nononcogenic Ad2 and the host cells they transform. This hypothesis is compatible with the previously summarized observations that Ad12 and Ad2 do not differ significantly in the efficiency with which they transform cells and that Ad12- and Ad2-transformed cells are both highly immunogenic. It appears that spontaneously cytolytic lymphoid cells and activated macrophages recognize transformed cells as different from nontransformed cells due to some as yet poorly defined change that occurs during transformation. It may be differ-

Table 7. Correlation between viral antigen expression and susceptibility to nonspecific effector cell-induced lysis among somatic cell hybrids formed from Ad2- and SV40-transformed Syrian hamster cell lines. (Adapted from Cook et al. 1983)

	Cell line	Viral T antigen[a]		Susceptibility to lysis by[b]	
		SV40	Ad2	Normal spleen cells	Activated macrophages
Parental cells	Ad2HE1	0	+	59.2 ± 5.9	88.0 ± 3.8
	SV40HE1	+	0	5.9 ± 1.1	19.7 ± 2.6
Hybrid cells	S1$^+$A1$^+$2.4[c]	+	+	51.5 ± 4.7	82.2 ± 5.0
	S1$^+$A1$^+$11.4	+	+	44.5 ± 1.8	90.4 ± 3.1
	S1$^+$A1$^-$8.2	+	0	2.3 ± 0.9	27.3 ± 3.8
	S1$^+$A1$^-$9.4	+	0	9.6 ± 1.6	26.9 ± 4.6
	S1$^+$A1$^-$10.3	+	0	12.3 ± 1.8	28.1 ± 4.3

[a] Indirect fluorescent antibody-reactive antigens detected in nonhybrid and hybrid cell lines. +, detectable virus-specific T antigen in nucleus and cytoplasm (Ad2 T) or nucleus (SV40 T) of more than 50% of cells; 0, no detectable virus-specific antigen
[b] Effector-cell-induced release of nuclear label (^{3}[H]-thymidine) in 48-h cytolysis assays. Mean ± SEM of nine experiments
[c] S1$^+$A1$^+$2.4, for example, is a line of hybrid cells formed by fusing an SV40HE1 thymidine-kinase-negative mutant (S1) with an Ad2HE1 hypoxanthine-guanine-phosphoribosyl-transferase-negative mutant (A1); 2 is the number of the clone of fused cells obtained from selective medium (clone 2); 0.4 is the number of the subclone from which the hybrid cell line was established (subclone 4); superscript + or − indicates the presence or absence of detectable SV40 or Ad2 T antigens in the hybrid cells

ences in the induction of cell surface changes during transformation that differentiate Ad12 from Ad2, or it may be some other transformed cell property that determines the ability of the cell to survive the injury inflicted by these effector cells. Whatever the transformed cell trait responsible for cytolytic susceptibility of Ad-transformed cells, the results of the somatic cell hybrid studies described above suggest that in the case of Ad2-transformed hamster cells, this transformed cell trait may be the result of the function of one or more of the Ad2 T antigens.

6 Summary and Conclusions

The reasons for the different tumor-inducing capacities among the Ad serotypes are unclear. One factor in determining the likelihood of tumor induction following Ad infection may be the permissiveness of the host cell for the specific Ad serotype. However, in cells from the same species, both highly oncogenic (e.g., Ad12) and nononcogenic (e.g., Ad2) Ad serotypes can transform cells which exhibit markedly different tumor-inducing capacities in the host. Thus, in addition to the permissiveness of the original infection, there must be other differences, expressed following transformation, which play a role in determining adenoviral oncogenicity.

The results of the studies summarized in Sect. 2 and 3 indicate that there is no significant difference in the efficiencies with which highly oncogenic Ad12 or nononcogenic Ad2 transform rat or hamster cells. Furthermore, there is no evidence that rodent cells transformed by these two Ad serotypes differ in their abilities to induce specific immune responses in the host. Studies of numerous in vitro properties observed among DNA-virus-transformed rodent cells have also failed to reveal a transformed cell trait that reliably predicts the ability of such cells to induce tumors in the immunocompetent host. The common shortcoming of these attempts at linking in vitro parameters of transformation with tumor-inducing capacity is that they have usually not accounted for interactions between transformed cells and the host defenses against such cells.

The importance of considering the host cellular immune defenses in attempting to understand differences in the tumor-inducing capacities of cells transformed by highly oncogenic Ad12 or nononcogenic Ad2 is demonstrated by the results of the rat and hamster studies reviewed in Sects. 4 and 5. In both animal models, in vivo data indicate that it is the interaction between host cellular immune defenses and Ad-transformed cells that is the key factor determining the outcome of transformed cell challenge. The results of bioassays of Ad-transformed cell immunogenicity, histopathological studies of early interactions between Ad tumor cells and host mononuclear inflammatory cells, and in vitro cytolysis assays using various host effector cell populations suggest that the most important components of the host cellular immune response to Ad-transformed cell challenge are early, immunologically nonspecific host effector cells.

Similar correlations between tumor-inducing capacity and the level of neoplastic cell susceptibility to lysis by spontaneously cytolytic host effector cells have been observed in other experimental models in which phenotypic variability among cell lines derived from chemically induced neoplasms has been examined. For example, in studies reviewed by HENNEY (1981) and by COLLINS et al. (1981), reduced susceptibility to lysis by spontaneously cytolytic host effector cells has been observed among cell variants derived after in vivo transplantation of susceptible tumor cell lines. The results of these studies suggest that changes in neoplastic cells resulting from in vivo selection caused the reduced cytolytic susceptibility observed among such variant cell lines. The task of defining the mechanisms by which such variations in susceptibility to host-effector-cell-induced lysis arises in such experimental models is formidable due to the nature of the original transforming agent and the complexity of the in vivo selection process. The results of the Ad-transformed rodent cell experiments reviewed in this chapter suggest that differences in susceptibility to spontaneous host-cell-mediated cytolysis arise following one-step in vitro transformation by different Ad serotypes in the absence of host selection pressure. Thus the Ad-transformed cell model may be useful in elucidating mechanisms by which differences in cytolytic susceptibility are induced.

As evidenced by the data reviewed in other chapters of this volume, there is a progressive increase in our understanding of the relationship between adenoviral gene function and the process of cell transformation. However, the results of the studies presented in this chapter suggest that the definition of transformed cell properties responsible for tumorigenicity will require a more thorough understanding of interactions between Ad-transformed cells and the host cellular immune response. Since both highly oncogenic Ad12 and nononcogenic Ad2 are capable of cell transformation, and since cells transformed by both Ad serotypes are highly immunogenic, it appears that properties other than those commonly associated with transformation are responsible for the success (Ad12) or failure (Ad2) of Ad-transformed cells in avoiding rejection by such host cellular defenses. Based upon our data and that of others presented herein, our hypothesis is that differences in the function of viral gene products encoded in cells transformed by highly oncogenic and nononcogenic Ad may be responsible for the induction of different levels of susceptibility or resistance to the lytic mechanisms of nonspecific host effector cells.

The expression of a specific level of susceptibility or resistance to cellular immune rejection would then be important in determining the tumor-inducing capacity of the Ad-transformed cell. This postulated regulation of the levels of cytolytic susceptibility by functional differences in Ad gene products expressed in transformed cells may ultimately provide an explanation at the molecular level for the observed range of tumor-inducing capacities among the various Ad subgroups.

Acknowledgments. We thank Drs. Raymond Gilden and Robert Huebner for the use of their unpublished studies of the lack of oncogenicity of Ad2 in rodents.

This work was supported by the Elsa U. Pardee Foundation and by Public Health Service Grant R23 CA31732 2 awarded by the National Cancer Institute, National Institutes of Health, DHHS.

References

Akagi T, Ogawa K (1972) Relationship among tumorigenicity, T antigen, and virus-specific transplantation antigen in adenovirus type 12 transformed and tumor cells. Gan 63:307–312

Allison AC, Berman LD, Levey RH (1967) Increased tumor induction by adenovirus type 12 in thymectomized mice and mice treated with anti-lymphocyte serum. Nature 215:185–187

Ankerst J, Sjögren HO (1969) Cross-reacting TSTAs in adeno 7 and 12 tumors demonstrated by ^{51}Cr-cytotoxicity and isograft rejection tests. Int J Cancer 4:279–287

Ankerst J, Sjögren HO (1970) Cross-reacting tumor-specific transplantation of antigens in tumors induced by adenoviruses 3, 14, and 12. Cancer Res 30:1499–1505

Berman LD (1967) On the nature of transplantation immunity in the adenovirus tumor system. J Exp Med 125:983–999

Billingham RE, Sawchuck GH, Silvers WK (1960) The induction of tolerance of skin homografts in Syrian hamsters. Transplant Bull 26:446–449

Challberg MD, Kelly TJ Jr (1982) Eukaryotic DNA replication: viral and plasmid model systems. Ann Rev Biochem 51:901–934

Collins JL, Patek PQ, Cohn M (1981) Tumorigenicity and lysis by natural killers. J Exp Med 153:89–106

Cook JL, Lewis AM Jr (1979) Host response to adenovirus 2-transformed hamster embryo cells. Cancer Res 39:1455–1461

Cook JL, Kirkpatrick CH, Rabson AS, Lewis AM Jr (1979a) Rejection of adenovirus 2-transformed cell tumors and immune responsiveness in Syrian hamsters. Cancer Res 39:4949–4955

Cook JL, Lewis AM Jr, Kirkpatrick CH (1979b) Age-related and thymus-dependent rejection of adenovirus 2-transformed cell tumors in the Syrian hamster. Cancer Res 39:3335–3340

Cook JL, Hibbs JB Jr, Lewis AM Jr (1980) Resistance of simian virus 40-transformed hamster cells to the cytolytic effect of activated macrophages: a possible factor in species-specific viral oncogenicity. Proc Natl Acad Sci USA 77:6773–6777

Cook JL, Hibbs JB Jr, Lewis AM Jr (1982) DNA virus-transformed hamster cell-host effector cell interactions: level of resistance to cytolysis correlated with tumorigenicity. Int J Cancer 30:795–803

Cook JL, Hauser J, Patch C, Lewis AM Jr, Levine AS (1983) Adenovirus 2 early gene expression promotes susceptibility to effector cell lysis of hybrids formed between adenovirus 2 and simian virus 40 transformed hamster cells. Proc Natl Acad Sci USA 80:5995–5999

Doerfler W (1982) Uptake, fixation, and expression of foreign DNA in mammalian cells: the organization of integrated adenovirus DNA sequencer. In: Graf T, Jaenisch R (eds) Tumor viruses, Neoplastic Transformations, and Differentiation. Springer, Berlin Heidelberg New York, pp 127–194 (Current topies in microbiology and immunology, vol 101)

Eddy BE, Grubbs GE, Young RD (1964) Tumor immunity in hamsters infected with adenovirus 12 or simian virus 40. Proc Soc Exp Biol Med 117:575–579

Flint SJ (1980a) Structure and organization of adenoviruses. In: Tooze J (ed) Molecular biology of tumor viruses. Part 2, DNA tumor viruses. Cold Spring Harbor Laboratory, Cold Spring Harbor, New York, pp 383–442

Flint SJ (1980b) Transformation by adenoviruses. In: Tooze J (ed) Molecular biology of tumor viruses. Part 2, DNA tumor viruses. Cold Spring Harbor Laboratory, Cold Spring Harbor, New York, pp 547–576

Foulds L (1969) Neoplastic development. Academic, London

Gallimore PH (1972) Tumour production in immunosuppressed rats with cells transformed in vitro by adenovirus type 2. J Gen Virol 16:99–102

Gallimore PH, Paraskeva C (1980) A study to determine the reasons for differences in the tumorigenicity of rat cell lines transformed by adenovirus 2 and adenovirus 12. Cold Spring Harbor Symp Quant Biol 44:703–713

Gallimore PH, McDougall JK, Chen LB (1977) In vitro traits of adenovirus-transformed cell lines and their relevance to tumorigenicity in nude mice. Cell 10:669–678

Gilden RV, Kern J, Freeman AE, Martin CE, McAllister RM, Turner HC, Huebner RJ (1968) T and tumor antigens of adenovirus group C-infected and transformed cells. Nature 219:517–518

Girardi AJ, Hilleman MR, Zwickey RE (1964) Tests in hamsters for oncogenic quality of ordinary viruses including adenovirus type 7. Proc Soc Exp Biol Med 115:1141–1150

Green M, Mackey JK, Wold WSM, Rigden P (1979) Thirty-one human adenovirus serotypes (Ad1-Ad31) from five groups (A-E) based upon DNA genome homologies. Virology 93:481–492

Haller O, Orn A, Gidlund M, Wigzell H (1980) In vivo activity of murine NK cells. In: Herberman RB (ed) Natural cell-mediated immunity against tumors. Academic, New York, pp 1105–1116

Harwood LMJ, Gallimore PH (1975) A study of the oncogenicity of adenovirus type 2 transformed rat embryo cells. Int J Cancer 16:498–508

Henney CS (1981) Do natural killer cells function through recognition of glycoconjugates on target cell membranes? In: Saunders JP, Daniels JC, Serrou B, Rosenfeld C, Denney CB (eds) Fundamental mechanisms in human cancer immunology. Elsevier/North Holland, New York, pp 465–475

Herberman R (1981) Overview of role of macrophages, natural killer cells, and antibody dependent cellular cytotoxicity as mediators of biological response modification. In: Chirigos MA, Mitchel M, Mastrangelo MJ, Krim M (eds) Mediation of cellular immunity in cancer by immune modifiers. Raven, New York, pp 261–267

Herberman RB, Ortaldo JR (1981) Natural killer cells: their role in defenses against disease. Science 214:24–30

Huebner RJ (1967) Adenovirus-directed tumor and T antigens. In: Pollard M (ed) Perspectives in virology, vol 5. Academic, New York, pp 147–166

Huebner RJ, Rowe WP, Lane WT (1962) Oncogenic effects in hamsters of human adenovirus types 12 and 18. Proc Natl Acad Sci USA 48:2051–2058

Huebner RJ, Lane WT, Welch AD, Calabresi P, McCollum RW, Prusoff WH (1963a) Inhibition by 5-iododeoxyuridine of the oncogenic effects of adenovirus type 12 in hamsters. Science 142:488–490

Huebner RJ, Rowe WP, Turner HC, Lane WT (1963b) Specific adenovirus complement-fixing antigens in virus-free hamster and rat tumors. Proc Natl Acad Sci USA 50:379–389

Kiessling R, Wigzell H (1979) An analysis of the murine NK cell as to structure, function, and biological relevance. Immunol Rev 44:165–208

Kirschstein RL, Rabson AS, Peters EA (1964) Oncogenic activity of adenovirus 12 in thymectomized BALB/c and C3H/HeN mice. Proc Soc Exp Biol Med 117:198–200

Kvist D, Östberg L, Persson H, Philipson L, Peterson PA (1978) Molecular association between transplantation antigens and cell surface antigen in adenovirus-transformed cell line. Proc Natl Acad Sci USA 75:5674–5678

Lewis AM Jr, Cook JL (1979) Association of tumor induction by ultraviolet light-inactivated adenovirus 2-simian virus 40 recombinants with a specific segment of simian virus 40 DNA. J Natl Cancer Inst 63:695–705

Lewis AM Jr, Cook JL (1980) Presence of allograft-rejection resistance in simian virus 40-transformed hamster cells and its possible role in tumor development. Proc Natl Acad Sci USA 77:2886–2889

Lewis AM Jr, Cook JL (1982) Spectrum of tumorigenic phenotypes among adenovirus 2, adenovirus 12, and simian virus 40-transformed Syrian hamster cells defined by host cellular immune-tumor cell interactions. Cancer Res 42:939–944

McAllister RM, MacPherson I (1968) Transformation of a hamster cell line by adenovirus 12. J Gen Virol 2:99–106

McAllister RM, Nicolson MO, Reed G, Kern J, Gilden RV, Huebner RJ (1969) Transformation of rodent cells by adenovirus 19 and other group D adenoviruses. J Natl Cancer Inst 43:917–922

Patch C, Hauser J, Lewis AM Jr, Levine AS (1983) Adenovirus 2 early gene expression reduces the tumor-inducing capacity of hybrid cells formed from simian virus 40- and adenovirus 2-transformed hamster embryo cells. Cancer Res 43:2571–2575

Persson H, Philipson L (1982) Regulation of adenovirus gene expression. In: Cooper M et al. (eds) Current topies in microbiology and immunology, vol 97. Springer, Berlin Heidelberg New York, pp 157–203

Persson H, Kvist S, Ostberg L, Peterson PA, Philipson L (1980) Adenoviral early glycoprotein E3-19K and its association with transplantation antigens. Cold Spring Harbor Symp Quant Biol 45:509–517

Persson H, Katze MG, Philipson L (1982) Purification of a native membrane-associated adenovirus tumor antigen. J Virol 42:905–917

Rabson AS, Kirschstein RL, Paul FJ (1964) Tumors produced by adenovirus 12 in mastomys and mice. J Natl Cancer Inst 32:77–87

Rask L, Lindblom JB, Peterson PA (1974) Subunit structure of H-2 alloantigens. Nature 249:833–835

Raska K Jr, Gallimore PH (1982) An inverse relation of the oncogenic potential of adenovirus transformed cells and their sensitivity to killing by syngeneic natural killer cells. Virology 123:8–18

Raska K Jr, Morrongiello MP, Fohring B (1980) Adenovirus type 12 tumor antigen. III. Tumorigenicity and immune response to syngeneic rat cells transformed with virions and isolated transforming fragment of adenovirus 12 DNA. Int J Cancer 26:79–86

Raska K Jr, Dougherty J, Gallimore PH (1982) Product of adenovirus type 2 early gene block E_1 in transformed cells elicits cytolytic response in syngeneic rats. Virology 117:530–535

Sehgal PB, Frazer NW, Darnell JE (1979) Early Ad2-transcription units: only promoter-proximal RNA continues to be made in the presence of DRB. Virology 94:185–191

Shiroki K, Shimojo H, Maeta Y, Hamada C (1979) Tumor-specific transplantation and surface antigen in cells transformed by the adenovirus 12 DNA fragments. Virology 99:188–191

Signas C, Katze MG, Persson H, Philipson L (1982) An adenovirus glycoprotein binds heavy chains of class I transplantation antigens from man and mouse. Nature 299:175–177

Silver J, Hood L (1974) Detergent-solubilized H-2 alloantigen is associated with a small molecular weight polypeptide. Nature 249:764–765

Sjögren HO, Ankerst J (1969) Effect of BCG and allogeneic tumor cells on adenovirus type 12 tumorigenesis in mice. Nature 221:863–864

Sjögren HO, Minowada J, Ankerst J (1967) Specific transplantation antigens of mouse sarcomas induced by adenovirus type 12. J Exp Med 125:689–701

Tevethia SS (1980) Immunology of simian virus 40. In: Klein G (ed) Viral oncology. Raven, New York, pp 581–602

Trentin JJ, Bryan E (1966) Virus-induced transplantation immunity to human adenovirus type 12 tumors of the hamster and mouse. Proc Soc Exp Biol Med 121:1216–1219

Trentin JJ, Yabe Y, Taylor G (1962) The quest for human cancer viruses. Science 137:835–841

Trentin JJ, Van Hoosier GL Jr, Samper L (1968) The oncogenicity of human adenoviruses in hamsters. Proc Soc Exp Biol Med 127:683–689

Vitetta ES, Uhr JW, Boyse EA (1975) Association of a β_2-microglobulin-like subunit with H-2 and TL alloantigens. J Immunol 114:252–254

Wadell G (1979) Classification of human adenoviruses by SDS-polyacrylamide gel electrophoresis of structural polypeptides. Intervirology 11:47–57

Wadell G, Hammarskjöld ML, Winberg G, Varsanyi TM, Sundell G (1980) Genetic variability of adenoviruses. Ann NY Acad Sci USA 354:16–42

Wilson MC, Fraeser NW, Darnell JE (1979) Mapping of RNA initiation sites by high doses of UV irradiation: evidence for three independent promoters within the left 11% of the Ad2 genome. Virology 94:175–184

Yabe Y, Trentin JJ, Grant T (1962) Cancer induction in hamsters by human type 12 adenovirus. Effect of age and of virus dose. Proc Soc Exp Biol Med 111:343–344

Yabe Y, Samper L, Grant T, Trentin JJ (1963) Cancer induction in hamsters by human type 12 adenovirus. Effect of route of injection. Proc Soc Exp Biol Med 113:221–224

Yabe Y, Samper L, Bryan E, Taylor G, Trentin J (1964) Oncogenic effect of human adenovirus type 12 in mice. Science 143:46–47

Yohn DS, Funk CA, Kalnins VI, Grace JT Jr (1965) Sex-related resistance in hamsters to adenovirus-12 oncogenesis. Influence of thymectomy at three weeks of age. J Natl Cancer Inst 35:617–624

Yohn DS, Funk CA, Grace JT (1968) Sex-related resistance in hamsters to adenovirus 12 oncogenesis. III. Influence of immunologic impairment by thymectomy or cortisone. J Immunol 100:771–780

Transformation and Oncogenicity
by Adenoviruses

A.J. VAN DER EB and R. BERNARDS

1 Introduction

Adenoviruses have attracted considerable attention since it was discovered by TRENTIN et al. (1962) and HUEBNER et al. (1962) that certain species (formerly called serotypes; WIGAND et al. 1982) are oncogenic when injected into newborn hamsters. Since then, adenoviruses have been used extensively as a model for studies on tumor induction in vivo and cell transformation in vitro. Together with the small papovaviruses, they have played an important role in fundamental cancer research and have provided invaluable tools for studies on the organization and expression of eukaryotic genes. The introduction of new techniques of DNA sequencing, molecular cloning, and DNA transfection in the past few

Department of Medical Biochemistry, Sylvius Laboratories, Wassenaarseweg 72, NL-2333 AL Leiden years have further contributed to a rapid development of adenovirus research in all its diverse aspects.

Adenoviruses are medium-sized viruses containing linear double-stranded DNA genomes. The DNA of the mammalian adenoviruses consists of 33–36 kilobase pairs (kb) (GREEN et al. 1967; VAN DER EB et al. 1969), whereas the avian adenoviruses have larger genomes, measuring about 45 kb (BELLETT and YOUNGHUSBAND 1972; LAVER et al. 1971). More than 80 different adenovirus species have been identified among vertebrates, 41 of which are of human origin (NORRBY et al. 1976; WADELL et al. 1980; WIGAND et al. 1982; DE JONG et al. 1983). HUEBNER (1967) originally classified the human adenoviruses into three subgroups (now called subgenera; WIGAND et al. 1982) A, B and C, on the basis of their oncogenicity in newborn hamsters. Subgenus A is highly oncogenic, inducing tumors with high frequency and after a short latency period; subgenus B is weakly oncogenic, causing tumors in a fraction of the injected animals after long latency periods; and subgenus C is nononcogenic. The species originally classified in subgenus C were later further subdivided into subgenera C, D, and E (GREEN et al. 1979; MCALLISTER et al. 1969a; WADELL et al. 1980). The recently discovered fastidious enteric adenoviruses may belong to a new subgenus F (WADELL et al. 1980). The adenoviruses belonging to subgenus F can only be grown with difficulty in a restricted number of cell culture systems, and up to now comprise two species, Ad40 and Ad41 (DE JONG et al. 1983; JOHANSSON et al. 1980; TAKIFF et al. 1981). The members within each subgenus are closely related with respect to GC content of the DNA and nucleotide sequence homology (PIÑA and GREEN 1965; GARON et al. 1973; MACKEY et al. 1979). Although only the members of subgenera A and B of human adenoviruses are oncogenic in hamsters and certain other rodents, all species of genera A–E are capable of morphologically transforming cultured rat or hamster cells. Little information is available about the transforming properties of the fastidious adenoviruses. Recently, Sussenbach observed transforming activity of Ad40 in cell culture (J.S. Sussenbach, personal communication).

Adenoviruses of nonhuman origin have been relatively little studied. Oncogenic viruses are found both among mammalian and avian adenoviruses (HULL et al. 1965; MCALLISTER et al. 1969b; PONOMAREVA et al. 1979; STRIZHACHENKO et al. 1975; ISHIBASHI et al. 1980). In all cases, oncogenic potential is defined as the ability of the virus to induce tumors after injection into newborn hamsters or other rodents.

Most of our current knowledge is based on studies of human Ad2 and Ad5 (both nononcogenic species of subgenus C) and Ad12 (an oncogenic species of subgenus A). This chapter will deal mainly with the transforming and oncogenic properties of these three adenoviruses.

2 Localization of the Transforming Genes

Human adenoviruses can transform a variety of cultured rodent cells, including fibroblasts from hamster (POPE and ROWE 1964), rat (FREEMAN et al. 1967), mouse (YOUNGHUSBAND et al. 1979; STARZINSKI-POWITZ et al. 1982), and rabbit (LEVINTHAL and PETERSON 1965). Nononcogenic Ad2 and Ad5 can replicate rather efficiently in hamster cells, and in order to achieve transformation of these cells it is necessary to use either UV-inactivated virus (LEWIS et al. 1974) or temperature-sensitive mutants (WILLIAMS 1973). Rat cells are semipermissive for Ad2 and Ad5 replication (GALLIMORE 1974), and transformation by these viruses is also most readily achieved when infectivity is reduced or abolished. In contrast, hamster and rat cells are completely nonpermissive to replication of oncogenic Ad12 (DOERFLER 1969; ZUR HAUSEN and SOKOL 1969), although this virus causes severe chromosomal damage in infected hamster cells, often resulting in cell death (ZUR HAUSEN 1968; STROHL 1969). Transformation is a rare event in all virus-cell combinations studied, the efficiency being as low as 1 focus-forming unit (FFU) per 10^4–10^6 PFU of virus, or a few transformed foci per 10^5–10^6 cells. Human cells, which are fully permissive to adenovirus replication, are extremely difficult to transform. Only two transformed human cell lines have been isolated by the time of writing: a human embryonic kidney cell line transformed in 1973 with sheared Ad5 DNA by Graham, known as the 293 line (GRAHAM et al. 1974a, 1977), and a human retinoblast line transformed with a cloned DNA fragment of Ad12 (BYRD et al. 1982). Both lines are completely permissive to adenovirus replication. The 293 line can complement Ad5 mutants with defects in their transforming genes, and this property has greatly facilitated the isolation of transformation-defective Ad5 mutants (GRAHAM et al. 1978; JONES and SHENK 1979a).

The discovery of restriction endonucleases and of a method to demonstrate biological activity of DNA in cultured cells made it possible in 1974 to localize the transforming activity of Ad2, Ad5, and Ad12 on the viral genome. Two different experimental approaches were used to achieve these results.

Analysis of the viral DNA sequences present in a series of Ad2-tranformed rat and hamster cells showed that the proportion of the viral genome retained in the cell lines varied considerably from one line to the other, but that all lines invariably contained the left-terminal 14% of the viral DNA. In all cell lines studied, about 50% of this terminal DNA segment was expressed as cytoplasmic RNA, transcribed from the viral r-strand (i.e., the DNA strand transcribed in the rightward direction). These results therefore indicated that the leftmost 14% of Ad2 DNA contained the viral genes required for transformation, or at least to maintain the cells in the transformed state (GALLIMORE et al. 1974; SHARP et al. 1974a, b; SAMBROOK et al. 1975; FLINT and SHARP 1976).

Direct proof that the transforming genes are located at the left end of the genome was obtained with DNA transfection experiments using the calcium phosphate technique (GRAHAM and VAN DER EB 1973). These studies showed that the transforming activity of Ad5 is located at the left-hand end of the viral genome (GRAHAM et al. 1974b) and that transformation could be obtained with purified restriction fragments originating from the left end of Ad5 DNA, as well as of Ad12 DNA (GRAHAM et al. 1974b). Rat cells transformed by a left-terminal 15% Ad5 DNA fragment were phenotypically indistinguishable from cells transformed by intact viral DNA or virions, while cells transformed by smaller DNA fragments exhibited aberrant transformed phenotypes (VAN DER EB et al. 1977). The left-hand 15% DNA segment is now known to contain the early region 1 (E1), one of the four early regions of the adenovirus genome which are transcribed in the early phase of the lytic infection (PETTERSSON et al. 1983). Subsequent studies confirmed the early observations and showed that the transforming genes of nononcogenic Ad2 and Ad5 (VAN DER EB et al. 1977, 1979), weakly oncogenic Ad3 and Ad7 (SEKIKAWA et al. 1978; DIJKEMA et al. 1979), highly oncogenic Ad12 and Ad31 (YANO et al. 1977; SHIROKI et al. 1977; JOCHEMSEN et al. 1982; SAWADA et al. 1981) and simian adenovirus SA7 (PONOMAREVA et al. 1979) are located at the left end of the genome. A similar position of the transforming genes has also been suggested for CELO virus, an avian adenovirus (YASUE and ISHIBASHI 1982). Since cells transformed by DNA segments containing only region E1 of Ad12 are oncogenic in immuno-competent animals (SHIROKI et al. 1977, 1979a; BERNARDS et al. 1983b) it can be concluded that oncogenicity is also determined, at least to a large extent, by region E1. This is further confirmed by the finding that injection of hamsters with Ad12 DNA or DNA fragments resulted in induction of tumors, albeit at a low frequency (JOCHEMSEN et al. 1982).

The patterns of integration of adenovirus DNA into the DNA of trans-formed cells have been studied in detail by several groups. Continuous expres-sion of viral transforming DNA sequences seems to be required for the mainte-nance of the transformed state, as was shown in recent experiments with *ts* mutants. Our current knowledge about the integration of adenovirus DNA sequences in transformed cells and the role of methylation on the expression of integrated viral genes is not considered in this chapter, as this subject is reviewed in detail by DOERFLER et al. (1983).

3   Organization of the Transforming Region

The transforming regions of the human adenoviruses that have been studied so far are structurally organized in a very similar way. As stated previously, the transforming region is identical to region E1, which has been completely sequenced for nononcogenic Ad5 and Ad2, weakly oncogenic Ad7, and highly oncogenic Ad12 (VAN ORMONDT et al. 1980; BOS et al. 1981; DIJKEMA et al. 1982; SUGISAKI et al. 1980; KIMURA et al. 1981). A detailed description of the organization and the nucleotide sequence of the E1 region of these viruses is presented by VAN ORMONDT and GALIBERT (this volume).

Studies of DNA:RNA hybrids as viewed by the electron microscope (CHOW et al. 1977, 1979) and by S1 nuclease analysis (BERK and SHARP 1978) and mapping studies of early viral promoters for RNA transcription (BERK and SHARP 1977; WILSON et al. 1979) have shown that region E1 consists of two adjacent transcriptional units, E1A (ca. 1.3–4.5%) and E1B (4.6–11.5%), each containing its own promoter. Region E1B harbors a second transcriptional unit, with an independent promoter, coding for the structural polypeptide IX (ALESTRÖM et al. 1980; WILSON et al. 1979). Polypeptide IX does not seem

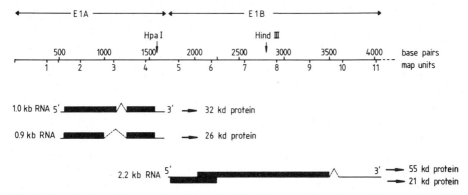

Fig. 1. Organization of the transforming region E1 of human adenovirus 5. The two subregions E1A and E1B are indicated, as well as the map positions of the mRNAs encoded by each of the subregions, as far as they are expressed in the transformed cells. *Dashed lines* in the mRNAs represent intervening sequences, while the *bars* indicate the RNA segments that are translated into protein. The molecular weights of the proteins represent the values predicted from the DNA sequence and the known positions of the intervening sequences

to play a role in transformation and hence will not be further considered in this chapter.

Region E1A of subgenus C adenoviruses codes for three major cytoplasmic RNAs of 0.5, 0.9, and 1.0 kb, transcribed from a single promoter. The three RNAs have common 5' and 3' ends, and differ in the amount of RNA sequences removed internally by splicing. The 1.0- and 0.9-kb RNAs are transcribed early in lytic infection, while the 0.5-kb RNA is synthesized almost exclusively late in the lytic cycle. In transformed cells only the 1.0- and 0.9-kb E1A RNAs have been detected.

Region E1B codes for three major cytoplasmic RNA species. Two of these transcripts, which measure 1.0 and 2.2 kb for Ad5, are transcribed from the same promoter and have identical 5' and 3' ends. The third RNA is transcribed from an independent promoter and codes for virion polypeptide IX. The 2.2-kb RNA is found both in the early and the late phase of lytic infection and in transformed cells, while the 1.0-kb RNA is synthesized predominantly late in infection and seems to be absent in transformed cells (VAN DEN ELSEN et al. 1983b).

The map positions of the RNA species transcribed in transformed cells from region E1 of Ad5 are shown in Fig. 1. A detailed description of the RNAs specified by the adenovirus early regions is presented by U. PETTERSSON (1983); RNA coordinates can be found in the contribution of VAN ORMONDT and GALIBERT (this volume).

The 1.0- and 0.9-kb RNAs from region E1A will specific polypeptides with predicted molecular weights of 32000 and 26000 respectively. For reasons that are not yet understood, the molecular weights of the E1A proteins, calculated from the electrophoretic mobility in SDS gels, are much higher than the predicted values. Moreover, the E1A polypeptides are resolved in SDS gels into at least four bands rather than two, while even more species are found in two-dimensional gels (HARTER and LEWIS 1978). The apparent molecular weights of the E1A polypeptides published in the literature vary considerably, most likely as a result of the use of different gel systems and molecular weight markers. The lowest reported values for in vitro synthesized Ad5 E1A proteins are 34, 36, 40 and 42 kd (JOCHEMSEN et al. 1981; LUPKER et al. 1981). Higher molecular weights published for Ad2 and Ad5 E1A proteins include: for the proteins specified by the 0.9-kb E1A, RNA values of 35 and 47 kd or 42 and 54 kd; and for the proteins specified by the 1.0-kb E1A, RNA values of 41 and 53 kd or 48 and 58 kd (HALBERT et al. 1979; ESCHE et al. 1980). Molecular weights of Ad5 E1A proteins precipitated from lytically infected or transformed cells with monospecific antisera or monoclonal antibodies are given as 45, 48.5, 50, and 52 kd (ROWE et al. 1983b) or 39, 41, 43 and 44 kd (A. Zantema, personal communication). Region E1A of Ad12 codes for polypeptides with apparent molecular weights ranging from about 40 to 22 kd (JOCHEMSEN et al. 1980; ESCHE and SIEGMANN 1982).

The 2.2-kb RNA encoded by region E1B specifies two major polypeptides which are translated from different, but partially overlapping reading frames (Bos et al. 1981). The predicted molecular weights for the Ad5 E1B polypeptides are 21 kd and 55 kd, for the Ad12 E1B polypeptides 19 kd and 54 kd. The apparent molecular weights of the Ad2 and Ad5 E1B proteins, calculated from their electrophoretic mobility in SDS gels, vary from 15 to 19 kd for the small polypeptide and from 52 to 65 kd for the large polypeptide (HALBERT et al. 1979; SCHRIER et al. 1979; JOCHEMSEN et al. 1980, 1982; ESCHE and SIEGMAN 1982). As predicted from nucleotide sequence studies and confirmed by (chymo)-tryptic peptide analysis, the two major E1B proteins are structurally unrelated (Bos et al. 1981; GREEN et al. 1980; HALBERT and RASKAS 1982; JOCHEMSEN et al. 1982). In this article, a molecular weight of 20 kd will be used for the small E1B polypeptide of both Ad5 and Ad12, and 55 kd for the large E1B polypeptide of both species.

Region E1B also produces a number of smaller polypeptides that appear to be related to the large E1B protein (ESCHE et al. 1982; MATSUO et al. 1982; VAN DEN ELSEN et al. 1982; P.I. SCHRIER, personal communication). A detailed discussion of early adenovirus proteins is presented by LEVINE (this volume).

4 Contribution of Regions E1A and E1B in Transformation

4.1 DNA Segments Smaller Than Region E1
Also Have Transforming Activity

As mentioned previously, cells transformed by DNA fragments comprising an intact region E1 are phenotypically very similar to cells transformed by total viral DNA or virions. This indicates that transformation and oncogenicity are exclusively or mainly functions of region E1, although RAŠKA et al. (1980) have shown that other regions of the Ad12 genome also may contribute to the oncogenic phenotype.

Studies with adenovirus DNA fragments which lack increasing parts from the right-hand end of region E1 have shown that such fragments still exhibit transforming activity, and that the smallest fragment capable of causing stable morphological transformation is the left-most 4.5%, which essentially comprises region E1A. This was found for nononcogenic Ad2 and Ad5 (HOUWELING et al. 1980; VAN DEN ELSEN et al. 1982), weakly oncogenic Ad3 and Ad7 (DIJKEMA et al. 1979), and highly oncogenic Ad12 (SHIROKI et al. 1979b). For Ad3 and Ad7, a 4% left-terminal fragment was also shown to contain transforming activity in primary BRK cells, although it has not been possible to establish cell lines from such foci.

Cells transformed by the leftmost 4.5% (region E1A) of the adenovirus genome exhibit a semitransformed phenotype and are unable to grow to high saturation densities (HOUWELING et al. 1980; SHIROKI et al. 1979b; VAN DEN ELSEN et al. 1982), suggesting that region E1B must have a role in morphological transformation. Rat kidney cells transformed by DNA fragments containing region E1A and about half of region E1B (fragments HindIII G of both Ad5 and Ad12 DNA, representing the left-terminal 8% and 7.5% respectively) appear almost completely transformed, although they generally reach somewhat lower saturation densities than cells transformed by the entire E1 region (VAN DER EB et al. 1977, 1979; JOCHEMSEN et al. 1982). Since cell lines transformed by the Ad5 or Ad12 HindIII G fragments do not produce an intact 55-kd E1B protein but always express the 20-kd E1B polypeptide (SCHRIER et al. 1979; JOCHEMSEN et al. 1982), it was initially concluded that the 20-kd protein must be responsible, directly or indirectly, for morphological transformation. Subsequent results, however (see Sect. 4.2), indicated that this conclusion may be incorrect and that the effect on transformation is more likely to be attributed to the action of a truncated 55-kd protein. HindIII G-transformed cells, in fact, still contain information for a 33-kd truncated product of the large E1B protein. Immunoprecipitation studies, using a monoclonal antibody against the 55-kd protein, have indeed shown that Ad5 HindIII G-transformed cells produce proteins of 19.5, 16.5, and 11 kd which specifically react with the antiserum (A. Zantema, personal communication).

4.2 Transformation by Plasmids Carrying Specific Mutations in the Transforming Genes

By using site-directed mutagenesis in cloned region E1 plasmids, it has been possible to investigate the contribution of the E1A- and E1B-encoded polypeptides in oncogenic transformation in more detail.

The mutations that have been introduced in region E1B were frame-shift mutations, resulting in the production of truncated proteins. Recombinant plasmids containing E1 regions of Ad5 or Ad12 in which the 20-kd E1B polypeptide was mutated had normal transforming activities in primary baby rat kidney cells, and the resulting transformed cells were morphologically very similar to cells transformed by intact E1 regions. These results suggested that the 20-kd E1B polypeptide may not have an important function in morphological transformation, in contrast to earlier conclusions (see Sect. 4.1). However, Ad12-transformed cells which lacked the 20-kd E1B polypeptide were nononcogenic in nude mice, indicating that the 20-kd E1B polypeptide does have a role in oncogenicity (BERNARDS et al. 1983a).

Plasmids containing Ad5 E1 regions with frame-shift mutations in the 55-kd E1B protein were also capable of transforming rat cells. The morphology of the transformed cells, however, was dependent on the position of the mutations: if the mutation was introduced at the HindIII site at 8 map units (nucleotide (nt) 2804) of the Ad5 sequence, the morphology was similar to that of cells transformed by intact E1 regions. If the mutation was introduced at the TthI site at 6.5 map units (nt 2395), the efficiency of transformation was greatly reduced and the morphology of the majority of the transformed cells was fibroblastic and resembled that of rat kidney cells transformed by Ad5 region E1A alone (R. Bernards, unpublished results). Since both mutant plasmids expressed the 20-kd E1B polypeptide normally but differed in the size of the truncated 55-kd product present in the cells (33 kd for the HindIII mutant and 9 kd for the TthI mutant), it is likely that the E1B gene responsible for normal morphological transformation is the 55-kd E1B protein, or a sufficiently large N-terminal product of it (which could still be present in cells transformed by the left-terminal 7.5% or 8% of the adenovirus genome). The assumption that an N-terminal truncated product of the 55-kd E1B protein is responsible for the manifestations of the fully transformed phenotype also seems to apply to other adenovirus species. In the Ad12 system it was found that the HindIII G fragment (0–7.5 map units) is also capable of causing morphological transformation of primary rat kidney cells (JOCHEMSEN et al. 1982), but that an E1 plasmid carrying a frame-shift mutation at the AosI site (nt 2089, 6 map units), resulting in the production of a 10-kd truncated product of the 55-kd E1B protein, does not transform primary rat kidney cells (BERNARDS et al. 1983a). (Region E1A of Ad12 does not have detectable transforming activity in primary rat cells, possibly due to a very low transforming efficiency.) Thus, expression of the 20-kd E1B gene in addition to E1A is apparently not sufficient for normal transformation.

In addition to a role in morphological transformation, the 55-kd E1B protein also contributes to the oncogenic potential of the transformed cells, since rat kidney cells transformed by the left-terminal 7.5% of Ad12 DNA, which express region E1A, the 20-kd E1B protein, and (at the most) a truncated 55-kd E1B polypeptide, are nononcogenic in nude mice (JOCHEMSEN et al. 1982). Thus both E1B polypeptides seem to be required for expression of the oncogenic phenotype, while morphological transformation seems to be dependent on the expression of the 55-kd E1B polypeptide only. Recent data, however, suggest that region E1A may have a major role in morphological transformation and that region E1B affects this process only indirectly. At least three points support this view: (a) region E1A alone is capable of transforming cells in culture; (b) region E1B alone has no detectable transforming activity (see Sect. 4.3); and (c) it has recently been shown that the morphology of transformed foci in primary cultures of baby rat kidney cells is determined by the identity of the E1A region, i.e., when region E1A is derived from Ad5, the colonies resemble

Ad5-transformed foci, and when E1A is derived from Ad12, the colonies resemble Ad12-transformed foci, even when region E1B is from Ad5 (VAN DEN ELSEN 1982). It is possible, therefore, that morphological transformation is determined to a large extent by region E1A. The reason that cells transformed by region E1A appear partially transformed may be that E1A is expressed in these cells at very low levels only (VAN DEN ELSEN et al. 1983b). Region E1B, and more specifically the 55-kd protein, may thus be required for efficient expression of region E1A (see also VAN DEN ELSEN et al. 1983c).

In this context, it is of interest to note that DNA extracted from complementation group II host-range mutants, which carry mutations in region E1B (see Sect. 5.1) is capable of transforming both rat and hamster cells (ROWE and GRAHAM 1983). Interestingly, hamster cell lines transformed with DNA from group II mutants induced tumors in hamsters, although the oncogenicity was rather low. The transformed hamster cells produced no detectable E1B protein (55-kd or 20-kd), which was interpreted to suggest that these proteins may not necessarily be essential for oncogenicity (ROWE and GRAHAM 1983). These results are at variance with those obtained with adenovirus-transformed rat cells, which already lose their oncogenicity in nude mice when either the small or the large E1B protein is mutated (JOCHEMSEN et al. 1982; BERNARDS et al. 1983a; VAN DER EB et al. 1983). The contradictory results can possibly be explained by the fact that transformed hamster cells more easily progress to more highly oncogenic phenotypes.

Using techniques similar to those described above for region E1B, attempts have been made to investigate the role of the E1A products in transformation in more detail. A number of specific Ad5 E1A mutant plasmids have been constructed and used to reassemble mutant viruses (see Sect. 5.4). In the Ad12 system, Bos et al. (1983) have shown that cloned E1 plasmids with a point mutation affecting the 1.0-kb E1A mRNA only, were incapable of transforming primary rat kidney cells. This defect could be overcome by inserting the SV40 enhancer region in the mutant plasmid. However, the resulting transformed cells, which exhibited the fully transformed phenotype, were nononcogenic, even in nude mice (Bos et al. 1983). Thus manifestation of the oncogenic phenotype requires simultaneous expression of the two E1B proteins as well as of the product of the 1.0-kb E1A mRNA.

4.3 Region E1B Alone Has No Transforming Activity

The demonstration that adenovirus region E1A can induce an incomplete or partial transformation in rat cells (SHIROKI et al. 1979b; HOUWELING et al. 1980) suggested that region E1B must have an essential role in morphological transformation. Ad5 group I host-range mutants, which contain defects in the 1.0-kb E1A mRNA but nevertheless express region E1B, are defective in transformation of primary rat kidney cells (CARLOCK and JONES 1981; SOLNICK 1981). This shows that expression of region E1B is not sufficient to cause morphological transformation, at least not in primary rat cells. A similar conclusion was reached from experiments in which the transforming activity was tested of Ad5

DNA fragments comprising region E1B only. In order to obtain expression of region E1B in the absence of E1A, plasmids were constructed in which region E1B of Ad5 was ligated to the SV40 promoter-enhancer segment. These plasmids were found to lack detectable transforming activity in primary rat kidney cells (VAN DEN ELSEN et al. 1983a). Since these rat kidney cultures have a very limited in vitro life span, the negative result could also have been caused by a lack of immortalizing activity of region E1B. However, experiments with the established rat cell line 3Y1 (KIMURA et al. 1975) also failed to reveal any transforming activity of the SV40-E1B hybrid region, although it was fully expressed in the cells. Complete transformation was readily obtained when rat kidney cells or 3Y1 cells were cotransfected with a mixture of the E1B-SV40 promoter plasmid and an E1A plasmid (VAN DEN ELSEN et al. 1982, 1983a). These results indicate that region E1B has no transforming activity, and stress once more the importance of region E1A in morphological transformation.

5 Adenovirus Mutants Defective in Transformation

5.1 *hr* and *dl* Mutants

A considerable number of mutants have been isolated mainly from nononcogenic Ad5, which carry defects in the transforming genes. One series (*hr* mutants) was isolated after chemical or UV mutagenesis of Ad5 virions (HARRISON et al. 1977) and a second set (*dl* mutants) was isolated as variants of Ad5 lacking the recognition site for the restriction enzyme *Xba*I at 4 map units in region E1A (JONES and SHENK 1979a). Both classes of mutants have been isolated as host-range mutants, i.e., they can be propagated efficiently in line 293 cells (the Ad5-transformed human embryonic kidney line; GRAHAM et al. 1977), but fail to grow in HeLa cells.

Based on complementation analyses, the Ad5 *hr* mutants were divided into group I and group II mutants (ROSS et al. 1980). Group I mutants have been mapped by marker rescue analysis in region E1A and group II mutants in region E1B (FROST and WILLIAMS 1978; GALOS et al. 1980). Owing to the defect in region E1A, group I mutants fail to express proteins of region E1B and other early regions (JONES and SHENK 1979b; ROSS et al. 1980). At high multiplicity of infection, however, the mutants express all early regions and even produce progeny virus in HeLa cells (JONES and SHENK 1979b; NEVINS 1981). Group I mutants are defective for transformation of rat embryo and rat embryo brain cells, but, interestingly, induce transformation in primary baby rat kidney cells with markedly increased efficiency (GRAHAM et al. 1978; RUBEN et al. 1982). Attempts to establish cell lines from group-I-transformed foci were unsuccessful, however, and transformed cells could only be obtained as polyclonal lines by passaging whole cultures. The cells produced the 20-kd and 55-kd Elb polypeptides but exhibited an abnormal fibroblastic morphology. The results are interpreted to indicate that group I mutants may be defective in maintenance of transformation and show that an intact region E1A is essential for normal transformation.

DNA sequence analysis of *hr*1, a group I mutant of Ad5, has shown that it contains a point mutation in the segment of region E1A which is unique to the 1.0-kb mRNA. As a result, a truncated polypeptide is produced from the 1.0-kb mRNA, while the product from the 0.9-kb mRNA is unchanged (RICCARDI et al. 1981). This implies that the polypeptide encoded by the 1.0-kb mRNA must play an essential and unique role, both in regulating expression of other early regions and in transformation.

Group II mutants produce greatly reduced amounts of E1B proteins, if any, and they are transformation defective in rodent cells (LASSAM et al. 1979a; ROSS et al. 1980; GRAHAM et al. 1978). Surprisingly, DNA extracted from group II mutants of Ad5 could transform rat cells in culture with the same efficiency as wild-type DNA (ROWE and GRAHAM 1983). This can possibly be explained by the fact that the group II mutants used still expressed sufficient genetic information from region E1B for transformation to occur normally. As discussed in Sect. 4.2, mutations in either the 20-kd or 55-kd protein do not necessarily interfere with transformation, at least when the cells are transfected with DNA. If intact virions are used the E1B mutations apparently prevent transformation.

The Ad5 host-range *dl* mutants isolated by JONES and SHENK (1979a) contain deletions and substitutions around the *Xba*I site at 4 map units (located at the right end of region E1A). Some of the mutants (*dl*311, *dl*312) have been shown to belong to host-range complementation group I, while others (*dl*313, *sub*315) belong to group II (ROSS et al. 1980). Both classes of *dl* mutants are defective in transformation of rat embryo cells (SHENK et al. 1979).

Recently, it has been reported that the group II mutant *dl*313 which lacks the entire region E1B and a small part of region E1A, can partially transform the established rat cell line 3Y1 and also, at high multiplicity of infection, primary rat kidney cells (SHIROKI et al. 1981; MAK and MAK 1983). This result appears to be in agreement with the demonstration that region E1A of human adenoviruses can incompletely transform rat cells (HOUWELING et al. 1980; DIJKEMA et al. 1979; SHIROKI et al. 1979b).

The observation that certain *hr* group I mutants can transform primary rat kidney cells with high efficiency, but that it has no been possible to establish cell lines from single transformed foci (GRAHAM et al. 1978), is difficult to explain. The fact that cell lines can be obtained only by passaging entire cultures containing primary foci suggests that the phenomenon may be related to a cell-density-dependent process. Ad5-transformed rat kidney cells, including cells transformed by region E1A, are known to produce growth factors which bind to EGF receptor (FISCHER et al. 1983; E.J.J. van Zoelen, personal communication). Binding of such growth factors stimulates cell proliferation and may induce expression of transformed properties. Mutation in region E1A could cause inappropriate production of growth factors by the transformed cells, which might only be adequate to maintain the transformed state when the cells are in sufficiently close mutual contact. Such conditions may not be present during isolation of a single transformed focus.

5.2 Cold-Sensitive Mutants

Despite extensive efforts in several laboratories, it has not been possible to isolate mutants with temperature(= heat)-sensitive defects in their transforming genes, comparable, for example, to the *ts*-A mutants of SV40. Recently, it has been observed, however, that certain Ad5 host-range mutants, namely *hr*1 and *hr*2, both group I mutants mapping in region E1A, are cold-sensitive for transformation in primary rat embryo fibroblasts. The mutants are transformation negative at 32° C (and 37° C; GRAHAM et al. 1978), but they transform efficiently at 38.5° C (Ho et al. 1982). *hr*1 transforms CREF cells, an established rat embryo line, even more efficiently at 37° C than wild-type Ad5, but is completely negative for transformation at 32° C (BABISS et al. 1983). Since wild-type Ad5 transforms CREF cells normally at 32° C, *hr*1 must be cold-sensitive for induction of transformation. Furthermore, CREF cells transformed by *hr*1 at 37° C lose part of their transformed properties after a shift to 32° C and show a significant decrease in immunofluorescence upon staining with anti-T sera. These findings indicate that the gene product affected by the *hr*1 mutation plays an important role, both in establishment of transformation and in expression of the transformed phenotype (BABISS et al. 1983).

DNA sequence analysis of cold-sensitive host-range mutants has recently revealed a mutational hotspot in the sequence *glu-his-pro-gly-his*, located in the 46-amino-acid segment unique to the product of the 1.0-kb E1A mRNA (H.S. Ginsberg, personal communication). This unique sequence may be specifically required for transformation, e.g., through an interaction with a cellular protein. Cold-sensitivity might be caused by the fact that the bond between the viral and the cellular protein is only sufficiently stable at high temperature.

Recently, a new series of host-range mutants with a cold-sensitive phenotype has been isolated from Ad5 (Ho et al. 1982). These *hr*^{cs} mutants grow well in HeLa cells at 38.5° C but show restricted growth at 32.5° C, whereas they grow equally well at both temperatures in line 293 cells. The *hr*^{cs} mutants mapping in E1A are cold-sensitive both for induction of transformation and for expression of the transformed phenotype in primary rat embryo cells. The *hr*^{cs} mutants mapping in region E1B are defective in transformation at both the low and the high temperature. The few foci that have been established as cell lines at 38.5° C show a cold-sensitive phenotype similar to that of cells transformed by *hr*^{cs} mutants mapping in region E1A.

These findings again indicate that regions E1A and E1B are simultaneously required both for initiation (induction) of transformation and expression of the transformed phenotype. (It seems doubtful whether the term "maintenance" can be used in the context of adenovirus transformation. It would seem that as soon as transformation is initiated and becomes phenotypically visible, i.e., after a few cell divisions, the transformed state is already maintained. Hence, initiation and maintenance of transformation could be basically synonymous.)

5.3 *cyt* Mutants

A different group of mutants, characterized by a reduced oncogenic potential and an increased cytolytic activity, has been isolated from highly oncogenic

Ad12 (TAKEMORI et al. 1968). These so-called *cyt* mutants cause extensive cytolysis effects in permissive cells and produce clear plaques in human embryonic kidney cells. Most *cyt* mutants are unable to transform hamster kidney cells and show a much reduced capacity to transform primary rat kidney cells (TAKEMORI et al. 1968; TAKEMORI 1972; MAK and MAK 1983). The defect has been localized in region E1B, most likely in the gene coding for the 20-kd polypeptide (LAI FATT and MAK 1982). Thus mutations in region E1B of Ad12 can markedly reduce tumorigenicity and transforming activity without inhibiting viral replication. The precise nature of the *cyt* mutations is not known.

5.4 Mutants with Specific Lesions in Region E1 Genes

The new developments in DNA technology have made it possible to introduce mutations at specific sites in DNA. A number of recent examples in which site-directed mutagenesis has been used to analyze transforming functions of adenoviruses will now be summarized.

CARLOCK and JONES (1981) have isolated an Ad5 host-range mutant containing a frame-shift mutation in the 1.0-kb E1 mRNA, as a result of which a truncated polypeptide is formed. The 0.9-kb mRNA remained unaffected, as the mutation (an insertion of an octanucleotide) was introduced into the region unique to the 1.0-kb mRNA. The mutant, H5in500, was defective for transformation of rat embryo and baby rat kidney cells, although region E1B and other early regions were expressed. A similar Ad5 mutant, *hr*440, was isolated by SOLNICK (1981). This mutant also produced a truncated polypeptide from the 1.0-kb mRNA, and in addition is defective in the splicing event required to generate the 0.9-kb mRNA. As expected, *hr*440 is also transformation-defective, even though region E1B is expressed (SOLNICK and ANDERSON 1982).

By using site-directed mutagenesis, MONTELL et al. (1982) have introduced a base change into the donor splice site of the 0.9-kb mRNA of Ad2 region E1A. Due to the degeneracy of the genetic code, the mutation (a U → G transversion) did not change the coding specificity of the affected triplet in the 1.0-kb mRNA. As a result, the 0.9-kb E1A mRNA and its product are not produced, but the 1.0-kb mRNA is present and its product unchanged. In contrast to the mutants mentioned previously, in which the 1.0-kb mRNA product is truncated, this mutant expressed all early functions and replicates normally in HeLa cells. In addition, the E1A region of this mutant (pEkpm975) was found to induce transformation in primary rat kidney cells (R. BERNARDS, unpublished).

From these data it can be concluded that the protein(s) encoded by the 1.0-kb mRNA contain all E1A functions required for efficient transcription of other early regions and for transformation. The finding that the mutant H5in500, which produces a normal polypeptide from the 0.9-kb mRNA but a truncated polypeptide from the 1.0-kb mRNA, is transformation defective but normal in expression of early regions shows that the 1.0-kb mRNA product(s) fulfill a specific role in transformation which can be dissociated from activation of region E1B.

6 Functional Properties of Regions E1A and E1B

6.1 Regulation of Expression of Region E1 Genes

Region E1B is the first early region to be expressed in lytically infected human cells (NEVINS et al. 1979). Transcripts from this region can be detected as early as 45 min post infection, the rate of transcription reaching a maximum at 3 h post infection and then remaining constant for at least 6 h. The other early regions become active 1.5–2 h post infection and reach maxima 2–4 h later (NEVINS et al. 1979). Transcription of region E1B begins at about 1.5 h and increases up to at least 9 h post infection.

By using host-range and deletion mutants of Ad5 carrying lesions in region E1A, it was shown that a product of E1A is required to obtain expression of region E1B and the other early regions (JONES and SHENK 1979b; BERK et al. 1979). Further experiments using inhibitors of protein synthesis have led to the conclusion that accumulation of mRNA from region E1B and other early regions in lytically-infected cells is normally inhibited by a cellular factor, presumably a protein. One or more of the region E1A products are somehow able to neutralize the inhibitory effect of the cellular factor, resulting in efficient expression of the other early regions (NEVINS 1981; PERSSON et al. 1981; KATZE et al. 1981). The regulation by region E1A of early mRNA accumulation appears to occur at the level of transcription (NEVINS 1981), involving either regulation of transcription from the promoters or stabilization of transcription complexes. Host-range or deletion mutants with defects in region E1A (group I mutants) are unable to replicate in HeLa cells. They do replicate efficiently in line 293 cells, which harbor a functional region E1 of Ad5 and can therefore complement the E1A defect of the mutants. Infection of HeLa cells with high multiplicities of Ad5 group I mutants results in transcription of regions E1B–E4 followed by replication of the mutant virus. A possible explanation of this phenomenon is that the large number of copies of early viral promoter regions (or transcription-initiation complexes) present in the cells causes binding of all, or most, of the cellular "repressor" molecules. As a result, transcription of regions E1B–E4 could proceed spontaneously in the absence of functional E1A products. Other explanations, involving a positive regulation effect of region E1A products on transcription of E1B–E4 are also possible.

Region E1A not only regulates expression of the other early regions in permissive cells but probably also in nonpermissive cells. This was demonstrated in an experiment in which the promoter/leader segment of region E1B of Ad12 was ligated to the coding region of the herpes virus thymidine kinase (tk) gene. Transfection of this hybrid plasmid into tk⁻ mouse cells resulted in the appearance of tk⁺ colonies only when a functional region E1A plasmid was included in the transfection mixture (BOS and TEN WOLDE-KRAAMWINKEL 1983). This experiment also showed that the DNA region within 135 b upstream from the E1B cap site is sensitive to regulation by region E1A.

6.2 Protein Kinase Activity

The demonstration that pp60^{src}, the product of the *src* gene of Rous sarcoma virus, has a protein kinase activity (COLLETT and ERIKSON 1978) with specificity for tyrosine, and that a similar enzymatic function was found to be associated with the middle T antigen of polyoma virus (SMITH et al. 1979), has led to a search for similar activities in adenovirus T antigen preparations. A protein kinase activity was indeed demonstrated in the proteins immunoprecipitated from Ad5-infected KB cells using sera from tumor-bearing animals (BRANTON et al. 1981; LASSAM et al. 1979b). The adenovirus-specific protein kinase phosphorylates the heavy chain of IgG, histone H3, and the viral 55-kd E1B polypeptide. Serine and threonine were phosphorylated but no phosphotyrosine was detected. A protein kinase activity was also found in proteins immunoprecipitated from Ad12-infected cells (BRANTON et al. 1981). Extracts of KB cells infected with representatives of transformation-defective group I and group II host-range mutants gave lower protein kinase activity than extracts from wild-type-infected cells (BRANTON et al. 1981). Kinase activity was also detected in Ad5- and Ad12-transformed rat cells but not in untransformed rat embryo fibroblasts (BRANTON et al. 1979).

The in vitro protein kinase activity phosphorylates a different set of peptides of the 55-kd protein than are phosphorylated under natural conditions in vivo. Thus the in vitro phosphorylation of the 55-kd protein does not mimic the phosphorylating activity occurring in vivo (MALETTE et al. 1983).

The finding that the kinase activity was lower in both group I and group II mutant-infected cells than in wild-type-infected cells suggests that the activity may not be an intrinsic property of one of the region E1 polypeptides, although no evidence was found for a specific trapping of the enzyme in immune complexes. More work will be needed to identify the origin of the kinase activity and to understand its role in productive infection or transformation.

6.3 The 55-kd E1B Protein (Ad5) Is Complexed to a Cellular 53-kd Protein

The 55-kd protein present in Ad5-transformed mouse cells has been found to be complexed to the same cellular protein previously shown to be associated with the SV40 large T antigen (SARNOW et al. 1982; LANE and CRAWFORD 1979; LINZER and LEVINE 1979). In both SV40- and Ad5-transformed cells the 53-kd protein is present in greater amounts than in untransformed cells. The Ad55-kd protein is not associated with the cellular protein in lytically infected cells. A 53-kd protein immunologically related to the one complexed to the SV40 large T antigen also occurs in increased amounts in EBV-transformed cells (LUKA et al. 1980), various other tumor cells (DE LEO et al. 1979), and embryonal carcinoma cells (LINZER and LEVINE 1979), suggesting that the elevated concentration is significant for the transformed state.

Association of the 53-kd protein with a viral protein is not a constant feature of virus-transformed cells, since no binding with viral antigens can be detected in Ad12-transformed rat cells, where the protein also occurs in elevated concentration (Schrier and Zantema, in preparation).

Rat cells partially transformed by region E1A of Ad5 also contain increased levels of the 53-kd protein. This shows that the presence of high concentrations of the protein is not restricted to fully transformed cells (Schrier and Zantema, in preparation). The fact that the same cellular protein is associated with the SV40 large T antigen and the Ad5 55-kd T antigen indicates that the two viral proteins may share some common functions.

7 Intracellular Localization
of Adenovirus-Transforming Proteins

Taking advantage of the availability of monoclonal or monospecific antibodies against Ad5-transforming proteins, attempts have been made to establish the intracellular localization of these proteins.

By using antisera raised against synthetic peptides corresponding to the C-terminals of the E1A gene products or the E1B 55-kd gene product of Ad5, the intracellular localization of the proteins in Ad5-infected KB cells was studied (YEE et al. 1983). The E1A proteins were found in discrete patches in the nucleus and in diffuse areas of the cytoplasm, whereas the 55-kd E1B protein occurred both in the nucleus and cytoplasm, but particularly in the perinuclear region. By using cell fractionation procedures followed by immunoprecipitation with hamster antitumor sera (ROWE et al. 1983a) it was found that the E1A 44-kd protein was recovered in equal amounts from the nucleoplasmic and cytoplasmic fractions. In the latter fraction, part of the protein was found to be associated with the cytoskeleton. A similar distribution was observed for the 55-kd E1B protein, but no affinity for the cytoskeleton was detected. At late times post infection the 55-kd antigen accumulated in the nucleus. The latter phenomenon may correlate with the finding that host cell mRNA also accumulates in the nucleus late in infection (BELTZ and FLINT 1979), suggesting a possible relationship between the two phenomena (ROWE et al. 1983a). The 20-kd protein was found almost exclusively associated with the membrane fraction of infected KB cells. Association of the 20-kd protein with membranes has also been reported by PERSSON et al. (1982), who used an antiserum raised against biochemically purified 20-kd protein. These authors also observed that when the membrane fraction was treated with trypsin prior to isolation and immunoprecipitation of the 20-kd protein, a fragment of 11–12 kd was recovered, suggesting that part of the 20-kd protein is protected by membrane components. The observation that the E1A proteins are associated with the cytoskeleton may be significant in connection with the finding that adenovirus mRNA is also associated with the cytoskeleton (VAN VENROOIJ et al. 1981). It may indicate that the E1 proteins possibly have a function on the post-transcriptional control of gene expression.

Using a monospecific antiserum specific for the 1.0-kb E1A mRNA product, it was found that this protein is associated with large cellular structures within both the nucleus and the cytoplasm. The nuclear form of the protein was found specifically associated with the nuclear matrix (FELDMAN and NEVINS 1983).

Immunofluorescence studies using monoclonal antibodies prepared against the Ad5 E1A and E1B proteins have shown that in rat kidney cells transformed by Ad5 region E1, the E1A proteins are localized in the nucleus, the E1B

20-kd protein particularly in the perinuclear area, and the E1B 55-kd protein also mainly in the perinuclear area, in a single discrete body close to the nucleus. The 20-kd and 55-kd proteins do not overlap in their localization. The bodies containing the 55-kd protein are usually well defined and can easily be recognized by phase-contrast microscopy (A. Zantema, personal communication). Immunoelectron microscopy has shown that the bodies containing the 55-kd E1B protein possibly consist of clusters of intermediate filaments (J.M. Fransen and L.A. Ginsel, personal communication). Immunofluorescence studies showed that the 53-kd cellular protein associated with the Ad5 55-kd E1B protein (SARNOW et al. 1982) is also located in Ad5-transformed cells in the same cytoplasmic body. Ad5 *Hind*III G-transformed rat cells, which contain only the information for the N-terminal half of the E1B 55-kd protein, do not show this cytoplasmic body. In these transformed cells, the E1B 20-kd protein and the cellular 53-kd protein are localized in the nucleus, like the E1A proteins, while no specific fluorescence was found for the truncated 55-kd product(s). Accumulation of the E1B 55-kd protein in a discrete body is not a general phenomenon for Ad-transformed cells, since no such accumulation was found for the 55-kd protein in Ad12-transformed rat cells. In the latter cells, the cellular 53-kd protein, which does not appear to be complexed to the Ad12 55-kd E1B protein, is localized in the nucleus.

8 Oncogenic Properties of Adenovirus-Transformed Cells

8.1 Introduction

As a general rule, cells transformed by nononcogenic subgenus C adenoviruses are nononcogenic in syngeneic animals, while cells transformed by subgenus A viruses are oncogenic. However, several exceptions to this rule have been reported in the literature, showing that subgenus-C-transformed cells may be oncogenic in immunocompetent animals, although always much less so than subgenus-A (Ad12)-transformed cells.

Ad2-transformed Syrian hamster cells were found to be often tumorigenic in newborn syngeneic animals, but tumorigenicity decreased when older hamsters were used (21 days or older). Similarly derived cell lines transformed by oncogenic Ad12 or SV40 were invariably tumorigenic in weanling hamsters (COOK and LEWIS 1979). Rejection of Ad2-transformed hamster cells was shown to require a T-cell-mediated immune response, which develops during the first 21 days of life (COOK et al. 1979). Ad2-transformed cell lines that were nononcogenic in newborn hamsters were usually highly tumorigenic in nude mice, or produced tumors in newborn hamsters when the animals were treated with antilymphocyte serum. The differences in tumor-inducing capacity between Ad2- and Ad12-transformed hamster cells have been attributed to differences in (inherent) resistance to the cellular immune response of the host (LEWIS and COOK 1982).

A variation in oncogenic spectrum has also been reported for rat cells transformed by nononcogenic Ad2 (AS and Hooded Lister rats). Rat-embryo-derived cell lines transformed by Ad2 were found to exhibit an oncogenic potential varying from tumorigenic in newborn rats to non-tumorigenic in nude mice (GALLIMORE et al. 1977). The heterogeneity in oncogenic phenotypes among Ad2-transformed cells was not due to the fact that they originated from different kinds of target cells in the uncloned population of rat embryo cells, since variability in oncogenic phenotype was also found among Ad2-transformed cells derived from a cloned rat liver cell line (PARASKEVA et al. 1982). There was no strict correlation between the ability to produce tumors and anchorage-independent growth, high protease activity, or ability to grow to high saturation density, but there was a clear inverse correlation between degree of oncogenicity and amount of fibronectin present in the cell cultures (GALLIMORE et al. 1977).

Ad5-transformed rat lines, derived from primary baby rat kidney cultures (Wag-Rij rats), were consistently nononcogenic in 4- to 6-day-old rats when tested at early passages. The cells were weakly oncogenic in nude mice, producing tumors in about 50% of the animals after a long latency period (BERNARDS et al. 1982). In contrast, Ad12-transformed rat kidney lines were always highly oncogenic in 4- to 6-day-old rats and nude mice.

As noted previously, the fact that many subgenus-C-transformed hamster cells, but not rat cells, are oncogenic in syngeneic animals suggests that the immunological defense mechanism of hamsters may be relatively poorly developed, at least compared to that of rats. An alternative explanation for this result is that transformed hamster cells are genetically less stable than rat cells, and could more easily derail to become more highly oncogenic.

Parameters that should also be taken into account when studying oncogenicity of transformed cells are the number of passages of propagation in vitro and the conditions of cell culture. The longer cell lines have been grown in vitro and the higher the cell densities during propagation in culture, the higher the risk that the cells have acquired an oncogenic potential which they did not originally possess.

8.2 The Role of Region E1A and E1B Oncogenesis

Taking advantage of the difference in oncogenic potential in rodents between Ad5 and Ad12, studies have been undertaken to establish which viral gene(s) are responsible for the observed differences in tumor-inducing capacity by these viruses. A series of hybrid recombinant plasmids have been constructed consisting of region E1A of Ad5 and E1B of Ad12, and vice versa (BERNARDS et al. 1982). Plasmids containing these hybrid E1 regions or intact E1 regions of Ad5 or Ad12 were used to transform primary rat kidney cells. It was found that plasmids containing region E1A of Ad5 induced transformation at relatively high frequency, irrespective of the origin of the E1B region. Plasmids containing region E1A of Ad12 had consistently lower transforming activities, in combination with both region E1B of Ad12 and region E1B of Ad5. This result showed

Table 1. Oncogenicity of adenovirus-transformed cells in immunocompetent and immunodeficient animals

Plasmid used for transformation	Expression in transformed cell		Oncogenicity of transformed cell (%)		
	E1A	E1B	Nude mice	Syngeneic rats	Nude rats
pAd5XhoC	5	5	50 (15/31)	0 (0/51)	n.d.
pAd12RIC	12	12	100 (23/23)	100 (18/18)[a]	n.d.
pAd512	5	12	100 (18/18)	0 (0/26)	100 (6/6)[c]
pAd125	12	5	10 (2/19)	10 (6/60)[b]	n.d.
p51212	5+12	12	100 (12/12)	0 (0/18)	n.d.

n.d., not done

[a] Average latent period 6 weeks
[b] Average latent period 4 months
[c] Average latent period 3 months

that the identity of the E1A region determines the frequency of transformation, and furthermore that regions E1A and E1B of Ad5 and Ad12 can complement each other in transformation. The latter conclusion is in agreement with earlier observations that Ad12 can complement host-range mutants of Ad5 in productive infection (ROWE and GRAHAM 1981). Transplantation studies showed that rat cells transformed by plasmids harboring region E1B of Ad12 were always highly oncogenic in nude mice, whereas cells containing region E1B of Ad5 were weakly oncogenic in these animals (Table 1). In immunocompetent syngeneic rats, Ad5-transformed cells were completely nononcogenic but Ad12-transformed cells were strongly oncogenic. Surprisingly, cells transformed by E1A of Ad5 plus E1B of Ad12, which induced tumors in 100% of injected nude mice, were completely nontumorigenic in immunocompetent rats, whereas cells transformed by E1A of Ad12 plus E1B of Ad5, which produced tumors in 10% of the nude mice, also produced tumors in 10% of the transplanted immunocompetent rats (BERNARDS et al. 1983b). The interpretation of these results was that transformed cells are not rejected by immunocompetent animals when they harbor the E1A region of Ad12, even when their in vivo growth potential in nude mice is low (e.g., in the case of cells transformed by Ad12 E1A plus Ad5 E1B). According to this view, the degree of oncogenicity of a transformed cell, as measured by its growth potential in athymic nude mice, is specified by the identity of region E1B, whereas the ability to resist or escape the T lymphocyte immune defense is determined by the identity of region E1A. Thus, the presence of region E1A of Ad12 apparently confers resistance to the immune surveillance of the host, while region E1A of Ad5 lacks this property.

Further studies using Ad5/Ad12 hybrid E1B regions showed that the high oncogenic potential in nude mice characteristic of Ad12-transformed cells is determined by the large 55-kd E1B protein, and not by the 19-kd E1B protein, although the presence of both proteins is required for oncogenicity (BERNARDS et al. 1983a; VAN DER EB et al. 1983).

By using recombinant plasmids containing two E1A regions, one derived from Ad5 and the other from Ad12, in addition to an E1B region, it was demonstrated that with respect to oncogenicity region E1A of Ad5 is dominant over E1A of Ad12; transformed rat cells carrying both E1A regions and E1B of Ad12 are nononcogenic in immunocompetent rats (BERNARDS et al. 1983b).

8.3 Interaction of Transformed Cells with the Host Immune System

The differences in oncogenic properties between cells transformed by oncogenic and nononcogenic adenoviruses, while primarily caused by differences in gene structure, may eventually be dependent on variations in cellular gene expression. In order to investigate whether oncogenic and nononcogenic adenovirus-transformed cells differ in the expression of cellular genes, Ad5- and Ad12-transformed rat kidney cells have been compared by immunological methods. By using antisera raised in mice against untransformed primary baby rat kidney cells, it was found that rat cells expressing Ad12 E1A lacked two cell-encoded proteins which were present both in untransformed cells and in transformed cells expressing Ad5 E1A. One of these proteins, of 45 kd in molecular weight, was identified as the heavy chain of the class I antigens encoded by the major histocompatibility complex (MHC; SCHRIER et al. 1983). The inactivating activity of the Ad12 E1A region was found to be encoded by the 1.0-kb mRNA – although the 0.9-kb mRNA may have a slight suppressing activity (BERNARDS et al. 1983b). The inhibition of class I heavy chain expression appeared to occur at the level of mRNA transcription, since no cytoplasmic mRNA of class I genes could be detected in cells expressing Ad12 E1A. The synthesis of the class I light chain, β_2-microglobulin, was not inhibited (SCHRIER et al. 1983). Since foreign antigens can only be recognized by the cellular immune system in the context of class I MHC antigens, one would expect that cells lacking class I antigens cannot be eliminated by the cellular immune defense. The results of the transplantation studies with Ad5- and Ad12-transformed rat cells (Table 1) indeed show that cells expressing Ad12 E1A are equally oncogenic in immunocompetent and immunodeficient animals. Thus it seems that cells expressing the E1A region of Ad5 may be nononcogenic because they are eliminated in immunocompetent animals by the cellular immune system, while cells expressing Ad12 E1A are oncogenic because they lack sufficient class I antigen to be recognized by the cellular immune defense. Evidence supporting this hypothesis was provided by the observation that cells expressing Ad12 E1A show a lower susceptibility to lysis by cytotoxic T lymphocytes (CTLs) in vitro than cells expressing Ad5 E1A (BERNARDS et al. 1983b). These results do not agree with those of others (RAŠKA et al. 1980; RAŠKA and GALLIMORE 1982; Föhring et al. to be published) who found that CTLs are reactive in vitro against Ad12-transformed cells, although the reported levels of killing were rather low. A possible explanation for these results is that inactivation of the class I genes by Ad12 E1A does not seem to be complete, since low levels of class I proteins could be detected in Ad12-transformed cells. Oncogenicity of Ad12-transformed cells, therefore, may not necessarily require the complete absence of class I antigens, but rather a sufficiently low level of expression to allow the cells to escape the CTL defense. An observation that might be of importance in this respect is that an Ad12-transformed cell line expressing regions E1, E3, and E4 was even more tumorigenic than cells expressing region E1 only (RAŠKA et al. 1980), suggesting that sequences from the right end of the Ad12 genome may further contribute to the resistance to the cellular immune defense. The observation that a 19-kd glycoprotein encoded by region E3 is associated with the class I antigens in transformed cells (SIGNÄS et al. 1982) may be relevant in this connection.

It has not been proven that the absence of class I antigens in cells expressing Ad12 E1A is caused by an inhibition of class I gene transcription. An alternative possibility is that Ad12 only transforms cells that have an intrinsically low level of expression of class I genes.

8.4 Intergenotypic Recombinant Viruses

In order to study the effect of hybrid E1 regions on the oncogenic potential of intact virions, recombinant adenoviruses have been constructed consisting of the genome of Ad5 or Ad12 in which either region E1A or E1B or both were replaced by the corresponding region of the heterologous virus.

In an initial study, SHIROKI et al. (1982) have isolated two recombinant Ad5 viruses containing (part of) region E1 of Ad12. Both viruses were defective for replication in human cells but were capable of transforming rat 3Y1 cells. Rat cells transformed by one of the recombinant viruses expressed only Ad12 region E1A and no Ad5 region E1 genes, whereas cells transformed by the other recombinant virus expressed region E1B of Ad5 and region E1 of Ad12. The latter cells were highly tumorigenic after transplantation into newborn rats, the former cells induced tumors inefficiently. The result that cells expressing only Ad12 E1A were oncogenic does not agree with the finding that mutation of either the 20-kd or the 55-kd Ad12 E1B protein abolished oncogenicity of transformed rat kidney cells, even in nude mice (BERNARDS et al. 1983a). The most probable explanation for this discrepancy is that different cell types were used for the isolation of transformed cells in the two studies.

SHIROKI et al. (1983) also isolated a nondefective Ad5 virus expressing E1A of Ad12 and E1B of Ad5. No data on oncogenicity of this virus have yet been reported. Recently, two additional nondefective Ad5–Ad12 recombinant viruses were constructed, one in which the Ad5 E1B region was replaced by the Ad12 E1B region (BERNARDS et al. 1983c) and another in which both E1A and E1B of Ad5 were replaced by the homologous transcriptional units of Ad12. Both viruses failed to induce tumors in newborn hamsters (BERNARDS et al. to be published). Therefore tumor induction in hamsters by infectious virus particles seems to require functions encoded outside the region E1, and is probably a more complex process than oncogenic transformation in vitro with isolated region E1 DNA fragments.

9 Summary

The data summarized in this chapter show that morphological transformation and oncogenesis by adenoviruses are brought about by the coordinated activity of regions E1A and E1B. Gene products of each of these subregions appear to fulfill distinct roles in oncogenic transformation, with the possible exception of the product(s) encoded by the 0.9-kb E1A mRNA. Also unclear is the function of the 20-kd E1B protein, which has a small role, if any, in morphological transformation, but appears to be essential for the development of the oncogenic phenotype, as defined by the ability of transformed cells to grow in immuno-deficient nude mice. The differences in biological properties of oncogenic and nononcogenic adenoviruses must be attributed to differences in the primary structure of the respective E1A and E1B gene products, in particular of the product(s) of the 1.0-kb E1A mRNA and of the 55-kd protein encoded by the 2.2-kb E1B mRNA. The availability of cold-sensitive adenovirus mutants has enabled us to conclude that the transformed phenotype is maintained as a result of continuous expression of at least region E1A gene products, and is therefore not the result of a hit-and-run mechanism.

Despite the progress in our understanding of adenovirus transformation and oncogenesis, virtually nothing is known about the precise mechanism by which the viral gene products bring about the neoplastic changes in cells. The only exception is the demonstration that Ad12 region E1A (1.0-kb RNA) appears to suppress the production of MHC class I antigen, which in turn may explain how Ad12-transformed cells can escape the immune surveillance of the host and then easily multiply to form a tumor.

In Table 2, an attempt has been made to summarize the roles of adenovirus region E1 gene products in oncogenic transformation and in lytic infection.

Table 2. Roles of adenovirus region E1 products in transformation and lytic infection

		Transformation	Lytic infection
E1A	0.9-kb mRNA	No known function	Inhibition of E2A late promoter[b]
	1.0-kb mRNA	Partial transformation (5 and 12) Immortalization (5) Suppression of MHC class I genes (12 only) Activation E1B-E4 (5 and 12)	Activation E1B-E4 (5 and 12)
E1B	20-kd protein	Required for expression of oncogenic phenotype (5 and 12) (only in combination with E1A)[a]	Cytocidal phenotype if deleted (12), but probably not essential for lytic infection
	55-kd protein	Required for complete morphological transformation (5 and 12) (N-terminal half is sufficient) Required for expression of oncogenic phenotype (12) (only in combination with E1A)	No known functions but probably essential for lytic infection

[a] After this manuscript was completed Chinnadurai reported (Cell 33, 759-766 (1983)) that mutation in the 20-kd E1B gene of Ad2 resulted in a considerable reduction of transforming activity of rat 3Y1 cells, when intact viral DNA or virions were used

[b] See Discussion in M. Rossini, Virology *131*, 49–58 (1983)

References

Aleström P, Akusjärvi G, Perricaudet M, Mathews MB, Klessig DF, Pettersson U (1980) The gene for polypeptide IX of adenovirus type 2 and its unspliced messenger RNA. Cell 19:671–681

Babiss LE, Ginsberg HS, Fischer PB (1983) Cold-sensitive expression of transformation by a host-range mutant of type 5 adenovirus. Proc Natl Acad Sci USA 80:1352–1356

Bellet AJD, Younghusband HB (1972) Replication of the DNA of chick embryo lethal orphan virus. J Mol Biol 72:691–709

Beltz GA, Flint SJ (1979) Inhibition of Hela cell protein synthesis during adenovirus infection: restriction of cellular messenger RNA sequences to the nucleus. J Mol Biol 131:353–373

Berk AJ, Sharp PA (1977) Ultraviolet mapping of adenovirus 2 early promoters. Cell 12:45–55

Berk AJ, Sharp PA (1978) Structure of adenovirus 2 early mRNAs. Cell 14:695–711

Berk AJ, Lee F, Harrison T, Williams J, Sharp PA (1979) Pre-early adenovirus 5 gene product regulates synthesis of early viral messenger RNAs. Cell 17:1935–1944

Bernards R, Houweling A, Schrier PI, Bos JL, Van der Eb AJ (1982) Characterization of cells transformed by Ad5/Ad12 hybrid early region 1 plasmids. Virology 120:422–432

Bernards R, Schrier PI, Bos JL, Van der Eb AJ (1983a) Role of adenovirus types 5 and 12 early region 1b tumor antigens in oncogenic transformation. Virology 127:45–54

Bernards R, Schrier PI, Houweling A, Bos JL, Van der Eb AJ, Zijlstra M, Melief CJM (1983b) Tumorgenicity of cells transformed by adenovirus type 12 by evasion of T-cell immunity. Nature 305:776–779

Bernards R, Vaessen MJ, Sussenbach JS, Van der Eb AJ (1983c) Construction and characterization of an adenovirus type 5/adenovirus type 12 recombinant virus. Virology 131:30–38

Bos JL, ten Wolde-Kraamwinkel HC (1983) The E1b promoter of Ad12 in mouse L tk⁻ cells is activated by adenovirus region E1a. EMBO J 2:73–76

Bos JL, Polder LJ, Bernards R, Schrier PI, Van den Elsen PJ, Van der Eb AJ, Van Ormondt H (1981) The 2.2 kb E1b mRNA of human Ad12 and Ad5 codes for two tumor antigens starting at different AUG triplets. Cell 27:121–131

Bos JL, Jochemsen AG, Bernards R, Schrier PI, Van Ormondt H, Van der Eb AJ (1983) Deletion mutants of region E1a of Ad12 E1 plasmids: Effect on oncogenic transformation. Virology 129:393–400

Branton PE, Lassam NJ, Graham FL, Mak S, Bailey ST (1979) T antigen-related protein kinase activity in cells infected and transformed by human adenoviruses. Cold Spring Harbor Symp Quant Biol 44:487–491

Branton PE, Lassam NJ, Downey JF, Yee S-P, Graham FL, Mak S, Bailey ST (1981) Protein kinase activity immunoprecipitated from adenovirus-infected cells by sera from tumor-bearing hamsters. J Virol 37:601–608

Byrd P, Brown KW, Gallimore PH (1982) Malignant transformation of human embryo retinoblasts by cloned adenovirus 12 DNA. Nature 298:69–71

Carlock LR, Jones NC (1981) Transformation-defective mutant of adenovirus type 5 containing a single altered E1a mRNA species. J Virol 40:657–664

Chow LT, Roberts JM, Lewis JB, Broker TR (1977) A map of cytoplasmic RNA transcripts from lytic adenovirus type 2, determined by electron microscopy of RNA:DNA hybrids. Cell 11:819–836

Chow LT, Broker TR, Lewis JB (1979) Complex splicing patterns of RNAs from the early regions of adenovirus 2. J Mol Biol 134:265–303

Collett MS, Erikson RL (1978) Protein kinase activity associated with the avian sarcoma virus src gene product. Proc Natl Acad Sci USA 75:2021–2024

Cook JL, Lewis AM (1979) Host response to adenovirus 2-transformed hamster embryo cells. Cancer Res 39:1455–1461

Cook JL, Lewis AM, Kirkpatrick CH (1979) Age-related and thymus-dependent rejection of adenovirus 2-transformed cell tumors in the Syrian hamster. Cancer Res 39:3335–3340

De Jong JC, Wigand R, Kidd AH, Wadell G, Kapsenberg G, Muzerie CJ, Wermenbol AG, Firtzlaff RG (1983) Candidate adenoviruses 40 and 41: fastidious adenoviruses from human infantile stool. J Med Virol 11:215–231

De Leo AB, Jay G, Apella E, Dubois GC, Law LW, Old LJ (1979) Detection of a transformation related antigen in chemically induced sarcomas and other transformed cells of the mouse. Proc Natl Acad Sci USA 76:2420–2424

Dijkema R, Dekker BMM, Van der Feltz MJM, Van der Eb AJ (1979) Transformation of primary rat kidney cells by fragments of weakly oncogenic adenoviruses. J Virol 32:943–950

Dijkema R, Dekker BMM, Van Ormondt H (1982) Gene organization of the transforming region of adenovirus type 7 DNA. Gene 18:143–156

Doerfler W (1969) Non-productive infection of baby hamster kidney cells with adenovirus type 12. Virology 38:587–606

Doerfler W, Gahlmann R, Stabel S, Deuring R, Lichtenberg U, Schulz M, Leisten R (1983) On the mechanism of recombination between adenoviral and cellular DNAs: the structure of junction sites. In: Doerfler W (ed) The molecular biology of adenoviruses 1. Current Topics in Microbiology and Immunology Vol 109. Springer Berlin Heidelberg New York Tokyo, pp 193–228

Esche H, Siegman B (1982) Expression of early viral gene products in adenovirus type 12-infected and -transformed cells. J Gen Virol 60:99–113

Esche H, Mathews MB, Lewis JB (1980) Proteins and messenger RNAs of the transforming region of wild-type and mutant adenoviruses. J Mol Biol 142:399–417

Feldman LT, Nevins JR (1983) Localization of the adenovirus E1a protein, a positive acting transcriptional factor in infected cells. Mol Cell Biol 3:829–838

Fischer PB, Boersig MR, Graham GM, Weinstein IB (1983) Production of growth factors by type 5 adenovirus-transformed rat embryo cells. J Cell Phys 114:365–370

Flint SJ, Sharp PA (1976) Adenovirus transcription. V. Quantitation of viral RNA sequences in adenovirus 2 infected and transformed cells. J Mol Biol 106:749–771

Freeman AE, Black PH, Vanderpool JH, Henby PH, Auston JB, Huebner RJ (1967) Transformation of primary rat embryo cells by adenovirus type 2. Proc Natl Acad Sci USA 58:1205–1212

Frost E, Williams J (1978) Mapping temperature-sensitive and host-range mutations of adenovirus type 5 by marker rescue. Virology 91:39–50

Gallimore PH (1974) Interactions of adenovirus type 2 with rat embryo cells: permissiveness, transformation and in vitro characterization of adenovirus type 2-transformed rat embryo cells. J Gen Virol 25:263–273

Gallimore PH, Sharp PA, Sambrook J (1974) Viral DNA in transformed cells: II. A study of the sequences of adenovirus 2 DNA in nine lines of transformed rat cells using specific fragments of the viral genome. J Mol Biol 89:49–72

Gallimore PH, McDougall JK, Chen LB (1977) In vitro traits of adenovirus-transformed cell lines and their relevance to tumorigenicity in nude mice. Cell 10:669–678

Galos RS, Williams J, Shenk T, Jones N (1980) Physical location of host-range mutations of adenovirus type 5: deletion and marker rescue mapping. Virology 104:510–513

Garon CF, Berry K, Hierholzer JC, Rose J (1973) Mapping of base sequence heterologies between genomes from different adenovirus serotypes. Virology 54:414–426

Graham FL, Van der Eb AJ (1973) A new technique for the assay of infectivity of human adenovirus DNA. Virology 52:456–467

Graham FL, Abrahams PJ, Mulder C, Heijneker HL, Warnaar SO, de Vries FAJ, Fiers W, Van der Eb AJ (1974a) Studies on in vitro transformation by DNA and DNA fragments of human adenoviruses and simian virus 40. Cold Spring Harbor Symp Quant Biol 39:637–650

Graham FL, Van der Eb AJ, Heijneker HL (1974b) Size and location of the transforming region in human adenovirus type 5 DNA. Nature 251:687–691

Graham FL, Smiley J, Russell WC, Nairu R (1977) Characterization of a human cell line transformed by DNA from human adenovirus type 5. J Gen Virol 36:59–72

Graham FL, Harrison T, Williams J (1978) Defective transforming capacity of adenovirus type 5 host-range mutants. Virology 86:10–21

Green M, Pina M, Kimes RC, Wensink PC, MacHattie LA, Thomas CA Jr (1967) Adenovirus DNA. I. Molecular weight and conformation. Proc Natl Acad Sci USA 57:1302–1309

Green M, Mackey JK, Wold WSM, Rigden P (1979) Thirty-one human adenovirus serotypes (Ad1–Ad31) form five groups (A–E) based upon DNA genome homologies. Virology 93:481–492

Green M, Wold WSM, Brackmann K, Cartas MA (1980) Studies of early proteins and transformation proteins of human adenoviruses. Cold Spring Harbor Symp Quant Biol 44:457–470

Halbert DN, Raskas HJ (1982) Tryptic and chymotryptic methionine peptide analysis of the in vitro translation products specified by the transforming region of adenovirus type 2. Virology 116:406–418

Halbert DN, Spector DJ, Raskas HJ (1979) In vitro translation products specified by the transforming region of adenovirus type 2. J Virol 31:621–629

Harrison T, Graham F, Williams J (1977) Host-range mutants of adenovirus type 5 defective for growth in HeLa cells. Virology 77:319–329

Harter ML, Lewis JB (1978) Adenovirus type 2 early proteins synthesized in vitro and in vivo: identification in infected cells of the 38000- to 50000-molecular-weight protein encoded by the left end of the adenovirus type 2 genome. J Virol 26:736–749

Ho Y-S, Galos R, Williams J (1982) Isolation of type 5 adenovirus mutants with a cold-sensitive host range phenotype: genetic evidence of an adenovirus transformation maintenance function. Virology 122:109–124

Houweling A, Van den Elsen PJ, Van der Eb AJ (1980) Partial transformation of primary rat cells by the leftmost 4.5% fragment of adenovirus 5 DNA. Virology 105:537–550

Huebner RJ (1967) Adenovirus-directed tumor and T antigens. In: Pollard M (ed) Perspectives in virology Vol 5. Academic, New York, pp 147–167

Huebner RJ, Rowe WP, Lane WT (1962) Oncogenic effects in hamsters of human adenovirus type 12 and 18. Proc Natl Acad Sci USA 48:2051–2058

Hull CN, Johnson IS, Culbertson CG, Reimer CB, Wright HF (1965) Oncogenicity of the simian adenovirus. Science 150:1044–1046

Ishibashi M, Yasue H, Fujinaga K, Kawamata J (1980) The oncogenicity of avian adenoviruses. I. An unusually large number of viral DNA molecules in some tumors and virus-specific T-antigenic proteins. Virology 106:349–360

Jochemsen H (1981) Studies on the transforming genes and their products of human adenovirus types 12 and 5. Thesis, University of Leiden, Netherlands

Jochemsen H, Daniëls GSG, Lupker JH, Van der Eb AJ (1980) Identification and mapping of early gene products of adenovirus type 12, Virology 105:551–563

Jochemsen H, Hertoghs JJL, Lupker JH, Davis A, Van der Eb AJ (1981) In vitro synthesis of adenovirus type 5 T antigens. II. Translation of virus-specific RNA from cells transformed by fragments of adenovirus type 5 DNA. J Virol 37:530–534

Jochemsen H, Daniëls GSG, Hertoghs JJL, Schrier PI, Van den Elsen PJ, Van der Eb AJ (1982) Identification of adenovirus type 12 gene products involved in transformation and oncogenesis. Virology 122:15–28

Johansson ME, Uhnoo I, Kidd AH, Madeley CR, Wadell G (1980) Direct identification of enteric adenovirus, a candidate new serotype associated with infantile gastroenteritis. J Clin Microbiol 12:95–100

Jones N, Shenk T (1979a) Isolation of adenovirus type 5 host range deletion mutants defective for transformation of rat embryo cells. Cell 17:683–689

Jones N, Shenk T (1979b) An adenovirus type 5 early gene functions regulates expression of other early viral genes. Proc Natl Acad Sci USA 76:3665–3669

Katze MG, Persson H, Phillipson L (1981) Control of adenovirus early gene expression: a post-transcriptional control mediated by region E1a products. Mol Cell Biol 1:807–813

Kimura G, Itagaki S, Summers J (1975) Rat cell line 3Y1 and its virogenic polyoma and SV40 transformed derivatives. Int J Cancer 15:694–706

Kimura T, Sawada Y, Shinawawa M, Shimizu Y, Shiroki K, Shimojo H, Sugisaki H, Takanami M, Uemizu Y, Fujinaga K (1981) Nucleotide sequence of the transforming region E1B of adeno-virus 12 DNA: structure and gene organization, and comparison with those of adenovirus type 5 DNA. Nucleic Acids Res 9:6571–6589

Lai Fatt RB, Mak S (1982) Mapping of an adenovirus function involved in the inhibition of DNA degradation. J Virol 42:969–977

Lane D, Crawford LV (1979) T antigen is bound to a host protein in SV40-transformed cells. Nature 278:261–263

Lassam NJ, Bayley ST, Graham FL (1979a) Tumor antigens of human Ad5 in transformed cells and in cells infected with transformation-defective host-range mutants. Cell 18:781–791

Lassam NJ, Bayley ST, Graham FL, Branton PE (1979b) Immunoprecipitation of protein kinase activity from adenovirus 5-infected cells using antiserum directed against tumour antigens. Nature 277:241–243

Laver WG, Younghusband HB, Wrigley NG (1971) Purification and properties of chick embryo lethal orphan virus (an avian adenovirus) Virology 45:598–614

Levinthal JD, Peterson W (1965) In vitro transformation and immunofluorescence with human adenovirus 12 in rat and rabbit kidney cells. Fed Proc 24:174

Lewis AM, Cook JL (1982) Spectrum of tumorigenic phenotypes among adenovirus 2-, adenovirus 12- and simian virus 40-transformed Syrian hamster cells defined by host cellular immune – tumor cell interactions. Cancer Res 42:939–944

Lewis AM, Rabson AS, Levine AS (1974) Studies on non-defective Ad2-SV40 hybrid viruses: transformation of hamster kidney cells by adenovirus 2 and the non-defective hybrid viruses. J Virol 13:1291–1301

Linzer DIH, Levine AJ (1979) Characterization of a 54 kdalton cellular SV40 tumor antigen present in SV40 transformed cells and uninfected embryonal carcinoma cells. Cell 17:43–52

Luka J, Jörnvall H, Klein G (1980) Purification and biochemical characterization of the Epstein-Barr virus-determined nucleic antigen and an associated protein with a 53000-dalton subunit. J Virol 35:592–602

Lupker JH, Davis A, Jochemsen H, Van der Eb AJ (1981) In vitro synthesis of adenovirus type 5 T antigens. I. Translation of early region 1-specific RNA from lytically infected cells. J Virol 37:524–529

Mackey J, Wold W, Rigden P, Green M (1979) Transforming region of group A. B and C adenoviruses: DNA homology studies with twenty-nine human adenovirus serotypes. J Virol 29:1056–1064

Mak I, Mak S (1983) Transformation of rat cells by cyt mutants of adenovirus type 12 and mutants of adenovirus type 5. J Virol 45:1107–1117

Malette P, Yee S-P, Branton PE (1983) Studies on the phosphorylation of the 58000 dalton early region 1B protein of human adenovirus type 5. J Virol 64:1069–1078

Matsuo T, Wold WSM, Hashimoto S, Rankin A, Symington J, Green M (1982) Polypeptides encoded by the transforming region E1b of human adenovirus 2. Immunoprecipitation from transformed and infected cells and cell-free translation of E1b-specific mRNA. Virology 118:456–465

McAllister RM, Nicolson MO, Lewis AM Jr, MacPherson I, Huebner RJ (1969a) Transformation of rat embryo cells by adenovirus type 1. J Gen Virol 4:29–36

McAllister RM, Riggs JL, Reed G, MacPherson I (1969b) Transformation of rodent cells by simian adenovirus SA-7. Proc Exp Biol Med 131:1442–1445

Montell C, Fisher EF, Caruthers MH, Berk AJ (1982) Resolving the functions of overlapping viral genes by site-specific mutagenesis at mRNA splice site. Nature 295:380–384

Nevins JR (1981) Mechanism of activation of early viral transcription by the adenovirus E1A gene products. Cell 26:213–220

Nevins JR, Ginsberg HS, Blanchard JM, Wilson MC, Darnell JE (1979) Regulation of the primary expression of early adenovirus transcription units. J Virol 32:727–733

Norrby E, Bartha A, Boulanger P, Dreizin RS, Ginsberg HS, Kalter SS, Kawamura H, Rowe HP, Russell WC, Schlesinger RW, Wigand R (1976) Adenoviridae. Intervirology 7:117

Paraskeva C, Brown KW, Gallimore PH (1982) Adenovirus-cell interaction early after infection. In vitro characteristics and tumorigenicity of adenovirus type 2-transformed rat liver epithelial cells. J Gen Virol 58:73–81

Persson H, Monstein H-J, Akusjärvi G, Phillipson L (1981) Adenovirus early gene products may control viral mRNA accumulation and translation in vivo. Cell 23:485–496

Persson H, Katze MG, Phillipson L (1982) An adenovirus tumor antigen associated with membranes in vivo and in vitro. J Virol 42:905–917

Petterson U, Virtanen A, Perricaudet M, Akusjärvi G (1983) The messenger RNAs from the transforming region of human adenoviruses. In: Doerfler W (ed) The molecular biology of adenoviruses 1. Current Topics in Microbiology and Immunology Vol. 109. Springer Berlin Heidelberg New York Tokyo, pp 107–123

Piña N, Green M (1965) Biochemical studies on adenovirus multiplication. IX. Chemical and base composition analysis of 28 human adenoviruses. Proc Natl Acad Sci USA 54:547–551

Ponomareva TI, Grodnitskaya NA, Goldberg EE, Chaplygina NM, Naroditsky BS, Tichonenko TI (1979) Biological activity of intact and cleared DNA of the simian adenovirus 7. Nucleic Acids Res 6:3119–3131

Pope JH, Rowe WP (1964) Immunofluorescent studies of adenovirus 12 tumors and of cells transformed or infected by adenoviruses. J Exp Med 120:577–588

Raška K, Gallimore PH (1982) An inverse relation of the oncogenic potential of adenovirus transformed cells and their sensitivity to killing by syngeneic natural killer cells. Virology 123:8–18

Raška K, Morongiello MP, Föhring B (1980) Adenovirus type 12 tumor antigen. III. Tumorigenicity and immune response to syngeneic rat cells transformed with virions and isolated transforming fragment of adenovirus 12 DNA. Int J Cancer 26:74–86

Riccardi RP, Jones RL, Cepko CL, Sharp PA, Roberts BE (1981) Expression of early adenovirus genes requires a viral encoded acidic polypeptide. Proc Natl Acad Sci USA 78:6121–6125

Ross SR, Levine AJ, Galos RS, Williams J, Shenk T (1980) Early viral proteins in HeLa cells infected with adenovirus type 5 host-range mutants. Virology 103:475–492

Rowe DT, Graham FL (1981) Complementation of adenovirus type 5 host-range mutants by adenovirus type 12 in coinfected HeLa and BHK-21 cells. J Virol 38:191–197

Rowe DT, Graham FL (1983) Transformations of rodent cells by DNA extracted from transformation defective adenovirus mutants. J Virol 46:1039–1044

Rowe DT, Graham FL, Branton PE (1983a) Intracellular localization of adenovirus type 5 tumor antigens in productively infected cells. Virology 129:456–468

Rowe DT, Yee S-P, Otis J, Graham FL, Branton PE (1983b) Characterization of human adenovirus type 5 early region 1A polypeptides using antitumor serum specific for the carboxy terminus. Virology 127:253–271

Ruben M, Bacchetti S, Graham FL (1982) Integration and expression of viral DNA in cells transformed by host-range mutants of adenovirus type 5. J Virol 41:674–685

Sambrook J, Botchan M, Gallimore P, Orzanne B, Pettersson U, Williams J, Sharp PA (1975) Viral DNA sequences in cells transformed by simian virus 40, adenovirus type 2 and adenovirus type 5. Cold Spring Harbor Symp Quant Biol 39:615–632

Sarnow P, Ho YS, Williams J, Levine AJ (1982) Adenovirus E1B-55kd tumor antigen and SV40 large tumor antigen are physically associated with the same 54kd cellular protein in transformed cells. Cell 28:387–394

Sawada Y, Yamashita T, Kanda F, Sekikawa K, Fujinaga K (1981) Mapping of restriction fragments and transforming ability of adenovirus 31. Tumor Res 16:7–17

Schrier PI, Van den Elsen PJ, Hertoghs JJL, Van der Eb AJ (1979) Characterization of tumor antigens in cells transformed by fragments of adenovirus type 5 DNA. Virology 99:372–385

Schrier PI, Bernards R, Vaessen RTMJ, Houweling A, Van der Eb AJ (1983) Expression of class I major histocompatibility antigens switched off by highly oncogenic adenovirus 12 in transformed rat cells. Nature 305:771–775

Sekikawa K, Shiroki K, Shimojo H, Ojima S, Fujinaga K (1978) Transformation of a rat cell line by an adenovirus 7 DNA fragment. Virology 88:1–7

Sharp PA, Pettersson U, Sambrook J (1974a) Viral DNA in transformed cells. I. A study of the sequences of adenovirus 2 DNA in a line of transformed rat cells using specific fragments of the viral genome. J Mol Biol 86:709–726

Sharp PA, Gallimore PH, Flint SJ (1974b) Mapping of adenovirus 2 RNA sequences in lytically infected cells and transformed cell lines. Cold Spring Harbor Symp Quant Biol 39:457–474

Shenk T, Jones N, Colby W, Fowlkes D (1979) Functional analysis of adenovirus type 5 host range deletion mutants defective for transformation of rat embryo cells. Cold Spring Harbor Symp Quant Biol 44:367–375

Shiroki K, Handa H, Shimojo H, Yano H, Ojima S, Fujinaga K (1977) Establishment and characterization of rat cell lines transformed by restriction endonuclease fragments of adenovirus 12 DNA. Virology 82:462–471

Shiroki K, Shimojo H, Maeta Y, Hamada C (1979a) Tumor-specific transplantation and surface antigen in cells transformed by the adenovirus 12 DNA fragments. Virology 98:188–191

Shiroki K, Shimojo H, Sawada Y, Uemizu Y, Fujinaga K (1979b) Incomplete transformation of rat cells by a small fragment of adenovirus 12 DNA. Virology 95:127–136

Shiroki K, Maruyama K, Saito I, Fukui Y, Shimojo H (1981) Incomplete transformation of rat cells by a deletion mutant of adenovirus type 5. J Virol 38:1048–1054

Shiroki K, Maruyama K, Saito I, Fukui Y, Yazaki K, Shimojo H (1982) Dependence of tumor-forming capacities of cells transformed by recombinants between adenovirus types 5 and 12 on expression of early region 1. J Virol 42:708–718

Shiroki K, Saito I, Maruyama K, Shimojo H (1983) Isolation of a non-defective recombinant between adenovirus type 5 and early region 1A of adenovirus type 12. J Virol 46:632–637

Signäs C, Katze MG, Persson H, Phillipson L (1982) An adenovirus glycoprotein is tightly bound to class I transplantation antigens. Nature 299:175–178

Smith AE, Smith R, Griffin B, Fried M (1979) Protein kinase activity associated with polyoma virus middle T. Cell 18:915–924

Solnick D (1981) An adenovirus mutant defective in splicing RNA from early region 1A. Nature 291:508–510

Solnick D, Anderson MA (1982) Transformation-deficient adenovirus mutant defective in expression of region E1A but not region E1B. J Virol 42:106–113

Starzinski-Powitz A, Schultz M, Esche H, Mukai N, Doerfler W (1982) The adenovirus 12 mouse cell system: permissivity and analysis of integration patterns of viral DNA in tumor cells. EMBO J 1:493–497

Strizhachenko NM, Graevskaya NA, Karmysheva VY, Syurin VN (1975) Studies on virus-specific antigenicity of tumour cells transformed by bovine adenovirus type 3. Arch Geschwulst Forsch 45:324–334

Strohl WA (1969) The response of BHK21 cells to infection with adenovirus 12. I. Cell killing and T antigen synthesis as correlated with viral genome function. Virology 39:642–652

Sugisaki H, Sugimoto K, Takanami M, Shiroki K, Saito I, Shimojo H, Sawada Y, Uemizu Y, Uesugi S, Fujinaga K (1980) Structure and gene organization in the transforming HindIII-G fragment of Ad12. Cell 20:777–786

Takemori N (1972) Genetic studies with tumorigenic adenoviruses III. Recombination in adenovirus type 12. Virology 47:157–167

Takemori N, Riggs JL, Aldrich C (1968) Genetic studies with tumorigenic adenoviruses I. Isolation of cytocidal (*cyt*) mutants of adenovirus type 12. Virology 36:575–586

Takiff HE, Straus SE, Garron CF (1981) Propagation and in vitro studies of previously non-cultivable enteral adenoviruses in 293 cells. Lancet II:832–834

Trentin JJ, Yabe Y, Taylor G (1962) The quest for human cancer viruses. Science 137:835–841

Van den Elsen PJ (1982) Studies on the contribution of early regions E1a and E1b of human adenoviruses in cell transformation. Thesis, University of Leiden, Netherlands

Van den Elsen PJ, de Pater S, Houweling A, Van der Veer J, Van der Eb AJ (1982) The relationship between region E1a and E1b of human adenoviruses in cell transformation. Gene 18:175–185

Van den Elsen PJ, Houweling A, Van der Eb AJ (1983a) Expression of region E1b of human adenoviruses in the absence of region E1a is not sufficient for complete transformation. Virology 128:377–390

Van den Elsen PJ, Klein B, Dekker BMM, Van Ormondt H, Van der Eb AJ (1983b) Analysis of virus-specific mRNAs present in cells transformed with restriction fragments of adenovirus type 5 DNA. J Gen Virol 64:1079–1090

Van den Elsen PJ, Houweling A, Van der Eb AJ (1983c) Morphological transformation of human adenoviruses is determined to a large extent by gene products of region E1a. Virology 131:242–246

Van der Eb AJ, Van Kesteren LW, Van Bruggen EFJ (1969) Structural properties of adenovirus DNAs. Biochim Biophys Acta 182:530–541

Van der Eb AJ, Mulder C, Graham FL, Houweling A (1977) Transformation with specific fragments of adenovirus DNAs. I. Isolation of specific fragments with transforming activity of adenovirus 2 and 5 DNA. Gene 2:115–132

Van der Eb AJ, Van Ormondt H, Schrier PI, Lupker JH, Jochemsen H, Van den Elsen PJ, DeLeys RJ, Maat J, Van Beveren CP, Dijkema R, de Waard A (1979) Structure and function of the transforming genes of human adenoviruses and SV40. Cold Spring Harbor Symp Quant Biol 44:383–399

Van der Eb AJ, Bernards R, Van den Elsen PJ, Bos JL, Schrier PI (1983) Studies on the role of adenovirus E1 genes in transformation and oncogenesis In: Harris CC, Autrup HN (eds) Human carcinogenesis. Academic, New York, pp 631–655

Van Ormondt H, Maat J, Van Beveren CP (1980) The nucleotide sequence of the transforming early region E1 of adenovirus type 5 DNA. Gene 11:299–309

Van Venrooij WJ, Sillekens PTG, Van Ekelen CAG, Reinders RJ (1981) On the association of mRNA with cytoskeleton in uninfected and adenovirus-infected human KB cells. Exp Cell Res 135:79–91

Wadell G, Hammerskjöld M-L, Winberg G, Varsanyi TW, Sundell G (1980) Genetic variability of adenoviruses. Ann NY Acad Sci 354:16–42

Wigand R, Bartha A, Dreizin RS, Esche H, Ginsberg HS, Green M, Hierholzer JC, Kalter SS,

McFerran JB, Pettersson U, Russell WC, Wadell G (1982) Adenoviridae, second report. Intervirology 18:169–176

Williams JF (1973) Oncogenic transformation of hamster embryo cells in vitro by adenovirus type 5. Nature 243:162–163

Wilson M, Fraser N, Darnell J (1979) Mapping of RNA initiation sites by high doses of UV irradiation. Evidence of three independent promoters within the left 11% of the Ad2 genome. Virology 94:175–184

Yano S, Ojima S, Fujinaga K, Shiroki K, Shimojo H (1977) Transformation of a rat cell line by an adenovirus type 12 DNA fragment. Virology 82:214–220

Yasue H, Ishibashi M (1982) The oncogenicity of avian adenoviruses. III. In situ DNA hybridization of tumor line cells localized a large number of a virocellular sequence in few chromosomes. Virology 116:99–115

Yee S-P, Rowe DT, Tremblay ML, McDermott M, Branton PE (1983) Identification of human adenovirus early region 1 products using antisera against synthetic peptides corresponding to the predicted carboxy termini. J Virol 46:1003–1013

Younghusband HB, Tyndall C, Bellett AJD (1979) Replication and interaction of virus DNA and cellular DNA in mouse cells infected by a human adenovirus. J Gen Virol 45:455–467

Zur Hausen H (1968) Chromosomal aberrations and cloning efficiency in adenovirus type 12-infected hamster cells. J Virol 2:915–917

Zur Hausen H, Sokol F (1969) Fate of adenovirus type 12 genomes in non-permissive cells. J Virol 4:255–263

Organization, Integration, and Transcription of Transforming Genes of Oncogenic Human Adenovirus Types 12 and 7

K. Fujinaga, K. Yoshida, T. Yamashita, and Y. Shimizu

1 Introduction

Thirty-one well-defined human adenovirus (Ad) serotypes are classified into five subgroups, A to E, according to their DNA-DNA homology (Green et al. 1979) as shown in Table 1. The members of subgroup A (Ad12, Ad18, and Ad31) are highly oncogenic, inducing tumors in newborn rodents at a high frequency within a few months; those of subgroup B (Ad3, Ad7, Ad14, Ad16, and Ad21) are weakly oncogenic, inducing tumors infrequently and only after longer periods; members of subgroups C to E are nononcogenic but transform rodent cells in culture (summarized by Green 1970; Tooze 1981). Transforming genes of the human adenoviruses Ad12 (Yano et al. 1977; Shiroki et al. 1977; Mak et al. 1979; Yamashita et al. 1982; Byrd et al. 1982), Ad31 (Yamashita and Fujinaga 1983), Ad3 (Dijkema et al. 1979), Ad7 (Sekikawa et al. 1978; Dijkema et al. 1979), Ad2 (Graham et al. 1974), Ad5 (Graham et al. 1974),

Department of Molecular Biology, Cancer Research Institute, Sapporo Medical College S-1, W-17, Chuo-ku, Sapporo 060, Japan

Table 1. Oncogenicity and grouping of adenoviruses by DNA homology

Group	Serotypes	DNA homology (%)		Oncogenicity	
		Within group	With other groups	In hamster	Cell transfor- mation
A	12, 18, 31	48–69	8–20	High	+
B	3, 7, 11, 14, 16, 21	89–94	9–20	Weak	+
C	1, 2, 5, 6	99–100	10–16	Nil	+
D	8, 9, 10, 13, 15, 17, 19, 20, 22, 23, 24, 25, 26, 27, 28, 29, 30	94–99	4–17	Nil[a]	+
E	4	100	4–23	Nil	+[b]

[a] Ad9 induces mammary fibroadenomas in rats
[b] Yamashita, Ueno, Suzuki, and Fujinaga (unpublished work)

and Ad4 (Yamashita, Nara, Suzuki, Ueno and Fujinaga, unpublished work) are located in the terminal region, early gene block E1 of the viral genome, and restriction DNA fragments containing these regions can transform rodent cells in culture. This review summarizes our studies on the organization, integration, and transcription of transforming genes of oncogenic Ad12 and Ad7.

2 Organization and Transcription of Transforming Genes

2.1 Transforming Genes and Their Nucleotide Sequences

Transformation of rat embryo cell line 3Y1 with the Ad12 *Eco*RI C fragment (YANO et al. 1977), the Ad12 *Hin*dIII G fragment (SHIROKI et al. 1977), and the Ad7 *Hin*dIII I·J fragment (SEKIKAWA et al. 1978) showed that transforming genes of oncogenic Ad12 and Ad7 reside in the leftmost 7–8% of the viral genome, within the early region E1 [Fig. 1; 0–11.2 map units (mu)]. Ad12 E1A (0–4.5 mu) and at least a part of Ad12 E1B (4.5–11.2 mu) are required for complete oncogenic transformation. Transformants induced by the Ad12 *Acc*I H fragment (0–4.6 mu) lack some of the characteristic phenotypes of transformation, such as efficient colony formation in soft agar culture and tumor production in newborn rodents (SHIROKI et al. 1979). Van der Eb and his co-workers showed that the Ad12 E1B region in addition to Ad5 or Ad12 E1A is required for highly oncogenic potential (VAN DEN ELSEN et al. 1982; BERNARDS et al. 1983; VAN DER EB et al. 1983).

The nucleotide sequences of the E1 region, the leftmost 11.2%, 3860 base pairs (bp) of the Ad12 Huie strain (SUGISAKI et al. 1980; KIMURA et al. 1981; Bos et al. 1981), the leftmost 7.8%, 2718 bp of the Ad7 Grider strain (Yoshida and Fujinaga, manuscript in preparation), and the leftmost 11.1%, 4010 bp of the Ad7 Gomen strain (DIJKEMA and DEKKER 1979; DIJKEMA et al. 1980a, b, 1981, 1982) have been determined by the Maxam-Gilbert method. Viral-

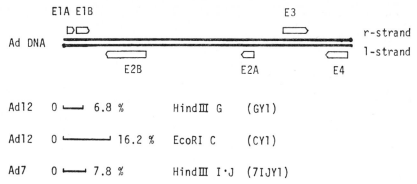

Fig. 1. Schematic illustration of adenovirus DNA fragments with transforming activities. The six early regions are designated E1A, E1B, E2A, E2B, E3 and E4, as indicated. Transformed rat cell lines CY1, GY1, and 7IJY1 were established by transfecting a clonal rat cell line, 3Y1, with the left-end fragments of the genome, Ad12 *Eco*RI C (16.2%), Ad12 *Hin*dIII G (6.8%), and Ad7 *Hin*dIII I·J (7.8%) respectively

specific mRNAs synthesized in infected KB cells and in transformed rat cells were mapped on Ad12 E1 (SAWADA and FUJINAGA 1980; SAITO et al. 1981; VIRTANEN et al. 1982) and on Ad7 E1 (YOSHIDA and FUJINAGA 1980; DIJKEMA et al. 1980b, 1981, 1982) by the Sl nuclease mapping technique and Northern blot hybridization, and their primary structures were deduced with reference to available information on specific or optimal sequences at or around sites of mRNA initiation, splicing and poly(A) addition as discussed in detail in Sect. 3. The amino acid sequences of possible polypeptides encoded thus became deducible.

2.2 Organization of Ad12 Transforming Genes and Their Transcriptions

In the Ad12 E1 region, there are two open stretches in E1A, one in reading frame 1 and the other in reading frame 3, and three open stretches in E1B, one in reading frame 2 and the other two in reading frame 1 (Fig. 2a). At least four major E1A and three major E1B mRNA species were mapped (Fig. 2b). In productively infected KB cells, mRNAs E1AI–IV and E1BI were synthesized early after infection (SAWADA and FUJINAGA 1980). In transformed rat cells (CY1; Fig. 1), mRNAs E1AI, E1A III, E1A IV and E1BI were present in appreciable amounts, but mRNAs E1AII, E1BII, E1BIII, and polypeptide IX (pIX) could hardly be detected (SAWADA and FUJINAGA 1980). The locations of translation initiation and termination codons and splice junctions (discussed in Sect. 2.3) determined the sizes and amino acid sequences of possible polypeptides to be encoded, as shown in Fig. 2c, d. In the E1A region, two polypeptide species of 29.7 and 26.0 kd can be encoded by mRNAs E1AI and E1AII and mRNAs E1AIII and E1AIV respectively by initiation at a common ATG initiation codon at nucleotide 502, shift from frame 1 to frame 3 by two different

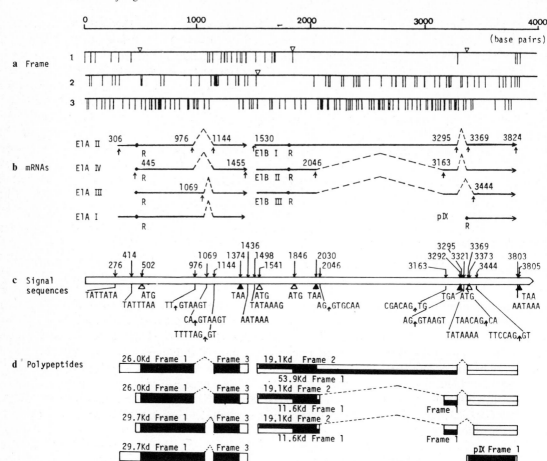

Fig. 2a–d. Diagrams of the transcription map and predicted coding regions in the early region E1 of Ad12 Huie strain DNA. **a** Occurrence of termination codons, left to right. The nonsense codons (TAA, TAG, TGA) in the l-strand of the E1 region of Ad12 DNA are arranged according to each of three possible reading frames and are indicated by *vertical lines*. In the long stop-codon-free stretches, *inverse triangles* indicate suspected initiation codons (ATG). **b** Transcription map in the early region E1 of Ad12 DNA (Sawada and Fujinaga 1980; Saito et al. 1981; Perricaudet et al. 1980; Virtanen et al. 1982). E1 mRNA species identified are numbered E1AI–IV and E1BI–III and indicated by lines below the corresponding early regions E1A and E1B. The *continuous lines* represent the areas found to anneal to mRNA, and the *interrupted lines* are the intron sequences. The *numbers* above the lines represent the coordinates of the 5′-ends, the splice points, and the 3′-ends. The *dots* marked *R* indicate potential ribosome-binding sites. **c** Signal sequences in the early region E1 of Ad12 DNA (Sugisaki et al. 1980; Kimura et al. 1981; Bos et al. 1981; Perricaudet et al. 1982). *Numbers above the line* represent nucleotide positions of assigned initiation and termination codons (*open and filled triangles*), splices, and specific or signal sequences at or around mRNA initiation and poly(A) addition. Their sequences are also shown *below the line*. *Numbers above the donor and acceptor sequences* for splices indicate positions of the end nucleotides of the exons. **d** Predicted coding regions on each mRNA (Sugisaki et al. 1980; Kimura et al. 1981; Bos et al. 1981). The assigned coding regions are indicated by *filled* or *half-filled bars* on the regions corresponding to mRNA sequences. The *half-filled bar* means that the mRNA E1BI can code for the 53.9-kd and/or the 19.1-kd polypeptides and the mRNAs E1BII and E1BIII can code for the 19.1-kd and/or 11.6-kd polypeptides. Their estimated *molecular weights* and their *coding frame numbers* are also shown near the bars

splicings (intron regions: nucleotides 977–1143, and nucleotides 1070–1143), and termination at a common termination codon TAA at nucleotide 1374 (Fig. 2c, d). In the E1B region, four polypeptides of 19.1, 53.9, 11.6, and 15.0 kd can be translated. Three mRNAs, E1BI–III, direct the synthesis of the 19.1-kd polypeptide, initiated at the first ATG at nucleotide 1541 and terminated at TAA at nucleotide 2030 without splicing. When the second ATG at nucleotide 1846 is also available for initiation in reading frame 1 (KIMURA et al. 1981; Bos et al. 1981; SAITO et al. 1983), mRNA E1BI can code the 53.9-kd polypeptide and mRNAs E1BII and E1BIII can code the 11.6-kd polypeptide, terminated with TAA at nucleotide 3292. The mRNA of pIX can code the 15.0-kd polypeptide, initiated with ATG at nucleotide 3373 and terminated with TAA at nuclotide 3803. This polypeptide corresponds to viral protein IX in Ad2 (CHOW et al. 1977; PETTERSSON and MATHEWS 1977).

2.3 Organization of Ad7 Transforming Genes and Their Transcriptions

The E1A region (0–4.5 mu) of Ad7 encodes three 5′- and 3′-coterminal mRNAs differing in the amounts of internal sequences removed by RNA splicing (YOSHIDA and FUJINAGA 1980; DIJKEMA et al. 1980a, b, 1981, 1982). The E1B region (4.5–11.2 mu) of Ad7 encodes two major 5′- and 3′-coterminal mRNAs with alternative splicing and mRNA of pIX (YOSHIDA and FUJINAGA 1980; DIJKEMA et al. 1982). In the nucleotide sequences of the leftmost 7.8% of the Ad7 Grider strain DNA (2718 bp), we assigned the initiation codon (ATG) and termination codon (TAA, TGA, TAG) in three reading frames and predicted possible polypeptides encoded (Fig. 3). In the mRNAs E1AI–III, reading frame 3 (Fig. 5A) is open for translating from initiation codon ATG at nucleotide 576. Beyond RNA splice points, polypeptides of 28.0 and 24.0 kd encoded by mRNAs E1AI and E1AII respectively could be translated in reading frame 1 (Fig. 3) and terminated at a stop codon TAA at nucleotide 1453. The 6.3-kd polypeptide specified by mRNA E1AIII is translated in reading frame 2 beyond the RNA splice point and terminated at a stop codon TAA at nucleotide 1349. The E1B region within the leftmost 7.8% of the Ad7 Grider strain DNA can code a polypeptide of 20.6 kd from nucleotide 1603 (ATG) to nucleotide 2137 (TAG) in reading frame 1 (Fig. 3).

Since the open reading frame for the polypeptide of 20.6 kd resides within the coding region of both mRNA E1BI and mRNA E1BII, it is possible that this polypeptide can be synthesized by translation of both messages. When the second ATG at nucleotide 1908 was used for translation initiation, presumed polypeptides of 55.0 kd and 9.0 kd, corresponding to those assigned in the nucleotide sequence of the E1B region of the Ad7 Gomen strain (DIJKEMA et al. 1982), could be synthesized by translation of mRNAs E1BI and E1BII respectively. Within the region of our sequence determination, N-terminal parts of presumed polypeptides of 55.0 kd and 9.0 kd were included (Fig. 3). A comparison of the nucleotide sequences (1–2718 bp) and the structural organization of the Ad7 Grider strain (Yoshida and Fujinaga, manuscript in preparation)

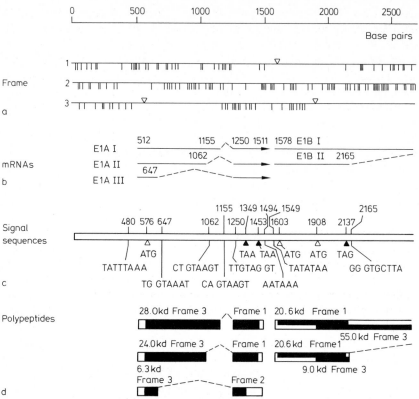

Fig. 3a–d. Diagrams of the transcription map and predicted coding regions in the leftmost 7.8% of Ad7 Grider strain DNA. **a** Occurrence of termination codons, left to right. The nonsense codons (TAA, TAG, TGA) in the l-strand of DNA are arranged according to each of three possible reading frames and indicated by *vertical lines*. In the long stop-codon-free stretches, *inverse triangles* indicate suspected initiation codons (ATG). **b** Transcription map of the leftmost 7.8% of Ad7 DNA (YOSHIDA and FUJINAGA 1980; DIJKEMA et al. 1980a, b, 1981, 1982). mRNA species identified are numbered E1AI-III and E1BI and E1BII and indicated by lines below the corresponding early regions E1A and E1B. The *continuous lines* represent the areas found to anneal to mRNA, and the *interrupted lines* are the intron sequences. The *numbers above the lines* represent the coordinates of the 5′-ends, the splice points, and the 3′-ends. **c** Signal sequences. *Numbers above the line* represent nucleotide positions of assigned initiation and termination codons (*open and filled triangles*), splices, and specific or signal sequences at or around mRNA initiation and poly(A) addition. Their sequences are also shown *below the line*. *Numbers above the donor and acceptor sequences* for splices indicate positions of the end nucleotides of the exons. **d** Predicted coding regions on each mRNA (DIJKEMA et al. 1980a, b, 1981, 1982; YOSHIDA and FUJINAGA 1980). The assigned coding regions are indicated by *filled* or *half-filled bars* on the regions corresponding to mRNA sequences. The *half-filled bar* means that the mRNA E1BI can code for the 55.0-kd and/or 20.6-kd polypeptides and the mRNA E1BII can code for the 20.6-kd and/or 9.0-kd polypeptides. Their estimated *molecular weights* and their *coding frame numbers* are also shown near the bars. Within the region of our sequence determination, N-terminal parts of presumed polypeptides of 55.0 kd and 9.0 kd are included

and its prototype, the Gomen strain (DIJKEMA et al. 1982), showed nucleotide substitutions at 33 sites and nucleotide insertion at a single site. The amino acid *gly* at the position 62 from the N-terminal in the E1A polypeptides of 28.0 and 24.0 kd in the Gomen strain is replaced by *glu* in the Grider strain.

Amino acids *arg, glu,* and *ile* at positions 48, 49 and 58 from the N-terminal in the E1B polypeptide of 20.6 kd in the Gomen strain were replaced by *ser, val,* and *ser* respectively in the Grider strain. A single nucleotide insertion occurs at nucleotide 1231 in the intron of the E1A region and results in the difference between the two strains in the reading frames for translations of polypeptides of both E1A and E1B. However, the overall gene organizations in the Grider and Gomen strains are essentially the same.

2.4 Comparison of Organizations of Ad12 Transforming Genes with Those of Ad2, Ad5, and Ad7

Comparison of the organizations and transcriptions of the transforming genes shows similarities among the highly oncogenic Ad12, weakly oncogenic Ad7, and nononcogenic Ad2 and Ad5. More pronounced homologies were found in predicted amino acid sequences deduced from nucleotide sequences (SUGISAKI et al. 1980; VAN ORMONDT et al. 1980a; KIMURA et al. 1981; BOS et al. 1981; DIJKEMA et al. 1982; VAN ORMONDT and HESPER 1983). Fig. 4 shows the amino acid sequence homologies of possible E1A and E1B polypeptides of Ad12 and Ad5. Two species of Ad12 E1A polypeptide of 29.7 and 26.0 kd and their

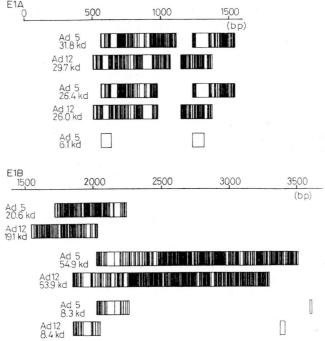

Fig. 4. Diagram showing the homologous amino acids occurring in the E1 polypeptides between Ad12 and Ad5 (SUGISAKI et al. 1980; PERRICAUDET et al. 1980; KIMURA et al. 1981; VIRTANEN et al. 1982). The E1 polypeptides are localized along the genome coordinate. *Black areas* represent homologies and *colourless areas* nonhomologies. *Ser* and *thr, leu* and *ile, arg* and *lys, asp* and *glu,* and *asn* and *gln* respectively were considered as homologous amino acids

counterpart Ad7 and Ad5 E1A polypeptides have high proline contents, are rich in highly acidic amino acids, and have widespread homologous amino acid sequences with the insertion and deletion of a unique 20- to 30-amino-acid sequence (VAN ORMONDT et al. 1978; SUGISAKI et al. 1980; VAN ORMONDT et al. 1980b; DIJKEMA et al. 1982; FUJINAGA et al. 1982). Ad12 E1B polypeptides of 53.9 kd and 19.1 kd and their counterpart Ad7 and Ad5 E1B polypeptides are neutral or slightly basic and show extensive homologies in amino acid sequences, except in 20% of the sequences near the N- and C-terminals of the larger and smaller species of polypeptides respectively (KIMURA et al. 1981; Bos et al. 1981; DIJKEMA et al. 1982; FUJINAGA et al. 1982; VAN ORMONDT and HESPER 1983).

2.5 Chimeric RNA Species and Possible Template

Further detailed mappings of mRNA species in the transforming regions of the Ad12 and Ad7 genomes suggested the presence of mRNA species unique to cells transformed by transforming DNA fragments, such as Ad12 HindIII G (GY1 cell line) and Ad7 HindIII I·J (7IJY1 cell line). These are chimeric RNA species with cellular-viral and viral-viral (E1B/E1A) hybrid-type sequences (SAWADA and FUJINAGA 1980; YOSHIDA and FUJINAGA 1980).

The presence and the structure of a chimeric RNA species of an E1B/E1A hybrid type in 7IJY1-l, a subline of 7IJY1 (SEKIKAWA et al. 1978), was confirmed by analyzing cDNA copies cloned in the pBR322 vector. As shown in Fig. 5, nucleotide 1913 in the E1B region joined nucleotide 154 in the E1A region

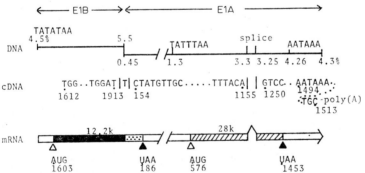

Fig. 5. Structure of the E1B/E1A chimeric mRNA deduced from analysis of the recombinant plasmid clone, CO8 DNA. Poly(A)-containing cytoplasmic RNAs were isolated from 7IJY1-1 cells. Their cDNA copies were synthesized by AMV reverse transcriptase and inserted into the *Pst*I site of the pBR322 plasmid after dG-dC tailing with terminal transferase, as described (PERRICAUDET et al. 1980). Colonies containing viral DNA sequences were identified by colony hybridization. The nucleotide sequences corresponding to the E1B/E1A chimeric mRNA in CO8, one of the clones containing viral DNA sequences, were determined by the Maxam-Gilbert procedure. The nucleotide sequences of the l-strand of the regions E1A and E1B in the Ad7 genome are taken from unpublished data (Yoshida and Fujinaga). Sequences around the 5'- and 3'-ends, the E1B/E1A junction, and the splice site are indicated. *Numbers* represent nucleotide positions on the genome. The *bar* denotes the polypeptides predicted from DNA sequences. The *caret* and *arrowhead* indicate the splice site and the 3'- end of mRNA respectively. (Yoshida and Fujinaga, manuscript in preparation)

in cDNA with an insertion of a T nucleotide between them. Such a chimeric mRNA molecule theoretically codes for polypeptides of a unique 12.2-kd species of the E1B/E1A fused type and of an authentic E1A 28-kd species (Fig. 3d) if the second initiation ATG at nucleotide 576 is also available. The significance and the role of the unique genetic information in cell transformation is unknown. The structures of viral-viral fused types in integrated viral DNAs were also determined by cleavage map analysis and DNA sequencing experiments on

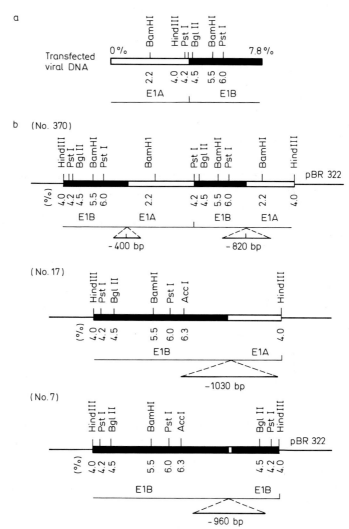

Fig. 6. a Physical map of the leftmost 7.8% DNA fragment of the Ad7 genome. **b** Physical maps of recombinant plasmid clones 370, 17, and 7. Cellular DNA prepared from transformed rat cells, 7IJY1-1, was cleaved with *Hind*III and fractionated in agarose gels. DNA fragments containing viral sequences were inserted into the *Hind*III site of the pBR322 plasmid. Colonies containing viral sequences were identified by colony hybridization. The physical maps were determined by cleavage of the plasmid DNA with various restriction enzymes followed by agarose gel electrophoresis. Deletions at the junction are shown (△). (Yoshida and Fujinaga, manuscript in preparation)

cellular genomic clones. As shown in Fig. 6, clone 370 contained two kinds of E1B/E1A joint. Clone 17 contained another E1B/E1A joint in a tandem head to tail, and clone 7 contained another E1B/E1B in a head-to-head manner. DNA sequence analysis revealed no specific features at or around the joints (Yoshida and Fujinaga, manuscript in preparation). Integration patterns of viral DNA sequences with head-to-tail (VISSER et al. 1979) and tail-to-tail (SAMBROOK et al. 1979) linked structures were also found in cells transformed by Ad2 or Ad5.

3 Specific Sequences for Transcription Signals

3.1 Specific Sequences for Transcription

Information on specific or optimal sequences at or around sites of mRNA initiation, splicing, and poly(A) addition in eukaryotes has accumulated from recent studies. These sequences are the Goldberg-Hogness box or TATA box (TATA$_T^A$AA) located about 30 bp upstream from the site of the transcription (PROUDFOOT 1979; GANNON et al. 1979), a poly(A) addition signal (AATAAA) 10–20 bp upstream from the poly(A) addition site (PROUDFOOT and BROWNLEE 1976; SEEBURG et al. 1977; MERREGAERT et al. 1978; MAAT and VAN ORMONDT 1979), and optimal sequences for the donor site (AG/GTAAGT) and the acceptor site (YYNYAG/; Y = pyrimidine, N = A, G, T, C) of splicing (BREATHNACH et al. 1978; SEIF et al. 1979; MOUNT 1982).

3.2 TATA-Box Sequences

The TATA-box sequence in eukaryotic genes resembles the Pribnow box in the prokaryotic promoter region (PRIBNOW 1975) and is considered to be essential for the faithful and efficient transcription of genes into mRNAs (OSBORNE et al. 1981; TSUJIMOTO et al. 1981). In Table 2, TATA box sequences in Ad12 and Ad7 transforming genes are shown with those of other adenovirus genes. T residues are often present at the fourth and/or fifth nucleotide of TATA-box sequences of adenovirus genes, and can be classified by nucleotide residues at positions 4 and 5 as shown in Table 2 (Sawada, Yaegashi, Shimizu, and Fujinaga, unpublished work). This classification seems consistent with the grouping of adenovirus genes by the time of gene expression after infection (i.e., early, intermediate, and late), except that the TATA box of early Ad12 E1B is classified into the late type. This exception may reflect the fact that the E1B gene of Ad12 is expressed only at a restricted rate as the major late gene in the early phase of infection and becomes fully expressed in the late phase of infection (Sawada, Yaegashi, Shimizu, and Fujinaga, unpublished work).

Table 2. TATA-box sequences in adenovirus genome

E1A type	Ad2 E1A	T A T T T T A T A C C C G G T G A G T T C C T C A A G A G G C C A*
	Ad7 E1A	T A T T T T A A A C C T G A C G A G T T C C G T C A A G A G G C C A*
	Ad12E1A	T A T T A T A G G C G C G G A A T A T T T A C C G A G G G C A*
	Ad12E1A	T A T T T T A A T G C C G C C G T G T T C G T C A A G A G G C C A*
E1B type	Ad2 E1B	T A T A T A A T G C G C C G T G G G C T A A T C T T G G T T A*C A*
	Ad7 E1B	T A T A T A A G T A G G A G C A G A T C T G T G T G G T T A G*
	Ad2 E3	G G T A T A A C T C A C C T G A A A A T C A G A G G G C G A G G*T A*
	Ad2 E4	T A T A T A T A C T C G C T C T G C A C T T G G C C C T*T*T*T*T*A*
	Ad2 pIX	T A T A T A A G G T G G G G G T C T T A T G T A G T T T T G*T A*
Late type	Ad2 major late	T A T A A A A G G G G G T G G G G G C G C G T T C G T C C T C A*
	Ad7 major late	T A T A A A A G G G G G C G G A C C T C T G T T C G T C C T C A*
	Ad2 E2A late	T A C A A A T T T G C G A A G G T A A G C C G A C G T C C A*C A*
	Ad12E1B	T A T A A A G C T G G G T T G G T G T T G C T T T G A A T A G*
	Ad12 pIX	T A T A A A A G G C T G G A A G T C A A C T A A A A A T T G*
Non-TATA type	Ad2 E2A	C C T T A A G A G T C A G C G C G C A G T A T T G C T G A A*G*
	Ad2 IVa2	T C G T G C T G G C C T G G A C G C G A G C C T T C G T C T*C A*
	Ad7 IVa2	T T G T G C T G G C C T G G A C A C G C G C T T T T G T A T*C A*
	Ad7 pIX	G G T A A G G T G G A C A A A T T G G G T A A A T T T T G T T A*

TATA-box sequences are underlined. Asterisks indicate cap sites for mRNAs

Data taken from ZIFF and EVANS (1978), BAKER and ZIFF (1979), BAKER et al. (1979), ALESTRÖM et al. (1980), DIJKEMA et al. (1980b, 1981, 1982), PERRICAUDET et al. (1980b), BAKER and ZIFF (1981), HASHIMOTO et al. (1981a, b), TOOZE (1981)

3.3 Optimal Sequences for Splicing

Specific sequences at splice junctions in adenovirus transforming gene regions are presented with those of the other adenovirus genes in Table 3.

The sites for splicings could be strongly suspected from sequence data and RNA mapping studies (see Sect. 2), and most of them were confirmed by sequencing cloned cDNA copies of each mRNA molecule (PERRICAUDET et al. 1979, 1980a, b; DIJKEMA et al. 1980b, 1981; VIRTANEN et al. 1982; Yoshida and Fujinaga, unpublished work). All the intron regions listed had GT residues at the 5′-terminal and AG residues at the 3′-terminal, consistent with the intron structure in other viral and eukaryotic genes known as the GT-AG rule or Chambon rule, and the consensus or optimal sequence for the donor site was AG/GTAAGT and that for the acceptor site was YYNCAG/GT. The positions of translation initiation (ATG) and termination (TGA, TAG and TAA) codons in three possible frames were assigned (Figs. 2b, 3b), and elucidation of splice

Table 3. Specific sequences for splicing of adenovirus mRNAs

		Donor	Acceptor
Ad2	E1A	A G / G T A C T G G G / G T G A G G C A / G T A A G T	T A A A A G / G T
	E1B	A G / G T G G C T A G / G T A C T G	T T G C A G / C A
	IVa2	A G / G T A A G A	G C G C A G / G G
	Major late	G G / G T G A G T .... C G / G T A A G A	C C A C A G / C T G T G T A G / G T
		A G / G T A G G C	C A A C A G / T T C G C C A G / A G
	E4	T G / G T A A G G	A T G C A G / G A A T A C A G / G T C A A G A G / T T C T T C A G / G A
		A G / G T C T T C	C G C A A G / T T
Ad7	E1A	T G / G T A A A T C T / G T A A G T C A / G T A A G T	T T G T A G / G T
	E1B	G G / G T G C T T A A / G T A A G T	T T G C A G / C T
	IVa2	A G / G T A A G T	A T G C A G / G G
Ad12	E1A	T T / G T A A G T C A / G T A A G T	T T T T A G / G T
	E1B	A G / G T G C A A	C G A C A G / T G
		A G / G T A A G T	T A A C A G / C A T T C C A G / G T

junctions made it possible to determine frame shifts and thus to determine the sizes and amino acid sequences of possible polypeptides encoded.

3.4 Poly(A) Addition Signal

Many eukaryotic mRNAs that have been characterized have the AAUAAA sequence approximately 10–20 nucleotides before the poly(A) tail at the 3′-terminal (PROUDFOOT and BROWNLEE 1976; SEEBURG et al. 1977; MERREGAERT et al. 1978; MAAT and VAN ORMONDT 1979). The sequence AATAAA was found in viral DNA sequences in regions upstream of poly(A) addition sites of different adenovirus mRNA molecules, as shown in Table 4.

Interestingly enough, Ad7 E1B had three AATAAA sequences upstream of the poly(A) addition site; when the E1B sequences of Ad2, Ad7, and Ad12 were arrayed to give maximum sequence homology, one of these sequences

Table 4. Poly(A) addition signal sequences and poly(A) addition sites

Ad2	E1A	*A A T A A A*GGGTGAGATAATGTTT*̇*AA
	E1B	*A A T A A A*AACCAGACTCTGTTTGGATTTTGATC*̇*AA
	E2	*A A T A A A*AACATTTGCCTTT*̇*ATTGAAAGTGTCTCCTAG
	E3	*A T T A A A*TGAGACATGATTCCTCGAGTTCCTCGAGTTCTTATATT
		*A A T A A A*TTACTTACTTAAAATCAGTCAGCAAATCTTTGTCCAGC
	E4	*A A T A A A*CACGTTGAAACATAACATGCAACAGGTTCACGATTCTT
	L2	*A A T A A A*AAGTCTGGACTCTC*̇*ACGCTCGCTTGGTCCTGTAACTAT
	L3	*A A T A A A*GGCAAATGTTTTTATTTGT*̇*ACACTCTCGGGT
	L4	*A A T A A A*TACAGAAATTAGAATCTACTGGGGCTCCTGT
	L5	*A A T A A A*GAATCGTGAACCTGTTGCATGTTATGTTTCAACGTGTT
	IVa2	*A A T A A A*GACAGCAAGACACTTGCTTGATCAAAATCC*̇*AAA
Ad7	E1A	*A A T A A A*AATTATGTCAGCT*̇*GC
	E1B	*A A T A A A*TAAAGAAATACTTGTTATAAAAAC*̇*AAA
Ad12	E1A	*A A T A A A*GGGTTTCGGTTG*̇*AA
	E1B	*A A T A A A*GAAAAAACTTAAATTGAGATGGTGTTATG*̇*AA

Data taken from AKUSJÄRVI and PETTERSSON (1979), PERRICAUDET et al. (1979), ZAIN et al. (1979), DIJKEMA et al. (1980b, 1981, 1982), PERRICAUDET et al. (1980a, b), VAN BEVEREN et al. (1981), FRAZER et al. (1982), VIRTANEN and PETTERSSON (1982), TOOZE (1981)

was found at the same position as in Ad12 E1B, the second at the same position as in Ad2 or Ad5 E1B, and the third overlapping the second and unique to Ad7 (VAN ORMONDT et al. 1980a; KIMURA et al. 1981; Bos et al. 1981; DIJKEMA et al. 1982; GINGERAS et al. 1982; VAN ORMONDT and HESPER 1983). Whether this reflects the molecular evolution of Ad2, Ad5, Ad7, and Ad12 is unknown.

4 Integrated Transforming Genes in Cells Transformed by Ad12 DNA Fragments

4.1 Integration of Viral Genome

Studies on the persistence of viral transforming genes in transformed cells, as well as the organizations and expressions of viral transforming genes, would provide essential information on the mechanism of viral transformation. In most tumors and transformed cell lines induced by adenoviruses, multiple copies of viral DNA and/or viral DNA fragments are found integrated into the host cell genome, arrayed colinearly with virion DNA and present in nonstoichiometric amounts (reviewed by DOERFLER 1982).

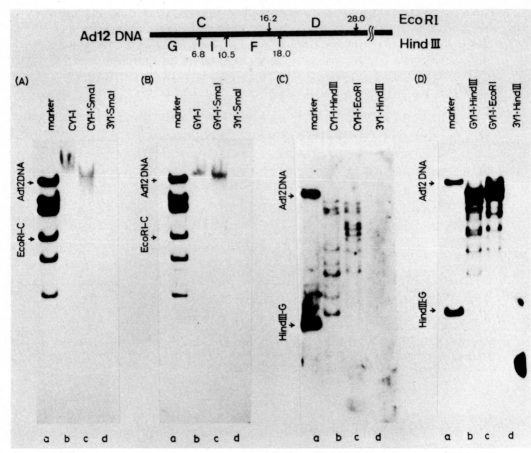

Fig. 7A–D. Viral DNA sequences in *Sma*I-, *Eco*RI- and *Hin*dIII-cleaved cellular DNAs from CY1-1 and GY1-1 cells. Cellular DNA fragments were subjected to electrophoresis on a 0.9% agarose gel, transferred to a nitrocellulose membrane filter, hybridized with in vitro ^{32}P-labeled Ad12 DNA (**A, B**) or ^{32}P-labeled Ad12 *Hin*dIII G fragment (**C, D**), and exposed to an X-ray film for 7 days (**A, B**), 14 days (**C**), or 4 days (**D**) according to the Southern technique (SOUTHERN 1975). (**A,** *a*) *Eco*RI-cleaved 3Y1 (10 µg), *Eco*RI-cleaved Ad12 DNA (0.5 ng), and uncleaved Ad12 DNA (0.5 ng); (**A,** *b*) uncleaved CY1-1 (10 µg); (**A,** *c*) *Sma*I-cleaved CY1 (10 µg); (**A,** *d*) *Sma*I-cleaved 3Y1 (10 µg). (**B,** *a*) *Eco*RI-cleaved 3Y1 (2.0 µg), *Eco*RI-cleaved Ad12 DNA (0.5 ng), and uncleaved Ad12 DNA (0.5 ng); (**B,** *b*) uncleaved GY1-1 (2.0 µg); (**B,** *c*) *Sma*I-cleaved GY1-1 (2.0 µg); (**B,** *d*) *Sma*I-cleaved 3Y1 (2.0 µg). (**C,** *a*) *Hin*dIII-cleaved 3Y1 (6.0 µg), *Hin*dIII-cleaved Ad12 DNA (0.34 ng), and uncleaved Ad12 DNA (0.34 ng); (**C,** *b*) *Hin*dIII-cleaved CY1-1 (6.0 µg); (**C,** *c*) *Eco*RI-cleaved CY1-1 (6.0 µg); (**C,** *d*) *Hin*dIII-cleaved 3Y1 (6.0 µg). (**D,** *a*) *Hin*dIII-cleaved 3Y1 (6.0 µg), *Hin*dIII-cleaved Ad12 DNA (1.0 ng), and uncleaved Ad12 DNA (1.0 ng); (**D,** *b*) *Hin*dIII-cleaved GY1-1 (6.0 µg); (**D,** *c*) *Eco*RI-cleaved GY1-1 (6.0 µg); (**D,** *d*) *Hin*dIII-cleaved 3Y1 (6.0 µg). (FUJINAGA et al. 1979)

The integration patterns differ in different transformed cell lines, and there is no evidence that specific or optimal sequences in either the viral or the host cell DNA are involved in the integration, although some patch homologies were found around junction sites between viral and host cell DNAs (DEURING et al. 1981; GAHLMANN et al. 1982; reviewed by DOERFLER 1982). Also, no information is available to answer the question of whether specific integration(s) is required for establishment and/or maintenance of transformed phenotypes. This is also still unknown with respect to the integrations of transforming gene sequences in cells transformed by specific Ad12 DNA fragments of *Eco*RI C (CY1; Fig. 1) and of *Hin*dIII G (GY1; Fig. 1). This section summarizes our results on viral DNA sequences integrated into these cell lines.

4.2 Copy Number and Fraction Integrated

The concentration (copy number) and nature of viral DNA sequences present in transformed cell lines have been estimated from the results of conventional reassociation kinetics (GELB et al. 1971) and early reassociation kinetics (FUJINAGA et al. 1974) of labeled viral DNA sequences in the presence of cellular DNAs. The accelerations of viral DNA reassociation reactions by transformed cell DNAs indicated the presence of Ad12 *Hin*dIII fragments G, I, and F, three components covering the Ad12 *Eco*RI C fragment (Fig. 7), at about the same frequencies of five to six copies per haploid quantity of cellular DNA in CY1-1 (SAWADA et al. 1979; FUJINAGA et al. 1979). Early reassociation kinetic analysis (FUJINAGA et al. 1974) showed that portions of the Ad12 *Hin*dIII G sequences were present at different frequencies and at least a portion as fragmented forms in GY1-1 and GY1-3, two sublines of GY1 (Table 5), although saturation hybridization revealed the presence of nearly all of the Ad12 *Hin*dIII G sequences in these cell lines (SAWADA et al. 1979).

4.3 Integration Pattern

Southern blot hybridizations (SOUTHERN 1975) were carried out to investigate integration patterns of viral DNA sequences in CY1-1 and GY1-1 cell lines (SAWADA et al. 1979; FUJINAGA et al. 1979). Only a bundle of cellular DNA

Table 5. Fraction of the DNA fragment and number of copies present per haploid cell DNA quantity of rat cell lines transformed by the Ad12 DNA *Hin*dIII G fragment (SAWADA et al. 1979)

Cell line	^{32}P-labeled probe	Number of copies per haploid cell	Proportion of probe sequence present in cells (%)	Proportion of Ad12 genome represented by integrated fragment (%)
GY1-1	*Hin*dIII G	74	46	3.3
	*Acc*I H	70	65	2.9
	*Acc*I J	139	17	0.5
GY1-3	*Hin*dIII G	468	28	2.0
	*Acc*I H	418	33	1.5
	*Acc*I J	376	12	0.4

Fraction and copy number were estimated by early reassociation kinetic analysis (FUJINAGA et al. 1974).

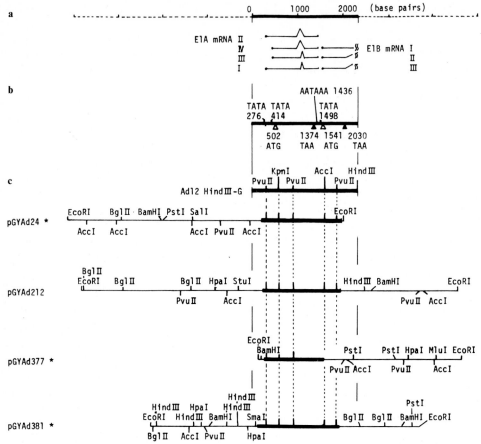

Fig. 8a–c. Cleavage maps of integrated viral and flanking cellular DNA regions cloned from GY1-3 cell DNA. Integrated viral DNA sequences with flanking cellular DNA sequences were cloned from GY1-3 cells into phage vector λgtWES·λB and recloned into plasmid pBR322 at the *Eco*RI site. Regions of integrated viral DNAs cloned were determined by restriction enzyme digestion analysis and Southern blot hybridization. Numbers represent nucleotide positions of Ad12 DNA. **a** Transcription map (see Fig. 2b). **b** Signal sequences of transcription and translation in the Ad12 genome (see Fig. 2c). **c** Cleavage maps of regions of integrated viral and flanking cellular DNAs in different recombinants. *Heavy* and *thin lines* represent viral and cellular DNA sequences respectively. Recombinant DNAs marked with *asterisks* showed transformation activity. (Sugisaki, Takanami, Yamashita, and Fujinaga, manuscript in preparation)

bands of more than 34 kb (size of Ad12 DNA) hybridized with the labeled Ad12 *Hind*III G fragment when cellular DNAs from CY1-1 and GY1-1 were cleaved with *Sma*I, which does not cut the Ad12 *Eco*RI C fragment (Fig. 7). *Eco*RI digestion of cellular DNAs generated eight or more cellular DNA bands containing viral DNA sequences (Fig. 7). These results indicate that viral DNA sequences are integrated at multiple sites into high-molecular-weight cellular DNAs in cells transformed by specific Ad12 DNA fragments containing viral transforming genes.

4.4 Analysis by Cloning

To investigate structures of integrated viral transforming gene sequences and flanking cellular DNA sequences in detail, viral DNA sequences in GY1-3 cells were cloned into phage vector λgtWES·λB with their flanking cellular sequences and recloned into plasmid pBR322 at the *Eco*RI site (Sugisaki, Takanami, Yamashita, and Fujinaga, manuscript in preparation). Restriction enzyme analysis revealed regions of integrated viral DNAs and their flanking cellular DNA sequences cloned into plasmids. The results showed that viral DNA sequences were integrated colinearly and no common DNA segment was linked to viral DNA sequences (Fig. 8). When rat embryo 3Y1 cells were transfected with *Eco*RI-digested recombinant DNAs, three of ten clones tested showed transforming activity (see Fig. 8 legend), and, in established transformants, viral DNA sequences with flanking cellular DNA sequences were integrated. Detailed analyses at the nucleotide level of viral DNAs, viral-cellular joints, and flanking cellular DNAs with their transcriptions and translations are now under way. We also hope that further analyses at the nucleotide level of regions of integrated viral DNAs and of regions around viral-cellular joints of integrated viral DNAs in relation to transforming activity will lead to an understanding of cell transformation by adenovirus transforming genes.

5 Summary

The organization and expression of Ad12 and Ad7 transforming genes have been analyzed at the nucleotide level. Sites of and sequences around mRNA initiations, splicings, and poly(A) additions and the regions coding for polypeptides were determined and compared with those of nononcogenic Ad2 or Ad5 transforming genes. High degrees of homology were found between most of the transforming gene products thus predicted for highly oncogenic Ad12 and nononcogenic Ad2 or Ad5.

Among the viral-specific mRNAs identified, not only species corresponding to those synthesized in infected KB cells during early stages of productive infection, but also unique chimeric ones containing sequences of the viral-viral or cellular-viral fused type, were detected in cells transformed by Ad12 and Ad7 transforming genes.

In cells transformed by specific Ad12 DNA fragments, transforming gene sequences were found integrated into high-molecular-weight cellular DNAs colinearly at multiple sites. Integrated Ad12 transforming gene with flanking cellular DNA sequences was cloned into plasmids and some of the cloned inserts showed transforming activity when transfected. Detailed analyses of the sequences around viral-cell joints and of cellular flanking sequences cloned into these plasmids are now under way.

Acknowledgments. We thank Dr. Hiroto Shimojo of the National Institute of Health, Tokyo and Dr. Mituru Takanami of the Institute for Chemical Research, Kyoto University for critical reading of the manuscript. The work was supported in part by grants for cancer research and scientific research from the Ministry of Education, Science and Culture, the Princess Takamatsu Fund for Cancer Research, and the Chiyoda Mutual Life Foundation.

References

Akusjärvi G, Pettersson U (1979) Sequence analysis of adenovirus DNA: complete nucleotide sequence of the spliced 5' noncoding region of adenovirus 2 hexon messenger RNA. Cell 16:841–850

Aleström P, Akusjärvi G, Perricaudet M, Mathews MB, Klessig D, Pettersson U (1980) The gene for polypeptide IX of adenovirus type 2 and its unspliced messenger RNA. Cell 19:671–681

Baker CC, Ziff EB (1979) Biogenesis, structure, and sites of encoding of the 5' termini of adenovirus-2 mRNAs. Cold Spring Harbor Symp Quant Biol 44:415–428

Baker CC, Ziff EB (1981) Promotors and heterogeneous 5' termini of the messenger RNAs of adenovirus serotype 2. J Mol Biol 149:189–221

Baker CC, Hérissé J, Courtois G, Gallibert F, Ziff E (1979) Messenger RNA for the Ad2 DNA binding protein: DNA sequences encoding the first leader and heterogeneity at the mRNA 5' end. Cell 18:569–580

Bernards R, Schrier PI, Bos JL, Van der Eb AJ (1983) Role of adenovirus type 5 and 12 early region 1b tumor antigens in oncogenic transformation. Virology 126:45–53

Bos JL, Polder LJ, Bernards R, Schrier PI, Van den Elsen PJ, Van der Eb AJ, Van Ormondt H (1981) The 2.2 kb E1B mRNA of human Ad12 and Ad5 codes for two tumor antigens starting at different AUG triplets. Cell 27:121–131

Breathnach R, Benoist C, O'Hare K, Gannon F, Chambon P (1978) Ovalbumin gene: evidence for a leader sequence in mRNA and DNA sequences at the exon-intron boundaries. Proc Natl Acad Sci USA 75:4853–4857

Byrd P, Chia W, Rigby PWJ, Gallimore PH (1982) Cloning of DNA fragments from the left end of the adenovirus type 12 genome: transformation by cloned early region 1. J Gen Virol 60:279–293

Chow LT, Roberts JM, Lewis JB, Broker TR (1977) A map of cytoplasmic RNA transcripts from lytic adenovirus type 2, determined by electron microscopy of RNA: DNA hybrids. Cell 11:819–836

Deuring R, Winterhoff U, Tamanoi F, Stabel S, Doerfler W (1981) Site of linkage between adenovirus type 12 and cell DNAs in hamster tumour line CLAC3. Nature 293:81–84

Dijkema R, Dekker BMM (1979) The inverted terminal repetition of the DNA of weakly oncogenic adenovirus type 7. Gene 8:7–15

Dijkema R, Dekker BMM, Van der Feltz MJM, Van der Eb AJ (1979) Transformation of primary rat kidney cells by DNA fragments of weakly oncogenic adenoviruses. J Virol 32:943–950

Dijkema R, Dekker BMM, Van Ormondt H (1980a) The nucleotide sequence of the transforming *Bgl*II-H fragment of adenovirus type 7 DNA. Gene 9:141–156

Dijkema R, Dekker BMM, Van Ormondt H, de Waard A, Maat J, Boyer HW (1980b). Gene organization of the transforming region of weakly oncogenic adenovirus type 7: the E1A region. Gene 12:287–299

Dijkema R, Maat J, Dekker BMM, Van Ormondt H, Boyer HW (1981) The gene for polypeptide IX of human adenovirus type 7. Gene 13:375–385

Dijkema R, Dekker BMM, Van Ormondt H (1982) Gene organization of the transforming region of adenovirus type 7 DNA. Gene 18:143–156

Doerfler W (1982) Uptake, fixation, and expression of foreign DNA in mammalian cells: the organization of integrated adenovirus DNA sequences. In: Graf T, Jaenisch R (eds) Tumorviruses, Neoplastic Transformation and Differentiation. Springer, Berlin Heidelberg New York, pp 127–194 (Current topics in microbiology and immunology, Vol 101)

Frazer NW, Baker CC, Moore MA, Ziff EB (1982) Poly(A) sites of adenovirus serotype 2 transcription units. J Mol Biol 155:207–233

Fujinaga K, Sekikawa K, Yamazaki H, Green M (1974) Analysis of multiple viral genome fragments in adenovirus 7-transformed hamster cells. Cold Spring Harbor Symp Quant Biol 39:633–636

Fujinaga K, Sawada Y, Uemizu Y, Yamashita T, Shimojo H, Shiroki K, Sugisaki H, Sugimoto K, Takanami M (1979) Nucleotide sequences, integration, and transcription of the adenovirus 12 transforming genes. Cold Spring Harbor Symp Quant Biol 44:519–532

Fujinaga K, Yoshida K, Sawada Y, Kimura T, Shimizu Y (1982) Organization and expression of oncogenic human adenovirus transforming genes. In: Proceedings of the 12th International Symposium of the Princess Takamatsu Cancer Research Fund. Primary and tertiary structure of nucleic acids and cancer research. Japan Scientific Society, Tokyo, pp 249–262

Gahlmann R, Leisten R, Vardimon L, Doerfler W (1982) Patch homologies and the integration of adenovirus DNA in mammalian cells. EMBO J 1:1101–1104

Gannon F, O'Hare K, Perrin F, LePennec JP, Benoist C, Cochet M, Breathnach R, Royal A, Garapin A, Cami B, Chambon P (1979) Organization and sequences at the 5' end of a cloned complete ovalbumin gene. Nature 278:428–434

Gelb LD, Kohne DE, Martin MA (1971) Quantitation of simian virus 40 sequences in African green monkey, mouse and virus-transformed cell genomes. J Mol Biol 57:129–145

Gingeras TR, Sciaky D, Gelinas RE, Bing-Dong J, Yen CE, Kelly MM, Bullock PA, Parsons BL, O'Neill KE, Roberts RJ (1982) Nucleotide sequences from the adenovirus-2 genome. J Biol Chem 257:13475–13491

Graham FL, Abrahams PJ, Mulder C, Heijnecker HL, Warnaar SO, de Vries FAJ, Fiers W, Van der Eb AJ (1974) Studies on in vitro transformation by DNA and DNA fragments of human adenoviruses and simian virus 40. Cold Spring Harbor Symp Quant Biol 39:637–650

Green M (1970) Oncogenic viruses. Annu Rev Biochem 39:701–756

Green M, Mackey JK, Wold WSM, Rigden P (1979) Thirty-one human adenovirus serotypes (Ad1-Ad31) form five groups (A–E) based upon DNA genome homologies. Virology 93:481–492

Hashimoto S, Pursley MH, Green M (1981a) Nucleotide sequences and mapping of novel heterogenous 5'-termini of adenovirus 2 early region 4 mRNA. Nucleic Acids Res 9:1645–1689

Hashimoto S, Wold WSM, Brackmann KH, Green M (1981b) Nucleotide sequence of 5' termini of adenovirus 2 early transforming region Ela and Elb messenger ribonucleic acids. Biochemistry 20:6640–6647

Kimura T, Sawada Y, Shinagawa M, Shimizu Y, Shiroki K, Shimojo H, Sugisaki H, Takanami M, Uemizu Y, Fujinaga K (1981) Nucleotide sequence of the transforming early region Elb of adenovirus type 12 DNA: structure and gene organization, and comparison with those of adenovirus type 5 DNA. Nucleic Acids Res 9:6571–6589

Maat J, Van Ormondt H (1979) The nucleotide sequence of the transforming HindIII-G fragment of adenovirus type 5 DNA. The region between map positions 4.5 (HpaI site) and 8.0 (HindIII site). Gene 6:75–90

Mak S, Mak I, Smiley JR, Graham FL (1979) Tumorigenicity and viral gene expression in rat cells transformed by Ad12 virions or by the EcoRI-C fragment of Ad12 DNA. Virology 98:456–460

Merregaert J, Van Emmelo J, Devos R, Porter A, Fellner P, and Fiers W (1978) The 3'-terminal nucleotide sequence of encephalomyocarditis virus RNA. Eur J Biochem 82:55–63

Mount SM (1982) A catalogue of splice junction sequences. Nucleic Acids Res 10:459–471

Osborne TF, Schell RE, Burch-Jaffe E, Berget SJ, Berk AJ (1981) Mapping a eukaryotic promotor: a DNA sequence required for in vivo expression of adenovirus pre-early functions. Proc Natl Acad Sci USA 78:1381–1385

Perricaudet M, Akusjärvi G, Virtanen A, Pettersson U (1979) Structure of two spliced mRNAs from transforming region of human subgroup C adenoviruses. Nature 281:694–696

Perricaudet M, le Moullec JM, Pettersson U (1980a) Predicted structure of two adenovirus tumor antigens. Proc Natl Acad Sci USA 77:3778–3782

Perricaudet M, le Moullec J-M, Tiollais P, Pettersson U (1980b) Structure of two adenovirus type 12 transforming polypeptides and their evolutionary implications. Nature 288:174–176

Pettersson U, Mathews MB (1977) The gene and messenger RNA for adenovirus polypeptide IX. Cell 12:741–750

Pribnow D (1975) Nucleotide sequence of an RNA polymerase binding site at an early T7 promoter. Proc Natl Acad Sci USA 72:784–788

Proudfoot NJ (1979) Eukaryotic promoters? Nature 279:376

Proudfoot NJ, Brownlee GG (1976) 3' Non-coding region sequences in eukaryotic messenger RNA. Nature 263:211–214

Saito I, Sato J, Handa H, Shiroki K, Shimojo H (1981) Mapping of RNAs transcribed from adenovirus type 12 early and VA RNA regions. Virology 114:379–398

Saito I, Shiroki K, Shimojo H (1983) mRNA species and proteins of adenovirus type 12 transforming regions: identification of proteins translated from multiple coding stretches in 2.2 kb region 1B mRNA in vitro and in vivo. Virology 127:272–289

Sambrook J, Greene R, Stringer J, Mitchison T, Hu S-L, Botchan M (1979) Analysis of the sites of integration of viral DNA sequences in rat cells transformed by adenovirus 2 or SV40. Cold Spring Harbor Symp Quant Biol 44:569–584

Sawada Y, Fujinaga K (1980) Mapping of adenovirus 12 mRNAs transcribed from transforming region. J Virol 36:639–651

Sawada Y, Ojima S, Shimojo H, Shiroki K, Fujinaga K (1979) Transforming DNA sequences in rat cells transformed by DNA fragments of highly oncogenic human adenovirus type 12. J Virol 32:379–385

Seeburg PH, Shine J, Martial JA, Baxter JD, Goodman HM (1977) Nucleotide sequence and amplification in bacteria of structural gene for rat growth hormone. Nature 270:486–494

Seif I, Khoury G, Dhar R (1979) BKV splice sequences based on analyses of preferred donor and acceptor sites. Nucleic Acids Res 6:3387–3398

Sekikawa K, Shiroki K, Shimojo H, Ojima S, Fujinaga K (1978) Transformation of rat cell line by an adenovirus 7 DNA fragment. Virology 88:1–7

Shiroki K, Handa H, Shimojo H, Yano S, Ojima S, Fujinaga K (1977) Establishment and characterization of rat cell lines transformed by restriction endonuclease fragments of adenovirus 12 DNA. Virology 82:462–471

Shiroki K, Shimojo H, Sawada Y, Uemizu Y, Fujinaga K (1979) Incomplete transformation of rat cells by a small fragment of adenovirus 12 DNA. Virology 95:127–136

Southern EM (1975) Detection of specific sequences among DNA fragments separated by gel electrophoresis. J Mol Biol 98:503–517

Sugisaki H, Sugimoto K, Takanami M, Shiroki K, Saito I, Shimojo H, Sawada Y, Uemizu Y, Uesugi S, Fujinaga K (1980) Structure and gene organization in the transforming HindIII-G fragment of Ad12. Cell 20:777–786

Tsujimoto Y, Hirose S, Tsuda M, Suzuki Y (1981) Promotor sequence of fibroin gene assigned by in vitro transcription system. Proc Natl Acad USA 78:4838–4842

Tooze J (ed) (1981) Molecular biology of tumor viruses, 2nd edn part 2. DNA tumor viruses. Cold Spring Harbor, New York

Van Beveren CP, Maat J, Dekker BMM, Van Ormondt H (1981) The nucleotide sequence of the gene for protein IVa 2 and of the 5′ leader segment of the major late mRNA of adenovirus type 5. Gene 16:179–189

Van den Elsen PJ, De Pater S, Houweling A, Van der Veer J, Van der Eb AJ (1982) The relationship between region E1a and E1b of human adenoviruses in cell transformation. Gene 18:175–185

Van der Eb AJ, Bernards R, Van den Elsen PJ, Bos JL, Schrier PI (1983) Studies on the role of adenovirus E1 genes in transformation and oncogenesis. Carcinogenesis (in press)

Van Ormondt H, Hesper B (1983) Comparison of the nucleotide sequences of early region E1b DNA of human adenovirus type 12, 7 and 5 (subgroups A, B and C). Gene 21:217–226

Van Ormondt H, Maat J, de Waard A, Van der Eb AJ (1978) The nucleotide sequence of the transforming HpaI-E fragment of adenovirus type 5 DNA. Gene 4:309–328

Van Ormondt H, Maat J, Van Bereren CP (1980a) The nucleotide sequence of the transforming early region E1 of adenovirus type 5 DNA. Gene 11:299–309

Van Ormondt H, Maat J, Dijkema R (1980b) Comparison of nucleotide sequences of the early E1a regions for subgroup A, B and C of human adenoviruses. Gene 12:63–76

Virtanen A, Pettersson U, le Moullec J-M, Tiollais P, Perricaudet M (1982) Different mRNAs from the transforming region of highly oncogenic and non-oncogenic human adenoviruses. Nature 295:705–707

Visser L, Van Maarschalkerweerd MW, Rozijn TH, Wassenaar ADC, Reemst AMCB, Sussenbach JS (1979) Viral DNA sequences in adenovirus-transformed cells. Cold Spring Harbor Symp Quant Biol 44:541–550

Yamashita T, Fujinaga K (1983) Establishment and characterization of rat cell lines transformed by the left-end fragments of adenovirus type 31. Gann 74:77–85

Yamashita T, Sugisaki H, Nara Y, Kanazawa S, Takanami M, Fujinaga K (1982) Transformation of rat 3Y1 cells by the cloned EcoRI-C fragment of human adenovirus type 12. Tumor Res 17:9–22

Yano S, Ojima S, Fujinaga K, Shiroki K, Shimojo H (1977) Transformation of a rat cell line by an adenovirus type 12 DNA fragment. Virology 82:214–220

Yoshida K, Fujinaga K (1980) Unique species of mRNA from adenovirus type 7 early region 1 in cells transformed by adenovirus type 7 DNA fragment. J Virol 36:337–352

Zain S, Sambrook J, Roberts RJ, Keller W, Fried M, Dunn AR (1979) Nucleotide sequence analysis of the leader segments in a cloned copy of adenovirus 2 fiber mRNA. Cell 16:851–861

Ziff EB, Evans RM (1978) Coincidence of the promotor and capped 5′ terminus of RNA from the adenovirus 2 major late transcription unit. Cell 15:1463–1475

Nucleotide Sequences of Adenovirus DNAs*

H. VAN ORMONDT[1] and F. GALIBERT[2]

1 Inverted Terminal Repetitions in the DNAs of Human and Animal (Mammalian, Avian) Adenoviruses

The forty-odd identified human adenoviruses have been classified into groups A–G on the basis of DNA homology. After denaturation and renaturation of Ad DNA, single-stranded circles can be detected by electron microscopy, indicating that Ad DNA contains an inverted terminal repetition (ITR) of the type

5′ a b c   . . . . . . .c′ b′ a′
3′ a′ b′ c′ . . . . . . .c b a

A number of these ITRs have been elucidated at the nucleotide level, belonging to human serotype groups A–E and also comprising sequences from simian, equine, canine, prosimian (tupaia), rodent (mouse) and avian adenoviruses (Table 1.1).

---

* The data presented in this chapter were collected from publications, from personal communications, and from a tape kindly provided by Drs. Hamm and Stüber of the EMBL DNA Sequence Data Bank

1 Department of Medical Biochemistry, University of Leiden, Leiden, The Netherlands

2 Laboratory of Experimental Hematology, Centre Hayem, Hôpital St. Louis, Paris, France

Table 1.1. ITRs in human and animal adenovirus DNAs

```
    Group A: Ad12 Huie (Sugisaki et al., 1980; Shinagawa and Padmanabhan,
                        1980; Byrd et al., 1982; J.L. Bos,personal communication)

    The Huie strain of Ad12 shows terminal heterogeneity; the variants
    observed by Shinagawa and Padmanabhan (1980), Byrd et al. (1982) and
    J.L. Bos (personal communication) are given in lower case under the
    sequence determined by Sugisaki et al. (1980).

         10        20        30        40        50        60
    CTATATATAT AATATACCTT ATACTGGACT AGTGCCAATA TTAAAATGAA GTGGGCGTAG

    catcatca   (Shinagawa and Padmanabhan, 1980)

    --tatcta   (Byrd et al., 1982)

    -ctatcta   (J.L. Bos, personal communication)

         70        80        90       100       110       120
    TGTGTAATTT GATTGGGTGG AGGTGTGGCT TTGGCGTGCT TGTAAGTTTG GGCGGATGAG

        130       140       150       160
    GAAGTGGGGC GCGGCGTGGG AGCCGGgCGC GCCGGaTGTG ACGT

    Residues G147 and A156 are absent in the sequence reported
    by Shinagawa and Padmanabhan (1980).
    ------------------------------------------------------------------------

    Group A: Ad18 (Garon et al., 1982)

         10        20        30        40        50        60
    CATCATCAAT AATATACCTT ATACTGGACT AGAGCCAATA TTAAAATGAA GTGGGTGTGG

         70        80        90       100       110       120
    CGATGTACTT TGATTGGGTG GAGGTGTGGC CTGGGCGTGT TTGTAAGTTT GGGCGGATGA

        130       140       150       160
    GGAAGTTGGG CGCGGCGTGG GAGCCGGCGC GCCGGTGTGA CGTGT

    ------------------------------------------------------------------------

    Group A: Ad31 (Stillman et al, 1982)

         10        20        30        40        50        60
    CATCATCAAT AATATACCTT ACACTGGACT TGAGCCAATA TTAAAATGAA GTGGGCGGAG

         70        80        90       100       110       120
    TGAATAGTTA ATTGACCGTA GGCGTGGTTT GCAAGTTTGC CGAAGCCGGA TGTGACGCGT

        130       140
    GTGGGAGCCG GGCGCGCCGG ATGTGACG

    ------------------------------------------------------------------------

    Group B: Ad3 (Tolun et al., 1979)

         10        20        30        40        50        60
    CTCTCTATAT AATATACCTT ATAGATGGAA TGGTGCCAAC ATGTAAATGA GGTAATTTAA

         70        80        90       100       110       120
    AAAAGTGCGC GCTGTGTGGT GATTGGCTGC GGGGTTAACG GCTAAAGGGG CGGCGCGACC

        130
    GTGGGAAAAT GACGT

    ------------------------------------------------------------------------

    Group B: Ad7 (strains Gomen (Dijkema and Dekker, 1979) and Greider
                  (Shinagawa and Padmanabhan, 1980)).
    The sequence given is that of the Gomen strain; different residues
    in the Greider strain are indicated in lower case.

         10        20        30        40        50        60
    CTCTCTATAT AATATACCTT ATAGATGGAA TGGTGCCAAC ATGTAAATGA GGTAATTTAA
         a                           t

         70        80        90       100       110       120
    AAAAGTGCGC GCTGTGTGGT GATTGGCTGT GGGGTGAATG ACTAACATGG GCGGGGCGGC
                                         c  g       a

        130
    CGTGGGAAAA TGACGT

    ------------------------------------------------------------------------

    Group B: Ad16 (M.L. Hammarskjöld and G. Winberg, personal communication)

         10        20        30        40        50        60
    CTATCTATAT AATATACCTT ATAGATGGAA TGGTGCCAAC ATGTAAATGA GGTAATTTAA

         70        80        90       100       110
    AAAAGTGCGC GCTGTGTGGT GATTGGCTGC GGGGTGAACG GCTAAAAGGG GCGG

    ------------------------------------------------------------------------
```

Table 1.1 (Continued)

```
--------------------------------------------------------------------------

   Group C: Ad2 (Arrand and Roberts, 1979; Shinagawa and Padmanabhan, 1979)
   This sequence is identical to that of Ad5; residue A8 is absent in the
   sequence reported by Arrand and Roberts)

          10        20        30        40        50        60
   CATCATCaAT AATATACCTT ATTTTGGATT GAAGCCAATA TGATAATGAG GGGGTGGAGT

          70        80        90       100
   TTGTGACGTG GCGCGGGGCG TGGGAACGGG GCGGGTGACG TAG

--------------------------------------------------------------------------


   Group C: Ad5 (Steenbergh et al., 1977)

          10        20        30        40        50        60
   CATCATCAAT AATATACCTT ATTTTGGATT GAAGCCAATA TGATAATGAG GGGGTGGAGT

          70        80        90       100
   TTGTGACGTG GCGCGGGGCG TGGGAACGGG GCGGGTGACG TAG

--------------------------------------------------------------------------


   Group D: Ad9 (Stillman et al., 1982)

          10        20        30        40        50        60
   CTATCTATAT AATATACCCC ACAAAGTAAA CAAAAGTTAA TATGCAAATG AGCTTTTGAA

          70        80        90       100       110       120
   TTTTAACGGT TTCGGGGCGG AGCCAACGCT GATTGGACGA GAGAAGACGA TGCAAATGAC

         130       140       150
   GTCACGACGC ACGGCTAACG GTCGCCGCGG AGGCGGGCC

--------------------------------------------------------------------------


   Group D: Ad10 (Stillman et al., 1982)
   The Ad10 ITR extends further than nucleotide 135; up to this point
   it is identical to that of Ad9.

          10        20        30        40        50        60
   CTTCATCAAT AATATACCCC ACAAAGTAAA CAAAAGTTAA TATGCAAATG AGCTTTTGAA

          70        80        90       100       110       120
   TTTTAACGGT TTCGGGGCGG AGCCAACGCT GATTGGACGA GAGAAGACGA TGCAAATGAC

         130
   GTCACGACGC ACGGC---

--------------------------------------------------------------------------


   Group E: Ad4 (Stillman et al., 1982)

          10        20        30        40        50        60
   CTCTCTCTAT AATATACCTT ATTTTTTTTG TGTGAGTTAA TATGCAAATA AGGCGTGAAA

          70        80        90       100       110
   ATTTGGGGAT GGGGCGCGCT GATTGGCTGT GACAGCGGCG TTCGTTAGGG GCGGGG

--------------------------------------------------------------------------


   Simian adenovirus SA7 (Tolun et al., 1979)

          10        20        30        40        50        60
   ----ATCAAT AATATACCTT ATTTGGGAAC GGTGCCAATA TGCTAATGAG GTGGGCGGAG

          70        80        90       100       110       120
   TTTGGTGACG TATGCGGAAA TGGGCGGAGT TAGGGGCGGG GTTTGGCGGT AGGCGTGGCT

--------------------------------------------------------------------------


   Simian adenovirus SA7P (B.M.M. Dekker and H. van Ormondt, unpublished)
   This virus was originally characterized as simian virus (SV) 20, but
   recently found to be a variant of SA7 (Denisova et al., 1982).


          10        20        30        40        50        60
   ---CATCAAT AATATACCTT ATTTGGGAAC GGTGCCAATA TGCTAATGAG GTGGGCGGAG

          70        80        90       100       110
   TTTGGTGACG TATGCGGAAG TGGGCGGAGC AAGGGGCGGG GCGAGAGGCG GAACTT

--------------------------------------------------------------------------


   Infectious canine hepatitis virus (ICHV; Shinagawa et al., 1983)

          10        20        30        40        50        60
   CATCATCAAT AATATACAGG ACAAAGAGGT GTGGCCTAAA TGTTGTTTTT TTTTAAAAAA

          70        80        90       100       110       120
   GTTTTTGTCT GATTGTTTTG ACAAGGTCAC ACCCTGTTCA GGGCGTTTCC CACGGGAAAG

         130       140       150       160
   ACCATGACGT CAATTGGGTG TTTTTGTGGA CTTTGGCCCG

--------------------------------------------------------------------------
```

Table 1.1 (Continued)

```
      Equine adenovirus EAd (Shinagawa et al., 1983)

           10        20        30        40        50        60
      CATCATCAAT AATATACAGG ACACACGGGC ATGGGGCCAA GAAAGGGGAG GAGTTGAGGC

           70        80        90       100
      GTGGCGGGAG GCGGGGGCGG AGGCGGGGCG GCGGGCGGGA GGC
```

```
      Tree shrew (tupaia) adenovirus (Brinckmann et al., 1983)

           10        20        30        40        50        60
      CATCATCAAT AATATACCTG ACACTTTTGA CGTAATGACG TCAGACGTAA GTTGCAAGTG

           70        80        90       100       110       120
      CCACGTCGTC GTGGGCGTGT CTTTTGTGAC CTTTGGACGG GCGTTTCGCT GGTCGGGTTC

          130       140       150       160
      CCAGTTTCGG GGTCGTTCCC GAGAACGTTG AGTCATGACA GCTGAC
```

```
      Murine adenovirus strain FL (Temple et al., 1981)

           10        20        30        40        50        60
      CATCATCAAT AATATACAGT TAGCAAAAAA TGGCGCCTTT GTTTGGCTTT GTTCCAACTG

           70        80        90
      TTTTTGGCCC GAGTTGGGTT TCGTTTTCCC GGG
```

```
      Avian adenovirus CELO (Aleström et al., 1982a; Shinagawa et al., 1983)

      The first 10 nucleotides of the sequence determined for the Ote strain
      by Shinagawa et al. (1983) are printed in lower case under the sequence
      determined by Aleström et al. (1982a).

           10        20        30        40        50        60
      GATGATGTAT AATAACCTCA AAAACTAACG CAGTCATAAC CGGCCATAAC CGCA
      c=tcatctat
```

```
      The sequence between nucleotides 9 and 22 is highly conserved in all

      human and simian ITRs studied sofar. Stillman et al. (1982) propose

      following consensus sequence:
```

```
                              10
                              T
                              ↑
                              |
  2,5,12,18,31    5' CATCATCA
                              \                     A        G A
                              ATAATATACCYYAY(N9-11)R GYYAAYAT N AATR(A)G
                              /                     T        T T
  4,7,9           5' CTATCTAT
                              ↓  ↓
                              C  C
                              4,7 4
```

2 DNA Sequence of Human Ad5 (Subgroup C) Between Coordinates 0.0 and 31.7

The sequence was determined by STEENBERGH et al. (1977), MAAT and VAN ORMONDT (1979), VAN ORMONDT et al. (1980b), VAN BEVEREN et al. (1981), BOS et al. (1981), and DEKKER and VAN ORMONDT (1984). The homology between the Ad5 and the corresponding Ad2 sequences (PERRICAUDET et al. 1979; ALE-STRÖM et al. 1980; GINGERAS et al. 1982; ALESTRÖM et al. 1982b) is about 99%. Therefore, there is no separate section here on the sequence of Ad2 DNA between coordinates 0 and 31. For the Ad2 data, the reader is referred to Sect. 9 which gives a comparison of the leftmost sequences of Ad5, Ad7 and Ad12, where the Ad2 residues which differ from those of Ad5 are printed in lower case above the Ad5 sequence.

The sequence (Table 2.1) is given in double-stranded format with 120 nucleotides per line, and the numbering (starting at the left terminus of Ad5 DNA) between the two strand sequences. Each number refers to the position above and below its last zero. The following features are marked (Table 2.2): the end of the ITR, RNA 5′ terminals (cap sites), splice donor and acceptor nucleotides, 3′-poly(A) addition sites, "TATA" boxes and 3′-poly(A) signals (AATAAA; underlined), and predicted or potential initiation and termination codons (underlined) (PERRICAUDET et al. 1979, 1980a; BAKER and ZIFF 1980, 1981; MAAT and VAN ORMONDT 1979; ALESTRÖM et al. 1980; VAN BEVEREN et al. 1981, AKUSJÄRVI and PETTERSSON 1979b; ZAIN et al. 1979; AKUSJÄRVI et al. 1980; JONES and SHENK 1980; AKUSJÄRVI and PERSSON 1981b; DEKKER and VAN ORMONDT 1984; VIRTANEN et al. 1982a; VIRTANEN and PETTERSSON 1983). Most of the Ad5 RNA coordinates have been derived from Ad2 data, but such an extrapolation is quite legitimate in view of the high degree of sequence homology between the two serotypes. Above or below the DNA sequence (sense strand) is given the predicted amino acid sequence (in one-letter code; see footnote to Table 2.1) for the E1A proteins (VAN ORMONDT et al. 1980a), the E1B proteins (Bos et al. 1981), protein IX (ALESTRÖM et al. 1980; VAN ORMONDT et al. 1980a), protein IVa2 (PERSSON et al. 1979; VAN BEVEREN et al. 1981), the 120K DNA polymerase (STILLMAN et al. 1982; FRIEFELD et al. 1983; DEKKER and VAN ORMONDT 1984), the precursor for the DNA terminal protein (pTP; SMART and STILLMAN 1982; DEKKER and VAN ORMONDT 1984), the Ad5 "agnoprotein" (VIRTANEN et al. 1982a; DEKKER and VAN ORMONDT 1984), and the N-terminal residues of the L1, 52K, 55K polypeptide (AKUSJÄRVI and PERSSON 1981b; DEKKER and VAN ORMONDT 1984). Apart from these identified proteins, a number of hitherto unidentified open reading frames (ORFs) have been found in the sequence; the amino acid sequences of their hypothetical translation products are also given.

Table 2.1. Ad5 DNA sequence 0–31.7%

```
                                                                                                          ┌end ITR
CATCATCAATAATATACCTTATTTTGGATTGAAGCCAATATGATAATGAGGGGGTGGAGTTTGTGACGTGGCGCGGGGCGTGGGAACGGGGCGGGTGACGTAGTAGTGTGGCGGAAGTGT
        10        20        30        40        50        60        70        80        90       100       110       120
GTAGTAGTTATTATATGGAATAAAACCTAACTTCGGTTATACTATTACTCCCCCACCTCAAACACTGCACCGCGCCCCGCACCCTTGCCCCGCCCACTGCATCATCACACCGCCTTCACA

GATGTTGCAAGTGTGGCGGAACACATGTAAGCGACGGATGTGGCAAAAGTGACGTTTTTGGTGTGCGCCGGTGTACACAGGAAGTGACAATTTTCGCGCGGTTTTAGGCGGATGTTGTAG
        130       140       150       160       170       180       190       200       210       220       230       240
CTACAACGTTCACACCGCCTTGTGTACATTCGCTGCCTACACCGTTTTCACTGCAAAAACCACACGCGGCCACATGTGTCCTTCACTGTTAAAAGCGCGCCAAAATCCGCCTACAACATC

TAAATTTGGGCGTAACCGAGTAAGATTTGGCCATTTTCGCGGGAAAACTGAATAAGAGGAAGTGAAATCTGAATAATTTTGTGTTACTCATAGCGCGTAATATTTGTCTAGGGCCGCGGG
        250       260       270       280       290       300       310       320       330       340       350       360
ATTTAAACCCGCATTGGCTCATTCTAAACCGGTAAAAGCGCCCTTTTGACTTATTCTCCTTCACTTTAGACTTATTAAAACACAATGAGTATCGCGCATTATAAACAGATCCCGGCGCCC

                                                                                                           "TATA" E1a
GACTTTGACCGTTTACGTGGAGACTCGCCCAGGTGTTTTTCTCAGGTGTTTTCCGCGTTCCGGGTCAAAGTTGGCGTTTTATTATTATAGTCAGCTGACGTGTAGTGTATTTATACCCGG
        370       380       390       400       410       420       430       440       450       460       470       480
CTGAAACTGGCAAATGCACCTCTGAGCGGGTCCACAAAAAGAGTCCACAAAAGGCGCAAGGCCCAGTTTCAACCGCAAAATAATAATATCAGTCGACTGCACATCACATAAATATGGGCC

          ┌5' E1a RNA                                                     start E1a 32K, 27K, 6K
          └                                                               M  R  H  I  I  C  H  G  G  V  I  T  E  E
TGAGTTCCTCAAGAGGCCACTCTTGAGTGCCAGCGAGTAGAGTTTTCTCCTCCGAGCCGCTCCGACACCGGGACTGAAAATGAGACATATTATCTGCCACGGAGGTGTTATTACCGAAGA
        490       500       510       520       530       540       550       560       570       580       590       600
ACTCAAGGAGTTCTCCGGTGAGAACTCACGGTCGCTCATCTCAAAAGAGGAGGCTCGGCGAGGCTGTGGCCCTGACTTTTACTCTGTATAATAGACGGTGCCTCCACAATAATGGCTTCT
```

One-letter code for amino acids: A, ala; C, cys; D, asp; E, glu; F, phe; G, gly; H, his; I, ile; K, lys; L, leu; M, met; N, asn; P, pro; Q, gln; R, arg; S, ser; T, thr; V, val; W, trp; Y, tyr

Table 2.1 (Continued)

```
                                          ┌ splice 9S RNA(6K)
 M   A   A   S   L   L   D   Q   L   I   E   E │ V   L   A   D   N   L   P   P   P   S   H   F   E   P   P   T   L   H   E   L   Y   D   L   D   V   T   A   P
AATGGCCGCCAGTCTTTTGGACCAGCTGATCGAAGAGGTACTGGCTGATAATCTTCCACCTCCTAGCCATTTTGAACCACCTACCCTTCACGAACTGTATGATTTAGACGTGACGGCCCC
      610         620         630         640         650         660         670         680         690         700         710         720
TTACCGGCGGTCAGAAAACCTGGTCGACTAGCTTCTCCATGACCGACTATTAGAAGGTGGAGGATCGGTAAAACTTGGTGGATGGGAAGTGCTTGACATACTAAATCTGCACTGCCGGGG


 E   D   P   N   E   E   A   V   S   Q   I   F   P   S   V   M   L   A   V   Q   E   G   I   D   L   L   T   F   P   P   A   P   G   S   P   E   P   P   H
CGAAGATCCCAACGAGGAGGCGGTTTCGCAGATTTTTCCCGACTCTGTAATGTTGGCGGTGCAGGAAGGGATTGACTTACTCACTTTTCCGCCGGCGCCCGGTTCTCCGGAGCCGCCTCA
      730         740         750         760         770         780         790         800         810         820         830         840
GCTTCTAGGGTTGCTCCTCCGCCAAAGCGTCTAAAAAGGGCTGAGACATTACAACCGCCACGTCCTTCCCTAACTGAATGAGTGAAAAGGCGGCCGCGGGCCAAGAGGCCTCGGCGGAGT


 L   S   R   Q   P   E   Q   P   E   Q   R   A   L   G   P   V   S   M   P   N   L   V   P   E   V   I   D   L   T   C   H   E   A   G   F   P   P   S   D   D
CCTTTCCCGGCAGCCCGAGCAGCCGGAGCAGAGAGCCTTGGGTCCGGTTTCTATGCCAAACCTTGTACCGGAGGTGATCGATCTTACCTGCCACGAGGCTGGCTTTCCACCCAGTGACGA
      850         860         870         880         890         900         910         920         930         940         950         960
GGAAAGGGCCGTCGGGCTCGTCGGCCTCGTCTCTCGGAACCCAGGCCAAAGATACGGTTTGGAACATGGCCTCCACTAGCTAGAATGGACGGTGCTCCGACCGAAAGGTGGGTCACTGCT


                     ┌ splice 12S RNA (27K)
 E   D   E   E │ G   E   E   F   V   L   D   Y   V   E   H   P   G   H   G   C   R   S   C   H   Y   H   R   R   N   T   G   D   P   D   I   M   C   S   L   C
CGAGGATGAAGAGGGTGAGGAGTTTGTGTTAGATTATGTGGAGCACCCGGGCACGGTTGCAGGTCTTGTCATTATCACCGGAGGAATACGGGGGACCCAGATATTATGTGTTCGCTTTG
      970         980         990        1000        1010        1020        1030        1040        1050        1060        1070        1080
GCTCCTACTTCTCCCACTCCTCAAACACAATCTAATACACCTCGTGGGGCCCGTGCCAACGTCCAGAACAGTAATAGTGGCCTCCTTATGCCCCTGGGTCTATAATACACAAGCGAAAC
                                                                                                                  *  T   N   A   K   S
                                                                                                              stop ORF 23K


 Y   M   R   T   C   G   M   F   V   Y │ S              ┌ splice 13S RNA(32K)
CTATATGAGGACCTGTGGCATGTTTGTCTACAGTAAGTGAAAATTATGGGCAGTGGGTGATAGAGTGGTGGGTTTGGTGTGGTAATTTTTTTTTTTAATTTTTACAGTTTTGTGGTTTAAA
     1090        1100        1110        1120        1130        1140        1150        1160        1170        1180        1190        1200
GATATACTCCTGGACACCGTACAAACAGATGTCATTCACTTTTAATACCCGTCACCCACTATCTCACCACCCAAACCACACCATTAAAAAAAAAAATTAAAAATGTCAAAACACCAAATTT
                                                     Y   S   S   R   H   C   T   Q   R   C   Y   T   F   I   I   P   L   P   H   Y   L   P   P   N   P   T   T   I   K   K   K   I   K   V   T   K   H   N   L   S


                 ┌ splice 9S, 12S, 13S RNAs
                 │ P   V   S   E   P   E   P   E   P   E   P   E   P   E   P   A   R   P   T   R   R   P   K   M   A   P   A   I   L   R    Ela 6K stop
                 │  V   L   C   L   N   L   S   L   S   P   S   Q   N   R   S   L   Q   D   L   P   A   V   L   K   W   R   L   L   S   *
GAATTTTGTATTGTGATTTTTTTTAAAAGGTCCTGTGTCTGAACCTGAGCCTGAGCCCGAGCCAGAACCGGAGCCTGCAAGACCTACCCGCCGTCCTAAAATGGCGCCTGCTATCCTGAGA
     1210        1220        1230        1240        1250        1260        1270        1280        1290        1300        1310        1320
CTTAAAACATAACACTAAAAAAATTTTCCAGGACACGACTTGGACTCGGACTCGGGCTCGGTCTTGGCCTCGGACGTTCTGGATGGGCGGCAGGATTTTACCGCGGACGATAGGACTCT
 N   Q   I   T   I   K   K   F   P   G   T   D   S   G   S   G   S   G   S   G   A   L   G   V   R   R   G   L   I   A   G   A   I   R   L   R


 R   P   T   S   P   V   S   R   E   C   N   S   S   T   D   S   C   D   S   G   P   S   N   T   P   P   E   I   H   P   V   V   P   L   C   P   I   K   P   V
CGCCCGACATCACCTGTGTCTAGAGAATGCAATAGTAGTACGGATAGCTGTGACTCCGGTCCTTCTTAACACACCTCCTGAGATACACCCGGTGGTCCCGCTGTGCCCCATTAAACCAGTT
     1330        1340        1350        1360        1370        1380        1390        1400        1410        1420        1430        1440
GCGGGCTGTAGTGGACACAGATCTCTTACGTTATCATCATGCCTATCGACACTGAGGCCAGGAAGATTGTGTGGAGGACTCTATGTGGGCCACCAGGGCGACACGGGGTAATTTGGTCA
 G   V   D   G   T   D   L   S   H   L   L   L   V   S   L   Q   S   E   P   G   E   L   V   G   G   S   I   C   G   T   T   G   S   H   G   M   L   G   T   A


 A   V   R   V   G   G   R   R   Q   A   V   E   C   I   E   D   L   L   N   E   P   G   Q   P   L   D   L   S   C   K   R   P   R   P   *   stop Ela 32K, 27K
GCCGTGAGAGTTGGTGGGCGTCGCCAGGCTGTGGAATGTATCGAGGACTTGCTTAACGAGCCTGGGCAACCTTTGGACTTGAGCTGTAAACGCCCCAGGCCATAAGGTGTAAACCTGTGA
     1450        1460        1470        1480        1490        1500        1510        1520        1530        1540        1550        1560
CGGCACTCTCAACCACCCGCAGCGGTCCGACACCTTACATAGCTCCTGAACGAATTGCTCGGACCCGTTGGAAACCTGAACTCGACATTTGCGGGGTCCGGTATTCCACATTTGGACACT
 T   L   T   P   P   R   R   W   A   T   S   H   I   S   S   K   S   L   S   G   P   C   G   K   S   K   L   Q   L   R   G   L   G   Y   P   T   F   R   H   N


                                                                   ┌ 3'-poly(A)                                                    'TATA' Elb
TTGCGTGTGTGGTTAACGCCTTTGTTTGCTGAATGAGTTGATGTAAGTTTAATAAAGGGTGAGATAATGTTTAACTTGCATGGCGTGTTAAATGGGGCGGGGCTTAAAGGGTATATAATG
     1570        1580        1590        1600        1610        1620        1630        1640        1650        1660        1670        1680
AACGCACACACCAATTGCGGGAAACAAACGACTTACTCAACTACATTCAAATTATTTCCCACTCTATTACAAATTGAACGTACCGCACAATTTACCCCGCCCCGAATTTCCCATATATTAC
 R   T   H   N   V   G   K   N   A   S   H   S   T   L   K   I   F   P   S   I   I   N   L   K   C   P   T   N   F   P   A   P   S   L   P   Y   I   I   R


        5' Elb RNAs ┐                start Elb 21K
                   ↓↓             M   E   A   W   E   C   L   E   D   F   S   A   V   R   N   L   L   E   Q   S   S   N   S   T   S   W   F   W   R
CGCCGTGGGCTAATCTTGGTTACATCTGACCTCATGGAGCCTTGGGAGTGTTTGGAAGATTTTTCTGCTGTGCGTAACTTGCTGGAACAGAGCTCTAACAGTACCTCTTGGTTTTGGAGG
     1690        1700        1710        1720        1730        1740        1750        1760        1770        1780        1790        1800
GCGGCACCCGATTAGAACCAATGTAGACTGGAGTACCTCCGAACCCTCACAAACCTTCTAAAAAGACGACACGCATTGAACGACCTTGTCTCGAGATTGTCATGGAGAACCAAAACCTCC
 R   P   S   I   K   T   V   D   S   R   M
                                     start ORF 23K


 F   L   W   G   S   S   Q   A   K   L   V   C   R   I   K   E   D   Y   K   W   E   F   E   E   L   L   K   S   C   G   E   L   F   D   S   L   N   L   G   H
TTTCTGTGGGGCTCATCCCAGGCAAAGTTAGTCTGCAGAATTAAGGAGGATTACAAGTGGGAATTTGAAGAGCTTTTGAAATCCTGTGGTGAGCTGTTTGATTCTTTGAATCTGGGTCAC
     1810        1820        1830        1840        1850        1860        1870        1880        1890        1900        1910        1920
AAAGACACCCCGAGTAGGGTCCGTTTCAATCAGACGTCTTAATTCCTCCTAATGTTCACCCTTAAACTTCTCGAAAACTTTAGGACACCACTCGACAAACTAAGAAACTTAGACCCAGTG


 Q   A   L   F   Q   E   K   V   I   K   T   L   D   F   S   T   P   G   R   A   A   A   A   A   V   A   F   L   S   F   I   K   D   K   W   S   E   E   T   H   L
                                                                                                                   M   E   R   R   N   P   S   E
CAGGCCGCTTTTCCAAGAGAAGGTCATCAAGCATTTGGATTTTTCCACACCGGGGCGCGCTGCGGCTGCTGTTGCTTTTTTGAGTTTTATAAAGGATAAATGGAGCGAAGAAACCCATCTG
     1930        1940        1950        1960        1970        1980        1990        2000        2010        2020        2030        2040
GTCCGCGAAAAGGTTCTCTTCCAGTAGTTCTGAAACCTAAAAAGGTGGCCCCGCGCGACGCCGACGACGAAAAAACTCAAAATATTTCCTATTTACCTCGCTTCTTTGGGTAGAC


                                                                            start Elb 55K, 8.3K
 S   G   G   Y   L   L   D   F   L   A   M   H   L   W   R   A   V   V   R   H   K   N   R   L   L   L   L   S   S   V   R   P   A   I   I   P   T   E   G   Q
 R   G   V   P   A   G   F   S   G   H   A   S   V   E   S   G   C   E   T   Q   E   S   P   A   T   V   V   F   R   P   P   G   D   N   T   D   G   G   A   A
AGCGGGGGGTACCTGCTGGATTTTCTGGACTTCGCTATGCATCTGTGGAGGAGCGGTTGTGAGACACAAGAATCGCCTGCTACTGTTGTCTTCCGCCCCGGCGATAATACCGACGGAGGACGAG
     2050        2060        2070        2080        2090        2100        2110        2120        2130        2140        2150        2160
TCGCCCCCCATGGACGACCTAAAAGACCGGTACGTAGACACCTCTCGCCAACACTCTGTGTTCTTAGCGGACGATGACAACAGAAGGCAGGCGGGCCGCTATTATGGCTGCCTCCTCGTC


                                                                          stop Elb 21K          splice ┐
 Q   Q   Q   Q   E   E   A   R   R   R   R   Q   E   Q   S   P   W   N   P   R   A   G   L   D   P   R   E   *                         (8.3K, 21K)
 A   A   A   G   G   S   Q   A   A   A   A   G   A   E   P   M   E   P   E   S   R   P   G   P   S │ M   N   V   V   Q   V   A   E │ L   Y   P   E   L   R
CAGCAGCAGCAGGAGGAAGCCAGGCGGCGGGCGGCAGGAGCAGAGCCCATGGAACCCGAGAGCCGGCCTGGACCCTCGGGAATGAAGTTGTACAGGTGGCTGAACTGTATCCAGAACTGA
     2170        2180        2190        2200        2210        2220        2230        2240        2250        2260        2270        2280
GTCGTCGTCGTCCTCCTTCGGTCCGCCGCCGCCGCGTCCTCGTCTCGGGTACCTTGGGCTCTCGGCCGGACCTGGGAGCCCTTACTTACAACATGTCCACCGACTTGACATAGGTCTTGACT
```

```
      R  I  L  T  I  T  E  D  G  Q  G  L  K  G  V  K  R  E  R  G  A  C  E  A  T  E  E  A  R  N  L  A  F  S  L  M  T  R  H  R
GACGCATTTTGACAATTACAGAGGATGGGCAGGGGCTAAAGGGGGTAAAGAGGGAGCGGGGGGGCTTGTGAGGCTACAGAGGAGGCTAGGAATCTAGCTTTTAGCTTAATGACCAGACACC
      2290      2300      2310      2320      2330      2340      2350      2360      2370      2380      2390      2400
CTGCGTAAAACTGTTAATGTCTCCTACCCGTCCCCGATTTCCCCCATTTCTCCCTCGCCCCCCGAACACTCCGATGTCTCCTCCGATCCTTAGATCGAAAATCGAATTACTGGTCTGTGG


      P  E  C  I  T  F  Q  Q  I  K  D  N  C  A  N  E  L  D  L  L  A  Q  K  Y  S  I  E  Q  L  T  T  Y  W  L  Q  P  G  D  D  F
GTCCTGAGTGTATTACTTTTCAACAGATCAAGGATAATTGCGCTAATGAGCTTGATCTGCTGGCGCAGAAGTATTCCATAGAGCAGCTGACCACTTACTGGCTGCAGCCAGGGGATGATT
      2410      2420      2430      2440      2450      2460      2470      2480      2490      2500      2510      2520
CAGGACTCACATAATGAAAAGTTGTCTAGTTCCTATTAACGCGATTACTCGAACTAGACGACCGCGTCTTCATAAGGTATCTCGTCGACTGGTGAATGACCGACGTCGGTCCCCTACTAA


      E  E  A  I  R  V  Y  A  K  V  A  L  R  P  D  C  K  Y  K  I  S  K  L  V  N  I  R  N  C  C  Y  I  S  G  N  G  A  E  V  E
TTGAGGAGGCTATTAGGGTATATGCAAAGGTGGCACTTAGGCCAGATTGCAAGTACAAGATCAGCAAACTTGTAAATATCAGGAATTGTTGCTACATTTCTGGGAACGGGGCCGAGGTGG
      2530      2540      2550      2560      2570      2580      2590      2600      2610      2620      2630      2640
AACTCCTCCGATAATCCCATATACGTTTCCACCGTGAATCCGGTCTAACGTTCATGTTCTAGTCGTTTGAACATTTATAGTCCTTAACAACGATGTAAAGACCCTTGCCCGGCTCCACC


      I  D  T  E  D  R  V  A  F  R  C  S  M  I  N  M  W  P  G  V  L  G  M  D  G  V  V  I  M  N  V  R  F  T  G  P  N  F  S  G
AGATAGATACGGAGGATAGGGTGGCCTTTAGATGTAGCATGATAAATATGTGGCCGGGGGTGCTTGGCATGGACGGGGTGGTTATTATGAATGTAAGGTTTACTGGCCCCAATTTTAGCG
      2650      2660      2670      2680      2690      2700      2710      2720      2730      2740      2750      2760
TCTATCTATGCCTCCTATCCCACCGGAAATCTACATCGTACTATTTATACACCGGCCCCACGAACCGTACCTGCCCCACCAATAATACTTACATTCCAAATGACCGGGGTTAAAATCGC


      T  V  F  L  A  N  T  N  L  I  L  H  G  V  S  F  Y  G  F  N  N  T  C  V  E  A  W  T  D  V  R  V  R  G  C  A  F  Y  C  C
GTACGGTTTTCCTGGCCAATACCAACCTTATCCTACACGGTGTAAGCTTCTATGGGTTTAACATACCTGTGTGGAAGCCTGGACCGATGTAAGGGTTCGGGGCTGTGCCTTTTACTGCT
      2770      2780      2790      2800      2810      2820      2830      2840      2850      2860      2870      2880
CATGCCAAAAGGACCGGTTATGGTTGGAATAGGATGTGCCACATTCGAAGATACCCAAATTGTTATGGACACACCTTCGGACCTGGCTACATTCCCAAGCCCCGACACGGAAAATGACGA


      W  K  G  V  V  C  R  P  K  S  R  A  S  I  K  K  C  L  F  E  R  C  T  L  G  I  L  S  E  G  N  S  R  V  R  H  N  V  A  S
GCTGGAAGGGGGTGGTGTGTCGCCCCAAAAGCAGGGCTTCAATTAAGAAATGCCTCTTTGAAAGGTGTACCTTGGGTATCCTGTCTGAGGGTAACTCCAGGGTGCGCCACAATGTGGCCT
      2890      2900      2910      2920      2930      2940      2950      2960      2970      2980      2990      3000
CGACCTTCCCCCACCACACAGCGGGGTTTTCGTCCCGAAGTTAATTCTTTACGGAGAAACTTTCCACATTGGAACCCATAGGACAGACTCCCATTGAGGTCCCACGCGGTGTTACACCGGA


      D  C  G  C  F  M  L  V  K  S  V  A  V  I  K  H  N  M  V  C  G  N  C  E  D  R  A  S  Q  M  L  T  C  S  D  G  N  C  H  L
CCGACTGTGGTTGCTTCATGCTAGTGAAAAGCGTGGCTGTGATTAAGCATAACATGGTATGTGGCAACTGCGAGGACAGGGCCTCTCAGATGCTGACCTGCTCGGACGGCAACTGTCACC
      3010      3020      3030      3040      3050      3060      3070      3080      3090      3100      3110      3120
GGCTGACACCAACGAAGTACGATCACTTTTCGCACCGACACTAATTCGTATTGTACCATACACCGTTGACGCTCCTGTCCCGGAGAGTCTACGACTGGACGAGCCTGCCGTTGACAGTGG


      L  K  T  I  H  V  A  S  H  S  R  K  A  W  P  V  F  E  H  N  I  L  T  R  C  S  L  H  L  G  N  R  R  G  V  F  L  P  Y  Q
TGCTGAAGACCATTCACGTAGCCAGCCACTCTCGCAAGGCCTGGCCAGTGTTTGAGCATAACATACTGACCCGCTGTTCCTTGCATTTGGGTAACAGGAGGGGGGTGTTCCTACCTTACC
      3130      3140      3150      3160      3170      3180      3190      3200      3210      3220      3230      3240
ACGACTTCTGGTAAGTGCATCGGTCGGTGAGAGCGTTCCGGACCGGTCACAAACTCGTATTGTATGACTGGGCGACAAGGAACGTAAACCCATTGTCCTCCCCCCACAAGGATGGAATGG


      C  N  L  S  H  T  K  I  L  L  E  P  E  S  M  S  K  V  N  L  N  G  V  F  D  M  T  M  K  I  W  K  V  L  R  Y  D  E  T  R
AATGCAATTTGAGTCACACTAAGATATTGCTTGAGCCCGAGAGCATGTCCAAGGTGAACCTGAACGGGGTGTTTGACATGACCATGAAGATCTGGAAGGTGCTGAGGTACGATGAGACCC
      3250      3260      3270      3280      3290      3300      3310      3320      3330      3340      3350      3360
TTACGTTAAACTCAGTGTGATTCTATAACGAACTCGGGCTCTCGTACAGGTTCCACTTGGACTTGCCCCACAAACTGTACTGGTACTTCTAGACCTTCCACGACTCCATGCTACTCTGGG


      T  R  C  R  P  C  E  C  G  G  K  H  I  R  N  Q  P  V  M  L  D  V  T  E  E  L  R  P  D  H  L  V  L  A  C  T  R  A  E  F
GCACCAGGTGCAGACCCTGCGAGTGTGGCGGTAAACATATTAGGAACCAGCCTGTGATGCTGGATGTGACCGAGGAGCTGAGGCCCGATCACTTGGTGCTGGCCTGCACCCGCGCTGAGT
      3370      3380      3390      3400      3410      3420      3430      3440      3450      3460      3470      3480
CGTGGTCCACGTCTGGGACGCTCACACCGCCATTTGTATAATCCTTGGTCGGACACTACGACCTACACTGGCTCCTCGACTCCGGGCTAGTGAACCACGACCGGACGTGGGCGCGACTCA
```

```
                                       ┌─ splice E1b                                          5' RNA IX      splice E1b
                           stop │E1b 55K                    "TATA"  IX                            │ │            │Q  P
      G  S  S  D  E  D  T  D  *
TTGGCTCTAGCGATGAAGATACAGATTGAGGTACTGAAATGTGTGGGCGTGGCTTAAGGGTGGGAAAGAATATATAAGGTGGGGGTCTTATGTAGTTTTTGTATCTGTTTTGCAGCAGCCG
      3490      3500      3510      3520      3530      3540      3550      3560      3570      3580      3590      3600
AACCGAGATCGCTACTTCTATGTCTAACTCCATGACTTTACACACCCGCACCGAATTCCCACCCTTTCTTATATATTCCACCCCCAGAATACATCAAAACATAGACAAAACGTCGTCGGC
```

```
         stop E1b 8.3K
         start IX
P  P  P  *
      M  S  T  N  S  F  D  G  S  I  V  S  S  Y  L  T  T  R  M  P  P  W  A  G  V  R  Q  N  V  M  G  S  S  I  D  G  R  P
CCGCCGCCATGAGCACCAACTCGTTTGATGGAAGCATTGTGAGCTCATATTTGACAACGCGCATGCCCCCATGGGCCGGGGTGCGTCAGAATGTGATGGGCTCCAGCATTGATGGTCGCC
      3610      3620      3630      3640      3650      3660      3670      3680      3690      3700      3710      3720
GGCGGCGGTACTCGTGGTTGAGCAAACTACCTTCGTAACACTCGAGTATAAACTGTTGCGCGTACGGGGGTACCCGGCCCCACGCAGTCTTACACTACCCGAGGTCGTAACTACCAGCGG
```

```
      V  L  P  A  N  S  T  T  L  T  Y  E  T  V  S  G  T  P  L  E  T  A  A  S  A  A  A  S  A  A  A  A  T  A  R  G  I  V  T  D
CCGTCCTGCCCGCAAACTCTACTACCTTGACCTACGAGACCGTGTCTGGAACGCCGTTGGAGACTGCAGCCTCCGCCGCCGCTTCAGCCGCTGCAGCCACCGCCCGCGGGATTGTGACTG
      3730      3740      3750      3760      3770      3780      3790      3800      3810      3820      3830      3840
GGCAGGACGGGCGTTTGAGATGATGGAACTGGATGCTCTGGCACAGACGTTGCGGCAACCTCTGACGTCGGAGGCGGCGGCGAAGTCGGCGACGTCGGTGGCGGGCGCCCTAACACTGAC
```

```
      F  A  F  L  S  P  L  A  S  S  A  A  S  R  S  S  A  R  D  D  K  L  T  A  L  L  A  Q  L  D  S  L  T  R  E  L  N  V  V  S
ACTTTGCTTTCCTGAGCCCGCTTGCAAGCAGTGCAGCTTCCCGTTCATCCGCCCGCGATGACAAGTTGACGGCTCTTTTGGCACAATTGGATTCTTTGACCCGGGAACTTAATGTCGTTT
      3850      3860      3870      3880      3890      3900      3910      3920      3930      3940      3950      3960
TGAAACGAAAGGACTCGGGCGAACGTTCGTCACGTCGAAGGGCAAGTAGGCGGGCGCTACTGTTCAACTGCCGAGAAAACCGTGTTAACCTAAGAAACTGGGCCCTTGAATTACAGCAAA
```

```
                                                                 stop IX                              ┌─3' poly(A)
      Q  Q  L  L  D  L  R  Q  Q  V  S  A  L  K  A  S  S  P  P  N  A  V  *                              │
CTCAGCAGCTGTTGGATCTGCGCCAGCAGGTTTCTGCCCTGAAGGCTTCCTCCCCTCCCAATGCGGTTTAAAACATAAATAAAAAACCAGACTCTGTTTGGATTTGGATCAAGCAAGTGT
      3970      3980      3990      4000      4010      4020      4030      4040      4050      4060      4070      4080
GAGTCGTCGACAACCTAGACGCGGTCGTCCAAAGACGGGACTTCCGAAGGAGGGGAGGGTTACGCCAAATTTTGTATTTATTTTTGGTCTGAGACAAACCTAAACCTAGTTCGTTCACA
                                                           3' poly(A) IVa2, E2b ┘
```

```
CTTGCTGTCTTTATTTAGGGGTTTTGCGCGCGCGGTAGGCCCGGGACCAGCGGTCTCGGTCGTTGAGGGTCCTGTGTATTTTTTCCAGGACGTGGTAAAGGTGACTCTGGATGTTCAGAT
      4090      4100      4110      4120      4130      4140      4150      4160      4170      4180      4190      4200
GAACGACAGAAATAAATCCCCAAAACGCGCGCGCCATCCGGGCCCTGGTCGCCAGAGCCAGCAACTCCCAGGACACATAAAAAAAGGTCCTGCACCATTTCCACTGAGACCTACAAGTCTA
                                                                          *  K  P  T  K  R  A  R  Y  A  R  S  W  R  D  R  D  N  L  T  R  H  I  K  E  L  V  H  Y  L  H  S  Q  I  N  L  Y
                                                                     stop IVa2
```

Table 2.1 (Continued)

```
ACATGGGCATAAGCCCGTCTCTGGGGTGGAGGTAGCACCACTGCAGAGCTTCATGCTGCGGGGTGGTGTTGTAGATGATCCAGTCGTAGCAGGAGCGCTGGGCGTGGTGCCTAAAAATGT
    4210      4220      4230      4240      4250      4260      4270      4280      4290      4300      4310      4320
TGTACCCGTATTCGGGCAGAGACCCCACCTCCATCGTGGTGACGTCTCGAAGTACGACGCCCCACCACAACATCTACTAGGTCAGCATCGTCCTCGCGACCCGCACCACGGATTTTTACA
  M  P  M  L  G  D  R  P  H  L  Y  C  W  Q  L  A  E  H  Q  P  T  T  N  Y  I  I  W  D  Y  C  S  R  Q  A  H  H  R  F  I  D
```

```
CTTTCAGTAGCAAGCTGATTGCCAGGGGCAGGCCCTTGGTGTAAGTGTTTACAAAGCGGTTAAGCTGGGATGGGTGCATACGTGGGGATATGAGATGCATCTTGGACTGTATTTTTAGGT
    4330      4340      4350      4360      4370      4380      4390      4400      4410      4420      4430      4440
GAAAGTCATCGTTCGACTAACGGTCCCCGTCCGGGAACCACATTCACAAATGTTTCGCCAATTCGACCCTACCCACGTATGCACCCTACTACTCTACGTAGAACCTGACATAAAAATCCA
  K  L  L  L  S  I  A  L  P  L  G  K  T  Y  T  N  V  F  R  N  L  Q  S  P  H  M  R  P  S  I  L  H  M  K  S  Q  I  K  L  N
```

```
TGGCTATGTTCCCAGCCATATCCCTCCGGGGATTCATGTTGTGCAGAACCACCAGCACAGTGTATCCGGTGCACTTGGGAAATTTGTCATGTAGCTTAGAAGGAAATGCGTGGAAGAACT
    4450      4460      4470      4480      4490      4500      4510      4520      4530      4540      4550      4560
ACCGATACAAGGGTCGGTATAGGGAGGCCCCTAAGTACAACACGTCTTGGTGGTCGTGTCACATAGGCCACGTGAACCCTTTAAACAGTACATCGAATCTTCCTTTACGCACCTTCTTGA
  A  I  N  G  A  M  D  R  R  P  N  M  N  H  L  V  L  V  T  Y  G  T  C  K  P  F  K  D  H  L  K  S  P  F  A  H  F  F  K
```

```
TGGAGACGCCCTTGTGACCTCCAAGATTTTCCATGCATTCGTCCATAATGATGGCAATGGGCCCACGGGCGGCGGCCTGGGCGAAGATATTTCTGGGATCACTAACGTCATAGTTGTGTT
    4570      4580      4590      4600      4610      4620      4630      4640      4650      4660      4670      4680
ACCTCTGCGGGAACACTGGAGGTTCTAAAAGGTACGTAAGCAGGTATTACTACCGTTACCCGGGTGCCCGCCGGCCGGCGCCGCTTCTATAAAGACCCTAGTGATTGCAGTATCAACACAA
  S  V  G  K  H  G  G  L  N  E  M  C  E  D  M  I  I  A  I  P  G  R  A  A  A  Q  A  F  I  N  R  P  D  S  V  D  Y  N  H  E
```

```
CCAGGATGAGATCGTCATAGGCCATTTTTACAAAGCGCGGGCGGAGGGTGCCAGACTGCGGTATAATGGTTCCATCCGGCCCAGGGGCGTAGTTACCCTCACAGATTTGCATTTCCCACG
    4690      4700      4710      4720      4730      4740      4750      4760      4770      4780      4790      4800
GGTCCTACTCTAGCAGTATCCGGTAAAAATGTTTCGCGCCCGCCTCCCACGGTCTGACGCCCATATTACCAAGGTAGGCCGGGTCCCCGCATCAATGGGAGTGTCTAAACGTAAAGGGTGC
  L  I  L  D  D  Y  A  M  K  V  F  R  P  R  L  T  G  S  Q  P  I  I  T  G  D  P  G  P  A  Y  N  G  E  C  I  Q  M  E  W  A
```

```
CTTTGAGTTCAGATGGGGGGATCATGTCTACCTGCGGGGCGATGAAGAAAACGGTTTCCGGGGTAGGGGAGATCAGCTGGGAAGAAAGCAGGTTCCTGAGCAGCTGCGACTTACCGCAGC
    4810      4820      4830      4840      4850      4860      4870      4880      4890      4900      4910      4920
GAAACTCAAGTCTACCCCCCTAGTACAGATGGACGCCCCGCTACTTCTTTTGCCAAAGGCCCCATCCCCTCTAGTCGACCCTTCTTTCGTCCAAGGACTCGTCGACGCTGAATGGCGTCG
  K  L  E  S  P  P  I  M  D  V  Q  P  A  I  F  F  V  T  E  P  T  P  S  I  L  Q  S  S  L  L  N  R  L  L  Q  S  K  G  C  G
```

```
CGGTGGGCCCGTAAATCACACCTATTACCGGGTGCAACTGGTAGTTAAGAGAGCTGCAGCTGCCGTCATCCCTGAGCAGGGGGGCCACTTCGTTAAGCATGTCCCTGACTCGCATGTTTT
    4930      4940      4950      4960      4970      4980      4990      5000      5010      5020      5030      5040
GCCACCCGGGCATTTAGTGTGGATAATGGCCCACGTTGACCATCAATTCTCTCGACGTCGACGGCAGTAGGGACTCGTCCCCCCGGTGAAGCAATTCGTACAGGGACTGAGCGTACAAAA
  T  P  G  Y  I  V  G  I  V  P  H  L  Q  Y  N  L  S  S  C  S  G  D  D  R  L  L  P  A  V  E  N  L  M  D  R  V  R  M  N  E
```

```
CCCTGACCAAATCCGCCAGAAGGCGCTCGCCGCCCAGCGATAGCAGTTCTTGCAAGGAAGCAAAGTTTTTCAACGGTTTGAGACCGTCCGCCGTAGGCATGCTTTTGAGCGTTTGACCAA
    5050      5060      5070      5080      5090      5100      5110      5120      5130      5140      5150      5160
GGGACTGGTTTAGGCGGTCTTCCGCGAGCGGCGGGTCGCTATCGTCAAGAACGTTCCTTCGTTTCAAAAAGTTGCCAAACTCTGGCAGGCGGCATCCGTACGAAAACTCGCAAACTGGTT
  R  V  L  D  A  L  L  R  E  G  G  L  S  L  L  E  Q  L  S  A  F  N  K  L  P  K  L  G  D  A  T  P  M  S  K  L  T  Q  G  L
```

```
GCAGTTCCAGGCGGTCCCACAGCTCGGTCACCTGCTCTACGGCATCTCGATCCAGCATATCTCCTCGTTTCGCGGGTTGGGGCGGCTTTCGCTGTACGGCAGTAGTCGGTGCTCGTCCAG
    5170      5180      5190      5200      5210      5220      5230      5240      5250      5260      5270      5280
CGTCAAGGTCGCCAGGGTGTCGAGCCAGTGGACGAGATGCCGTAGAGCTAGGTCGTATAGAGGAGCAAAGCGCCCAACCCCGCCGAAAGCGACATGCCGTCATCAGCCACGAGCAGGTC
L  E  L  R  D  W  L  E  T  V  Q  E  V  A  D  R  D  L  M  D  G  R  K  A  P  Q  P  P  K  R  Q  V  A  T  T  P  A  R  G  S
         *  P  M  E  I  W  C  I  E  E  N  R  P  N  P  R  S  E  S  Y  P  L  L  R  H  E  D  L
               stop E2b 120K
```

```
ACGGGCCAGGGTCATGTCTTTCCACGGGCGCAGGGTCCTCGTCAGCGTAGTCTGGGTCACGGTGAAGGGGTGCGCTCCGGGCTGCGCGCTGGCCAGGGTGCGCTTGAGGCTGGTCCTGCT
    5290      5300      5310      5320      5330      5340      5350      5360      5370      5380      5390      5400
TGCCCGGTCCCAGTACAGAAAGGTGCCCGCGTCCCAGGAGCAGTCGCATCAGACCCAGTCGCACTTCCCCACGCGAGGCCCGACGCGCGACCGGTCCCACGCGAACTCCGACCAGGACGA
  R  A  L  T  M  D  K  W  P  R  L  T  R  T  L  T  T  Q  T  V  T  F  P  H  A  G  P  Q  A  S  A  L  T  R  K  L  S  T  R  S
P  G  P  D  H  R  E  V  P  A  P  D  E  D  A  Y  D  P  D  R  H  L  P  A  S  R  A  A  R  Q  G  P  H  A  Q  P  Q  D  Q  Q
                                                    *  P  S  P  T  R  E  P  S  R  A  P  W  P  A  S  S  A  P  G  A  P
                                                       stop ORF 12.2K
```

```
GGTGCTGAAGCGCTGCCGGTCTTCGCCCTGCCGCGTCGGCCAGGTAGCATTTGACCATGGTGTCATAGTCCAGCCCCTCCGCGGCGTGGCCCTTGGCGCGCAGCTTGCCCTTGGAGGAGGC
    5410      5420      5430      5440      5450      5460      5470      5480      5490      5500      5510      5520
CCACGACTTCGCGACGGCCAGAAGCGGGACGCGCAGCCGGTCCATCGTAAACTGGTACCACAGTATCAGGTCGGGGAGGCGCCGCACCGGGAACCGCGCGTCGAACGGGAACCTCCTCCG
  T  S  F  R  Q  R  D  E  G  Q  A  D  A  L  Y  C  K  V  M  T  D  Y  D  L  G  E  A  A  H  G  K  A  R  L  K  G  K  S  S  A
  H  Q  L  A  A  P  R  R
  A  S  A  S  G  T  K  A  R  R  T  P  W  T  A  N  S  W  P  T  M  T  W  G  R  R  P  T  A  R  P  A  C  S  A  R  P  P  P  A
                    splice IVa2 RNA
```

```
GCCGCACGAGGGGCAGTGCAGACTTTTGAGGGCGTAGAGCTTGGGCGCGAGAAATACCGATTCGGGGAGTAGGCATCCGCGCCGCAGGCCCCGCAGACGGTCTCGCATTCCACGAGCCA
    5530      5540      5550      5560      5570      5580      5590      5600      5610      5620      5630      5640
CGGCGTGCTCCCCGTCACGTCTGAAAACTCCCGCATCTCGAACCCGCGCTCTTTATGGCTAAGGCCCCTCATCCGTAGGCGCGGCGTCCGGGGCGTCTGCCAGACGTAAGGTGCTCGGT
  G  C  S  P  C  H  L  S  K  L  A  Y  L  K  P  A  L  F  V  S  E  P  S  Y  A  D  A  G  C  V  T  E  C  E  V  L  W
  A  R  P  A  T  C  V  K  S  P  T  S  S  P  R  S  F  Y  R  N  R  P  T  P  M  R  A  A  P  G  A  S  P  R  A  N  W  S  G  P
```

```
GGTGAGCTCTGGCCGTTCGGGGTCAAAAACCAGGTTTCCCCCATGCTTTTTGATGCGTTTCTTACCTCTGGTTTCCATGAGCCGGTGTCCACGCTCGGTGACGAAAAGGCTGTCCGTGTC
    5650      5660      5670      5680      5690      5700      5710      5720      5730      5740      5750      5760
CCACTCGAGACCGGCAAGCCCCAGTTTTTGGTCCAAAGGGGGTACGAAAAACTACGCAAAGAATGGAGACCAAAGGTACTCGGCCACAGGTGCGAGCCACTGCTTTTCCGACAGGCACAG
  T  L  E  P  R  E  P  D  F  V  L  N  G  G  H  K  K  I  R  K  K  G  R  T  E  M  L  R  H  G  R  E  T  V  F  L  S  D  T  D
  S  S  Q  G  N  P  T  L  F  W  T  E  G  M
                              start ORF 12.2K
                                 splice IVa2 RNA    start IVa2
```

```
CCCGTATACAGACTTGAGAGGCCTGTCCTCGAGCGGTGTTCCGCGGTCCTCCTCGTATAGAAACTCGGACCACTCTGAGACAAAGGCTCGCGTCCAGGCCAGCACGAAGGAGGCTAAGTG
    5770      5780      5790      5800      5810      5820      5830      5840      5850      5860      5870      5880
GGGCATATGTCTGAACTCTCCGGACAGGAGCTCGCCACAAGGCGCCAGGAGGAGCATATCTTTGAGCCTGGTGAGACTCTGTTTCCGAGCGCAGGTCCGGTCGTGCTTCCTCCGATTCAC
  G  Y  V  S  K  L  P  R  D  E  L  P  T  G  R  D  E  E  Y  L  F  E  S  W  E  S  V  F  A  R  T  W  A  L  V  F  S  A  L  H
                                                    5' IVa2 RNA
```

```
GGAGGGGTAGCGGTCGTTGTCCACTAGGGGGTCCACTCGCTCCAGGGTGTGAAGACATCATGTCGCCCCTCTTCGGCATCAAGGAAGGTGATTGGTTTGTAGGTGTAGGCCACGTGACCGGG
    5890      5900      5910      5920      5930      5940      5950      5960      5970      5980      5990      6000
CCTCCCCATCGCCAGCAACAGGTGATCCCCCAGGTGAGCGAGGTCCCACACTTCTGTGTACAGCGGGAGAAGCCGTAGTTCCTTCCACTAACCAAACATCCACATCCGGTGCACTGGCCC
  S  P  Y  R  D  N  D  V  L  P  D  V  R  E  L  T  H  L  C  M  D  G  E  E  A  D  L  F  T  I  P  K  Y  T  Y  A  V  H  G  P
```

```
                 "TATA" major late RNAs       ┌ 5' 1st late leader                              ┌splice
TGTTCCTGAAGGGGGGCTATAAAAGGGGGTGGGGGCGCGTTCGTCCTCACTCTCTTCCGCATCGCTGTCTGCGAGGGCCAGCTGTTGGGGTGAGTACTCCCTCTGAAAAGCGGGCATGAC
     6010      6020      6030      6040      6050      6060      6070      6080      6090      6100      6110      6120
ACAAGGACTTCCCCCCGATATTTTCCCCCACCCCCGCGCAAGCAGGAGTGAGAGAAGGCGTAGCGACAGACGCTCCCGGTCGACAACCCCACTCATGAGGGAGACTTTTCGCCCGTACTG
  T  G  S  P  P  S  Y  F  P  T  P  A  R  E  D  E  S  E  E  A  D  S  D  A  L  A  L  Q  Q  P  S  Y  E  R  Q  F  A  P  M  V

TTTCTGCGCTAAGATTGTCAGTTTCCAAAAACGAGGAGGATTTGATATTCACCTGGCCCGCGGTGATGCCTTTGAGGGTGGCCGCATCCATCTGGTCAGAAAAGACAATCTTTTTGTTGTC
     6130      6140      6150      6160      6170      6180      6190      6200      6210      6220      6230      6240
AAGACGCGATTCTAACAGTCAAAGGTTTTTGCTCCTCCTAAACTATAAGTGGACCGGGCGCCACTACGGAAACTCCCACCGGCGTAGGTAGACCAGTCTTTTCTGTTAGAAAAACAACAG
  E  A  S  L  N  D  T  E  L  F  S  S  S  K  I  N  V  Q  G  A  T  I  G  K  L  T  A  A  D  M  Q  D  S  F  V  I  K  K  N  D

                                         start ORF 11.7K
                                           M  E  R  R  V  W  F  L  S  R  S  A  R  S  L  A  A  M  F  S  C  T  Y  S
AAGCTTGGTGGCAAACGACCCGTAGAGGGCGTTGGACAGCAACTTGGCGATGGAGCGCAGGGTTTGGTTTTTGTCGCGATCGGCGCGCTCCTTGGCCGCGATGTTTAGCTGCACGTATTC
     6250      6260      6270      6280      6290      6300      6310      6320      6330      6340      6350      6360
TTCGAACCACCGTTTGCTGGGCATCTCCCGCAACCTGTCGTTGAACCGCTACCTCGCGTCCCAAACCAAAAACAGCGCTAGCCGCGCGAGGAACCGGCGCTACAAATCGACGTGCATAAG
  L  K  T  A  F  S  G  Y  L  A  N  S  L  L  K  A  I  S  R  L  T  Q  N  K  D  R  D  A  R  E  K  A  A  I  N  L  Q  V  Y  E

  R  A  T  H  R  H  S  G  K  T  V  V  R  S  S  G  T  R  C  T  R  Q  P  R  L  C  R  V  T  R  S  T  L  V  A  T  S  P  R  R
GCGCGCAACGCACCGCCATTCGGGAAAGACGGTGGTGCGCTCGTCGGGCACCAGGTGCACGCGCCAACCGCGGTTGTGCAGGGTGACAAGGTCAACGCTGGTGGCTACCTCTCCGCGTAG
     6370      6380      6390      6400      6410      6420      6430      6440      6450      6460      6470      6480
CGCGCGTTGCGTGGCGGTAAGCCCTTTCTGCCACCACGCGAGCAGCCCGTGGTCCACGTGCGCGGTTGGCGCCAACACGTCCCACTGTTCCAGTTGCGACCACCGATGGAGAGGCGCATC
  R  A  V  C  R  W  E  P  F  V  T  T  R  E  D  P  V  L  H  V  R  W  G  R  N  H  L  T  V  L  D  V  S  T  A  V  E  G  R  L
                                                                                          *  R  Q  H  S  G  R  R  T  P
                                                                                          stop ORF 12.8K

  R  S  L  V  Q  Q  R  R  P  P  L  R  E  Q  N  G  G  R  G  S  S  C  V  S  S  G  G  S  A  S  T  V  K  T  P  G  S  R  R  A
GCGCTCGTTGGTCCAGCAGAGGCGGCCGCCCTTGCGCGAGCAGAATGGCGATGGCGGTAGGGGGTCTAGCTGCGTCTCGTCCGGGGGTCTGCGTCCACGGTAAAGACCCCGGGCAGCAGGCGCGC
     6490      6500      6510      6520      6530      6540      6550      6560      6570      6580      6590      6600
CGCGAGCAACCAGGTCGTCTCCGCCGGCGGGAACGCGCTCGTCTTACCGCCATCCCCCAGATCGACGCAGAGCAGGCCCCCCAGACGCAGGTGCCATTTCTGGGGCCCGTCGTCCGCGCG
  R  E  N  T  W  C  L  G  K  R  S  C  F  P  P  L  P  D  L  Q  T  E  D  P  P  D  A  D  V  T  F  V  G  P  L  L  R  A
  A  R  Q  D  L  L  P  P  R  G  Q  A  L  L  I  A  T  P  P  R  A  A  D  R  G  P  P  R  R  G  R  Y  L  G  R  A  A  P  A  R

     stop ORF 11.7K
  S  K  *
GTCGAAGTAGTCTATCTTGCATCCTTGCAAGTCTAGCGCCTGCTGCCATGCGCGGGCGGCAAGCGCGCGCTCGTATGGGTTGAGTGGGGGACCCCATGGCATGGGGTGGGTGAGCGCGGA
     6610      6620      6630      6640      6650      6660      6670      6680      6690      6700      6710      6720
CAGCTTCATCAGATAGAACGTAGGAACGTTCAGATCGCGGACGACGGTACGCGCCCGCCGTTCGCGCGCGAGCATACCCAACTCACCCCCTGGGGTACCGTACCCCACCCACTCGCGCCT
  D  F  Y  D  I  K  C  G  Q  L  D  L  A  Q  Q  W  A  R  A  A  L  A  R  E  Y  P  N  L  P  P  G  W  P  M  P  H  T  L  A  S
  R  L  L  R  D  Q  M  R  A  L  R  A  G  A  A  M  R  P  R  C  A  R  A  R  I  P  Q  T  P  S  G  M  A  H  P  P  H  A  R  L

GGCGTACATGCCGCAAATGTCGTAAACGTAGAGGGGCTCTCTGAGTATTCCAAGATATGTAGGGTAGCATCTTCCACCGCGGATGCTGGCGCGCACGTAATCGTATAGTTCGTGCGAGGG
     6730      6740      6750      6760      6770      6780      6790      6800      6810      6820      6830      6840
CCGCATGTACGGCGTTTACAGCATTTGCATCTCCCCGAGAGACTCATAAGGTTCTATACATCCCATCGTAGAAGGTGGCGCCTACGACCGCGCGTGCATTAGCATATCAAGCACGCTCCC
  A  Y  M  G  C  I  D  Y  V  Y  L  P  E  R  L  I  G  L  Y  T  N  W  S  I  Y  P  L  *
  R  V  H  R  L  H  R  L  R  L  P  A  R  Q  T  N  W  S  I  Y  P  Y  C  R  G  G  R  I  S  A  R  V  Y  D  Y  L  E  H  S  P
                                                                 start ORF 12.8K

AGCGAGGAGGTCGGGACCGAGGTTGCTACGGGCGGGCTGCTCTGCTCGGAAGACTATCTGCCTGAAGATGGCATGTGAGTTGGATGATATGGTTGGACGCTGGAAGACGTTGAAGCTGGC
     6850      6860      6870      6880      6890      6900      6910      6920      6930      6940      6950      6960
TCGCTCCTCCAGCCCTGGCTCCAACGATGCCCGCCCGACGAGACGAGCCTTCTGATAGACGGACTTCTACCGTACACTCAACCTACTATACCAACCTGCGACCTTCTGCAACTTCGACCG
  A  L  L  D  P  G  L  N  S  R  A  P  Q  E  A  R  F  V  I  Q  R  F  I  A  H  S  N  S  S  I  T  P  R  Q  F  V  N  F  S  A

GTCTGTGAGACCTACCGCGTCACGCACGAAGGAGGCGTAGGAGTCGCGCAGCTTGTTGACCAGCTCGGCGGTGACCTGCACGTCTAGGGCGCAGTAGTCCAGGGTTTCCTTGATGATGTC
     6970      6980      6990      7000      7010      7020      7030      7040      7050      7060      7070      7080
CAGACACTCTGGATGGCGCAGTGCGTGCTTCCTCCGCATCCTCAGCGCGTCGAACAACTGGTCGAGCCGCCACTGGACGTGCAGATCCCGCGTCATCAGGTCCCAAAGGAACTACTACAG
  D  T  L  G  V  A  D  R  V  F  S  A  Y  S  D  R  L  K  N  V  L  E  A  T  V  Q  V  D  L  A  C  Y  D  L  T  E  K  I  I  D

                       splice ┬─5'               2nd major late leader                            3'┬─splice
ATACTTATCCTGTCCCTTTTTTTTCCACAGCTCGCGGTTGAGGACAAACTCTTCGCGGTCTTTCCAGTACTCTTGGATCGGAAACCCGTCGGCCTCCGAACGGTAAGAGCCTAGCATGTA
     7090      7100      7110      7120      7130      7140      7150      7160      7170      7180      7190      7200
TATGAATAGGACAGGGAAAAAAAAGGTGTCGAGCGCCAACTCCTGTTTGAGAAGCGCCAGAAAGGTCATGAGAACCTAGCCTTTGGGCAGCCGGAGGCTTGCCATTCTCGGATCGTACAT
  Y  K  D  Q  G  K  K  K  W  L  E  R  N  L  V  F  E  E  R  D  K  W  Y  E  Q  I  P  F  G  D  A  E  S  R  Y  S  G  L  V  Y

                                                                                                      start ORF 9.4K
                                                                                                        M  T  L  R
GAACTGGTTGACGGCCTGGTAGGCGCAGCATCCCTTTTCTACGGGTAGCGCGTATGCCTGCGCGGCCTTCCGGAGCGAGGTGTGGGTGAGCGCAAAGGTGTCCCTGACCATGACTTTGAG
     7210      7220      7230      7240      7250      7260      7270      7280      7290      7300      7310      7320
CTTGACCAACTGCCGGACCATCCGCGTCGTAGGGAAAAGATGCCCATCGCGCATACGGACGCGCCGGAAGGCCTCGCTCCACACCCACTCGCGTTTCCACAGGGACTGGTACTGAAACTC
  F  Q  N  V  A  Q  Y  A  C  C  G  K  E  V  P  L  A  Y  A  Q  A  A  K  R  L  S  T  H  T  L  A  F  T  D  R  V  M  V  K  L

  Y  W  Y  L  K  S  V  S  S  H  P  P  C  S  Q  S  K  K  K  S  V  R  F  L  E  R  G  F  G  R  A  K  V  T  S  L  K  S  I  F  P
GTACTGGTATTTGAAGTCAGTGTCGTCGCATCCGCCCTGCTCCCAGAGCAAAAAGTCCGTGCGCCGTTTTTGGAACGCGGATTTGGCAGGGCGAAGGTGACATCGTTGAAGAGTATCTTTCC
     7330      7340      7350      7360      7370      7380      7390      7400      7410      7420      7430      7440
CATGACCATAAACTTCAGTCACAGCAGCGTAGGCGGGACGAGGGTCTCGTTTTTCAGGCACGCGAAAAACCTTGCGCCTAAACCGTCCCGCTTCCACTGTAGCAACTTCTCATAGAAAGG
  Y  Q  Y  K  F  D  T  D  D  C  G  G  Q  E  W  L  L  F  D  T  R  K  K  S  R  P  N  P  L  A  F  T  V  D  N  F  L  I  K  G

                                                                                              ORF 9.4K stop
  A  R  G  I  K  L  R  V  M  R  K  G  P  G  T  S  E  R  L  L  I  T  W  A  A  S  T  I  S  S  K  P  L  M  L  W  P  T  M  *
CGCGCGGAGGCATAAAGTTGCGTGTGATGCGGAAGGGTCCCGGCACCTCGGAACGGTTGTTAATTACCTGGGCGGCGAGCACGATCTCGTCAAAGCCGTTGATGTTGTGGCCCACAATGTA
     7450      7460      7470      7480      7490      7500      7510      7520      7530      7540      7550      7560
GCGCGCTCCGTATTTCAACGCACACTACGCCTTCCCAGGGCCGTGGAGCCTTGCCAACAATTAATGGACCCGCCGCTCGTGCTAGAGCAGTTCGGCAACTACAACACCGGGTGTTACAT
  A  R  P  M  F  N  R  T  I  R  F  P  G  P  V  E  S  R  N  N  I  V  Q  A  A  L  V  I  E  D  F  G  N  I  H  G  V  I  Y

AAGTTCCAAGAAGCGCGGGATGCCCTTGATGGAAGGCAATTTTTTAAGTTCCTCGTAGGTGAGCTCTTCAGGGGAGCTGAGCCCGTGCTCTGAAAGGGCCCAGTCTGCAAGATGAGGGTT
     7570      7580      7590      7600      7610      7620      7630      7640      7650      7660      7670      7680
TTCAAGGTTCTTCCGCGCCCTACGGGAACTACCTTCCGTTAAAAAATTCAAGGAGCATCCACTCGAGAAGTCCCCTCGACTCGGGCACGAGACTTTCCCGGGTCAGACGTTCTACTCCCAA
  L  E  L  F  R  P  I  G  K  I  S  P  L  K  K  L  E  E  Y  T  L  E  E  P  S  S  L  G  H  E  S  L  A  W  D  A  L  H  P  N
```

Table 2.1 (Continued)

```
GGAAGCGACGAATGAGCTCCACAGGTCACGGGCCATTAGCATTTGCAGGTGGTCGCGAAAGGTCCTAAACTGGCGACCTATGGCCATTTTTTCTGGGGTGATGCAGTAGAAGGTAAGCGG
     7690      7700      7710      7720      7730      7740      7750      7760      7770      7780      7790      7800
CCTTCGCTGCTTACTCGAGGTGTCCAGTGCCCGGTAATCGTAAACGTCCACCAGCGCTTTCCAGGATTTGACCGCTGGATACCGGTAAAAAAGACCCCACTACGTCATCTTCCATTCGCC
  S   A   V   F   S   S   W   L   D   R   A   M   L   M   Q   L   H   D   R   F   T   R   F   Q   R   G   I   A   M   K   E   P   T   I   C   Y   F   T   L   P

GTCTTGTTCCCAGCGGTCCCATCCAAGGTTCGCGGCTAGGTCTCGCGCGGCAGTCACTAGAGGCTCATCTCCGCCGAACTTCATGACCAGCATGAAGGGCACGAGCTGCTTCCCAAAGGC
     7810      7820      7830      7840      7850      7860      7870      7880      7890      7900      7910      7920
CAGAACAAGGGTCGCCAGGGTAGGTTCCAAGCGCCGATCCAGAGCGCGCCGTCAGTGATCTCCGAGTAGAGGCGGCTTGAAGTACTGGTCGTACTTCCCGTGCTCGACGAAGGGTTTCCG
  D   Q   E   W   R   D   W   G   L   N   A   A   L   D   R   A   A   T   V   L   P   E   D   G   G   F   K   M   V   L   M   F   P   V   L   Q   K   G   F   A

                 splice ┌ 5' i-leader                    start agnoprotein 16.6K
                        │                                M   R   A   D   R   E   E   L   D   L   P   P   P   I   G   G   V   A   I   D   V
CCCCATCCAAGTATAGGTCTCTACATCGTAGGTGACAAAGAGACGCTCGGTGCGAGGATGCGAGCCGATCGGGAAGAACTGGATCTCCCGCCACCAATTGGAGGAGTGGCTATTGATGTG
     7930      7940      7950      7960      7970      7980      7990      8000      8010      8020      8030      8040
GGGGTAGGTTCATATCCAGAGATGTAGCATCCACTGTTTCTCTGCGAGCCACGCTCCTACGCTCGGCTAGCCCTTCTTGACCTAGAGGGCGGTGGTTAACCTCCTCACCGATAACTACAC
  G   M   W   T   Y   T   E   V   D   Y   T   V   F   L   R   E   T   R   P   H   S   G   I   P   F   F   Q   I   E   R   W   W   N   S   S   H   S   N   I   H

  V   K   V   E   V   P   A   T   G   R   T   L   V   L   A   F   V   K   T   C   A   V   L   A   A   V   H   G   L   Y   I   L   H   E   V   D   L   T   T   A
GTGAAAGTAGAAGTCCCTGCGACGGGCCGAACACTCGTGCTGGCTTTTGTAAAAACGTGCGCAGTACTGGCACGGTGCACGGGCTGTACATCCTGCACGAGGTTGACCTGACGACCGCCG
     8050      8060      8070      8080      8090      8100      8110      8120      8130      8140      8150      8160
CACTTTCATCTTCAGGGACGCTGCCCGGCTTGTGAGCACGACCGAAAACATTTTTGCACGCGTCATGACCGTCGCCACGTGCCCGACATGTAGGACGTGCTCCAACTGGACTGCTGGCGC
  H   F   Y   F   D   R   R   A   S   C   E   H   Q   S   K   Y   F   R   A   C   Y   Q   C   R   H   V   P   Q   V   D   Q   V   L   N   V   Q   R   G   R

  H   K   E   A   E   W   E   F   E   P   L   A   W   R   V   W   L   V   V   F   Y   F   G   C   L   S   L   T   V   W   L   L   E   G   S   Y   G   G   S   D
CACAAGGAAGCAGAGTGGGAATTTGAGCCCCTCGCCTGGCGGGTTTGGCTGGTGGTCTTCTACTTCGGCTGCTTGTCCTTGACCGTCTGGCTGCTCGAGGGGAGTTACGGTGGATCGGAC
     8170      8180      8190      8200      8210      8220      8230      8240      8250      8260      8270      8280
GTGTTCCTTCGTCTCACCCTTAAACTCGGGGAGCGGACCGCCCAAACCGACCACCAGAAGATGAAGCCGACGAACAGGAACTGGCAGACCGACGAGCTCCCCTCAATGCCACCTAGCCTG
  V   L   F   C   L   P   F   K   L   G   E   G   P   P   N   P   Q   H   D   E   V   E   A   A   Q   G   Q   G   D   P   Q   E   L   P   T   V   T   S   R   V

                                                                                            i-leader 3' ┌ splice
  H   H   A   A   R   A   Q   S   P   D   V   R   A   R   R   S   E   L   D   D   N   I   A   Q   M   G   A   V   H   G   L   E   L   P   R   R   Q │
CACCACGCCGCGCGAGCCCAAAGTCCAGATGTCCGCGCGCGGCGGTCGGAGCTTGATGACAACATCGCGCAGATGGGAGCTGTCCATGGTCTGGAGCTCCCGCGGCGTCAGGTCAGGCGG
     8290      8300      8310      8320      8330      8340      8350      8360      8370      8380      8390      8400
GTGGTGCGGCGCGCTCGGGTTTCAGGTCTACAGGCGCGCGCCGCCGCCAGCCTCGAACTACTGTTGTAGCGCGTCTACCCTCGACAGGTACCAGACCTCGAGGGCGCCGCAGTCCAGTCCGCC
  V   V   G   R   S   G   L   T   W   I   D   A   R   P   P   R   L   K   I   V   V   D   R   L   H   S   S   D   M
                                                                                      start E2b 120K

GAGCTCCTGCAGGTTTACCTCGCATAGACGGGTCAGGGCGCGGGCTAGATCCAGGTGATACCTAATTTCCAGGGGCTGGTTGGTGGCGGCGTCGATGGCTTGCAAGAGGCCGCATCCCCG
     8410      8420      8430      8440      8450      8460      8470      8480      8490      8500      8510      8520
CTCGAGGACGTCCAAATGGAGCGTATCTGCCCAGTCCCGCGCCGGATCTAGGTCCACTATGGATTAAAGGTCCCCGACCAACCACCGCCGCAGCTACCGAACGTTCTCCGGCGTAGGGGC
         *   N   G   P   A   P   Q   H   R   R   R   H   S   A   L   P   R   M   G   A
  stop ORF 20.8K

CGGCGCGACTACGGTACCGCGGCGGGCGGTGGGCCGCGGGGGTGTCCTTGGATGATGCATCTAAAAGCGGTGACGCGGGCGAGCCCCCGGAGGTAGGGGGGGCTCCGGACCCGCCGGG
     8530      8540      8550      8560      8570      8580      8590      8600      8610      8620      8630      8640
GCCGCGCTGATGCCATGGCGCGCCGCCCGCCACCCGGCGCCCCCACAGGAACCTACTACGTAGATTTCGCCACTGCGCCCGCTCGGGGGCGTCCATCCCCCCCGAGGCCTGGGCGGCCC
  A   R   S   R   Y   R   A   A   P   P   P   G   R   P   H   G   Q   I   I   C   R   F   A   T   V   R   A   L   G   R   L   Y   P   P   S   R   V   R   S
                                                               *   F   R   H   R   P   R   A   G   P   L   P   P   E   P   G   A   P   L
                                                              stop pTP 75K

AGAGGGGGCAGGGGCACGTCGGCGCCGCGCGCGGGCAGGAGCTGGTGCTGCGCGCGTAGGTTGCTGGCGAACGCGACGACGCGGCGGTTGATCTCCTGAATCTGGCGCCTCTGCGTGAAG
     8650      8660      8670      8680      8690      8700      8710      8720      8730      8740      8750      8760
TCTCCCCCGTCCCCGTGCAGCCGCGGCGCGCGCCCGTCCTCGACCACGACGCGCGCATCCAACGACCGCTTGCGCTGCTGCGCCGCCAACTAGAGGACTTAGACCGCGGAGACGCACTTC
  L   P   C   P   C   T   P   A   A   R   P   C   S   S   T   S   R   A   Y   T   A   P   S   R   S   A   A   T   S   R   R   F   R   A   G   R   R   S   S
  P   P   L   P   V   D   A   G   R   A   P   L   L   Q   H   Q   A   R   L   N   S   A   F   A   V   V   R   R   N   I   E   Q   I   R   R   Q   T   F   V

ACGACGGGCCCGGTGAGCTTGAGCCTGAAAGAGAGTTCGACAGAATCAATTTCGGTGTCGTTGACGGCGGCCTGGCGCAAAATCTCCTGCACGTCTCCTGAGTTGTCTTGATAGGCGATC
     8770      8780      8790      8800      8810      8820      8830      8840      8850      8860      8870      8880
TGCTGCCCGGGCCACTCGAACTCGGACTTTCTCTCAAGCTGTCTTAGTTAAAGCCACAGCAACTGCCGCCGGACCGCGTTTTAGAGGACGTGCAGAGGACTCAACAGAACTATCCGCTAG
  S   P   G   S   L   K   L   R   F   S   L   E   V   S   D   I   E   T   D   N   V   A   A   Q   R   L   I   E   Q   V   D   G   S   N   D   Q   Y   A   I   E
  V   P   G   T   L   K   L   R   F   S   L   E   V   S   D   I   E   T   D   N   V   A   A   Q   R   L   I   E   Q   V   D   G   S   N   D   Q   Y   A   I   E

TCGGCCATGAACTGCTCGATCTCTTCCTCCTGGAGATCTCCGCGTCCGGCTCGCTCCACGGTGGCGGCGAGGTCGTTGGAAATGCGGGCCATGAGCTGCGAGAAGGCGTTGAGGCCTCCC
     8890      8900      8910      8920      8930      8940      8950      8960      8970      8980      8990      9000
AGCCGGTACTTGACGAGCTAGAGAAGGAGGACCTCTAGAGGCGCAGGCCGAGCGAGGTGCCACCGCCGCTCCAGCAACCTTTACGCCCGGTACTCGACGCTCTTCCGCAACTCCGGAGGG
  P   W   S   S   S   R   K   R   S   I   E   A   D   P   E   S   W   P   P   S   T   T   P   F   A   P   W   S   S   R   S   P   T   S   A   E   R
  A   M   F   Q   E   I   E   E   E   Q   L   D   G   R   A   R   E   V   T   A   A   L   D   N   S   I   R   A   M   L   G   S   F   A   N   L   G   G   E

TCGTTCCAGACGCGGCTGTAGACCACGCCCCCTTCGGCATCGCGGGCGCGCATGACCACCTGCGCGAGATTGAGCTCCACGTGCCGGGCGAAGACGGCGTAGTTTCGCAGGCGCTGAAAG
     9010      9020      9030      9040      9050      9060      9070      9080      9090      9100      9110      9120
AGCAAGGTCTGCGCCGACATCTGGTGCGGGGGAAGCCGTAGCGCCCGCGCGTACTGGTGGACGCGCTCTAACTCGAGGTGCACGGCCCGCTTCTGCCGCATCAAAGCGTCCGCGACTTTC
  T   G   S   A   A   T   S   W   A   G   K   P   M
  N   W   V   R   S   Y   V   V   G   G   E   A   D   R   A   R   M   V   V   Q   A   L   N   L   E   V   H   R   A   F   V   A   Y   N   R   L   R   Q   F   L
                                                                                                    start ORF 20.8K

AGGTAGTTGAGGGTGGTGGCGGTGTGTTCTGCCACGAAGAAGTACATAACCCAGCGTCGCAACGTGGATTCGTTGATATCCCCCAAGGCCTCAAGGCGCTCCATGGCCTCGTAGAAGTCC
     9130      9140      9150      9160      9170      9180      9190      9200      9210      9220      9230      9240
TCCATCAACTCCCACCACCGCCACACAAGACGGTGCTTCTTCATGTATTGGGTCGCAGCGTTGCACCTAAGCAACTATAGGGGGTTCCGGAGTTCCGCGAGGTACCGGAGCATCTTCAGG
  Y   N   L   T   T   A   T   H   E   A   V   F   F   Y   M   V   W   R   R   L   T   S   E   N   I   D   G   L   A   E   L   R   E   M   A   E   Y   F   D   V

                                  start ORF 17.7K
                                  M   S   S   A   T   V   S   R   T   S   R   S   K   A   T   G   A   S   S
ACGGCGAAGTTGAAAAACTGGGAGTTGCGCGCCGACACGGTTAACTCCTCCTCCAGAAGACGGATGAGCTCGGCGACAGTGTCGCGCACCTCGCGCTCAAAGGCTACAGGGGCCTCTTCT
     9250      9260      9270      9280      9290      9300      9310      9320      9330      9340      9350      9360
TGCCGCTTCAACTTTTTGACCCTCAACGCGCGGCTGTGCCAATTGAGGAGGAGGTCTTCTTGCCTACTCGAGCCGCTGTCACAGCGCGTGGAGCGCGAGTTTCCGATGTCCCCGGAGAAGA
  A   F   N   F   F   Q   S   N   R   A   S   V   T   L   E   E   E   L   L   R   I   L   E   A   V   T   D   R   V   E   R   E   F   A   V   P   A   E   E   E
```

```
   S  S  S  I  S  S  S  I  R  A  S  P  S  S  S  S  G  G  G  G  G  G  G  G  T  R  R  R  R  R  R  T  G  R  R  S  T  K  R  S  I
TCTTCTTCAATCTCCTCTTCCATAAGGGCCTCCCCTTCTTCTTCTTCTGGCGGCGGTGGGGGAGGGGGGACACGGCGGCGACGACGGCGCACCGGGAGGCGGTCGACAAAGCGCTCGATC
   9370       9380       9390       9400       9410       9420       9430       9440       9450       9460       9470       9480
AGAAGAAGTTAGAGGAGAAGGTATTCCCGGAGGGGAAGAAGAAGAAGACCGCCGCCACCCCCTCCCCCCTGTGCCGCCGCTGCTGCCGCGTGGCCCTCCGCCAGCTGTTTCGCGAGCTAG
    E  E  I  E  E  E  M  L  A  E  G  E  E  E  E  P  P  P  P  P  P  P  P  V  R  R  R  R  R  R  V  P  L  R  D  V  F  R  E  I  M

   I  S  P  R  R  R  R  M  V  S  V  T  A  R  P  F  S  R  G  R  S  W  K  T  P  P  V  M  S  R  L  W  V  G  G  G  L  P  C  G
ATCTCCCCGCGGCGACGGCGCATGGTCTCGGTGACGGCGCGGCCGTTCTCGCGGGGGCGCAGTTGGAAGACGCCGCCGTCATGTCCCGGTTATGGGTTGGCGGGGGGCTGCCATGCGGC
   9490       9500       9510       9520       9530       9540       9550       9560       9570       9580       9590       9600
TAGAGGGGCGCCGCTGCCGCGTACCAGAGCCACTGCCGCGCCGCCAAGAGCGCCCCGCGTCAACCTTCTGCGGCGGGGCAGTACAGGGCCAATACCCAACCGCCCCCCGACGGTACGCCG
    E  G  R  R  R  R  R  M  T  E  T  V  A  R  G  N  E  R  P  R  L  Q  F  V  G  G  T  M  D  R  N  H  T  P  P  P  S  G  H  P  L

                                                   splice ┌─ 5' 3rd major late leader
                                                          │                  stop agnoprotein 16.6K
   R  D  T  A  L  T  M  H  L  N  N  C  C  V │G  T  P  P  P  R  D  L  S  E  S  A  S  T  G  S  E  N  L  S  R  K  A  S  N  Q
                                           │   V  L  R  R  R  G  T  *
AGGGATACGGCGCTAACGATGCATCTCAACAATTGTTGTGTAGGTACTCCGCCGCCGAGGGACCTGAGCGAGTCCGCATCGACCGGATCGGAAAACCTCTCGAGAAAGGCGTCTAACCAG
   9610       9620       9630       9640       9650       9660       9670       9680       9690       9700       9710       9720
TCCCTATGCCGCGATTGCTACGTAGAGTTGTTAACAACACATCCATGAGGCGGCGGCTCCCTGGACTCGCTCAGGCGTAGCTGGCCTAGCCTTTTGGAGAGCTCTTTCCGCAGATTGGTC
    S  V  A  S  V  I  C  R  L  L  Q  Q  T  P  V  G  G  G  L  S  R  L  S  D  A  D  V  P  D  S  F  R  E  L  F  A  D  L  W  D

3rd leader 3' ┌── splice                                                                         stop ORF 17.7K
   S  Q  S  Q │G  R  L  S  T  V  A  G  G  S  G  R  R  S  G  L  F  L  A  E  V  L  L  M  M  *
TCACAGTCGCAAGGTAGGCTGAGCACCGTGGCGGGCGGCAGCGGGCGGCGGCGGTCGGGGTTGTTTCTGGCGGAGGTGCTGCTGATGATGTAATTAAAGTAGGCGGTCTTGAGACGGCGATG
   9730       9740       9750       9760       9770       9780       9790       9800       9810       9820       9830       9840
AGTGTCAGCGTTCCATCCGACTCGTGGCACCGCCCGCCGTCGCCGCCGCCAGCCCCAACAAAGACCGCCTCCACGACGACTACTACATTAATTTCATCCGCCAGAACTCTGCCGCCTAC
    C  D  C  P  L  S  L  V  T  A  P  P  L  P  R  R  D  P  N  N  R  A  S  T  S  S  I  I  Y  N  F  Y  A  T  K  L  R  R  I  T

GTCGACAGAAGCACCATGTCCTTGGGTCCGGCCTGCTGAATGCGCAGGCGGTCGGCCATGCCCCAGGCTTCGTTTTGACATCGGCGCAGGTCTTTGTAGTAGTCTTGCATGAGCCTTTCT
   9850       9860       9870       9880       9890       9900       9910       9920       9930       9940       9950       9960
CAGCTGTCTTCGTGGTACAGGAACCCAGGCCGGACGACTTACGCGTCCGCCAGCCGGTACGGGGTCCGAAGCAAAACTGTAGCCGCGTCCAGAAACATCATCAGAACGTACTCGGAAAGA
    S  L  L  V  M  D  K  P  G  A  Q  Q  I  R  L  R  D  A  M  G  W  A  E  N  Q  C  R  R  L  D  K  Y  Y  D  Q  M  L  R  E  V

ACCGGCACTTCTTCTTCTCCTTCCTCTTGTCCTGCATCTCTTGCATCTATCGCTGCGGCGGCGGCGGAGTTTGGCGTAGGTGGCGCCCTCTTCCTCCCATGCGTGTGACCCCGAAGCCC
   9970       9980       9990       10000      10010      10020      10030      10040      10050      10060      10070      10080
TGGCCGTGAAGAAGAAGAGGAAGGAGAACAGGACGTAGAGAACGTAGATAGCGACGCCGCCGCCGCCTCAAACCGGCATCCACCGCGGGAGAAGGAGGGTACGCACACTGGGGCTTCGGG
    P  V  E  E  E  G  E  E  Q  G  A  D  R  A  D  I  A  A  A  A  A  S  N  P  R  L  H  R  G  R  G  G  M  R  T  V  G  F  G  R

CTCATCGGCTGAAGCAGGGCTAGGTCGGCGACAACGCGCTCGGCTAATATGGCCTGCTGCACCTGCGTGAGGGTAGACTGGAAGTCATCCATGTCCACAAAGCGGTGGTATGCGCCCGTG
   10090      10100      10110      10120      10130      10140      10150      10160      10170      10180      10190      10200
GAGTAGCCGACTCGTCCCGATCCAGCCGCTGTTGCGCGAGCCGATTATACCGGACGACGTGGACGCACTCCCATCTGACCTTCAGTAGGTACAGGTGTTTCGCCACCATACGCGGGCAC
    M  P  Q  L  L  A  L  D  A  V  V  R  E  A  L  I  A  Q  Q  V  Q  T  L  T  S  Q  F  D  D  M  D  V  F  R  H  Y  A  G  T  N

TTGATGGTGTAAGTGCAGTTGGCCATAACGGACCAGTTAACGGTCTGGTGACCCGGCTGCGAGAGCTCGGTGTACCTGAGACGCGAGTAAGCCCTCGAGTCAAATACGTAGTCGTTGCAA
   10210      10220      10230      10240      10250      10260      10270      10280      10290      10300      10310      10320
AACTACCACATTCACGTCAACCGGTATTGCCTGGTCAATTGCCAGACCACTGGGCCGACGCTCTCGAGCCACATGGACTCTGCGGCTCATTCGGGAGCTCAGTTTATGCATCAGCAACGTT
    I  T  Y  T  C  N  A  M  V  S  W  N  V  T  Q  H  G  P  Q  S  L  E  T  Y  R  L  R  S  Y  A  R  S  D  F  V  Y  D  N  C  T

                                                                                         ORF 14.4K start
                                                                                              M  I  S  V
GTCCGCACCAGGTACTGGTATCCCACCAAAAAGTGCGGCGGCGGCTGGCGGTAGAGGGGCCAGCGTAGGGTGGCCGGGGCTCCGGGGCGGAGATCTTCCAACATAAGGCGATGATATCCG
   10330      10340      10350      10360      10370      10380      10390      10400      10410      10420      10430      10440
CAGGCGTGGTCCATGACCATAGGGTGGTTTTTCACGCCGCCGCCGACCGCCATCTCCCCGGTCGCATCCCACCGGCCCCGAGGCCCCCGCTCTAGAAGGTTGTATTCCGCTACTATAGGC
    R  V  L  Y  Q  Y  G  V  L  F  H  P  P  P  Q  R  Y  L  P  W  R  L  T  A  P  A  G  P  A  L  D  E  L  M  L  R  H  Y  G  Y

   D  V  P  G  H  P  G  D  A  G  G  G  G  G  G  A  R  K  V  A  D  A  V  P  D  V  A  Q  R  Q  K  V  L  H  G  R  D  A  L  A
TAGATGTACCTGGACATCCAGGTGATGCCGGCGGCGGTGGTGGAGGCGGCGGGAAAGTCGGCAGCGCGGTTCCAGATGTTGCGCAGCGGCAAAAAGTGCTCCATGGTCGGGACGCTCTGG
   10450      10460      10470      10480      10490      10500      10510      10520      10530      10540      10550      10560
ATCTACATGGACCTGTAGGTCCACTACGGCCGCCGCCACCACCTCCGCGCGCCTTTCAGCGCCTGCGCCAAGGTCTACAACGCGTCGCCGTTTTCACGAGGTACCAGCCCTGCGAGACC
    I  Y  R  S  M  W  T  I  G  A  A  T  T  S  A  R  P  F  D  R  V  R  N  W  I  N  R  L  P  L  F  H  E  M
                                                                                            start pTP 75K?

                                                        ┌─ 5' VA1 RNA
   G  Q  A  R  A  I  V  D  A  L  D  R  A  K  G  E  P  V  S │G  H  S  S  V  V  W  W  I  N  S  Q  G  Y  H  G  G  R  P  G  F
CCGGTCAGGCGCGCGCAATCGTTGACGCTCTAGACCGTGCAAAAGGAGAGCCTGTAAGCGGGCACTCTTCCGTGGTCTGGTGGATAAATTCGCAAGGGTATCATGGCGGACGACCGGGGT
   10570      10580      10590      10600      10610      10620      10630      10640      10650      10660      10670      10680
GGCCAGTCCGCGCGCGTTAGCAACTGCGAGATCTGGCACGTTTTCCTCTCGGACATTCGCCCGTGAGAAGGCACCAGACCACCTATTTAAGCGTTCCCATAGTACCGCCTGCTGGCCCCA
    E  P  R  I  R  P  S  A  V  I  H  A  V  T  A  R  V  S  N  P  G  V  R  R  Q  T  T  G  E  C  S  F  W  L  P  S  R  R  G  G

                                                                                            3' VA1 RNA ┬┬┬┬
TCGAGCCCCGTATCCGGCCGTCCGCCGTGATCCATGCGGTTACCGCCGCGTGTCGAACCCAGGTGTGCGACGTCAGACAACGGGGGAGTGCTCCTTTTGGCTTCCTTCCAGGCGCGGCG
   10690      10700      10710      10720      10730      10740      10750      10760      10770      10780      10790      10800
AGCTCGGGGCATAGGCCGGCAGGCGGCACTAGGTACGCCAATGGCGGGCGCACAGCTTGGGTCCACACGCTGCAGTCGTTGCCCCTCACGAGGAAAACCGAAGGAAGGTCCGCGCCGC
    E  P  R  I  R  P  S  A  V  I  H  A  V  T  A  R  V  S  N  P  G  V  R  R  Q  T  T  G  E  C  S  F  W  L  P  S  R  R  G  G

                 stop ORF 14.4K                                        ┌─ 5' VA2 RNA
   C  C  A  S  F  F  G  H  W  P  R  A  A  *
GCTGCTGCGCTAGCTTTTTTGGCCACTGGCCGCGCGCAGCGTAAGCGGTTAGGCTGGAAAGCGAAAGCATTAAGTGGCTCGCTCCCTGTAGCCGGAGGGTTATTTTCCAAGGGTTGAGTC
   10810      10820      10830      10840      10850      10860      10870      10880      10890      10900      10910      10920
CGACGACGCGATCGAAAAAACCGGTGACCGGCGCGCGTCGCATTCGCCAATCCGACCTTTCGCTTTCGTAATTCACCGAGCGAGGGACATCGGCCTCCCAATAAAAGGTTCCCAACTCAG

                                                                                            3' VA2 RNA ┬┬┬┬
GCGGGACCCCCGGTTCGAGTCTCGGACCGGCCGGACTGCGGCGAACGGGGGTTTGCCTCCCCGTCATGCAAGACCCCGCTTGCAAATTCCTCCGGAAACAGGGACGAGCCCCTTTTTTGC
   10930      10940      10950      10960      10970      10980      10990      11000      11010      11020      11030      11040
CGCCCTGGGGGCCAAGCTCAGAGCCTGGCCGGCCTGACGCCGCTTGCCCCCAAACGGAGGGGCAGTACGTTCTGGGGCGAACGTTTAAGGAGGCCTTTGTCCCTGCTCGGGGAAAAACG

splice ┌── 5' main body L1 RNA
       │start L1 55,52K?
       │ M  H  P  V  L  R  Q  M  R  P  P  P  Q  Q  R  Q  E  Q  E  Q  R  Q  T  C  R  A  P  S  P  P  P  T  A  S  G  G  A
TTTTCCCAGATGCATCCGGTGCTGCGGCAGATGCGCCCCCTCCTCAGCAGCGGCAAGAGACAAGAGCAGCGGCAGACATGCAGGGCACCCTCCCCTCCTCCTACCGCGTCAGGAGGGGCG
   11050      11060      11070      11080      11090      11100      11110      11120      11130      11140      11150      11160
AAAAGGGTCTACGTAGGCCACGACGCCGTCTACGCGGGGGAGGAGTCGTCGCCGTTCTCGTTCTCGTCGTCCGTCTGTACGTCCCGTGGGAGGGGAGGAGGATGGCGCAGTCCTCCCCGC
```

Table 2.1 (Continued)

```
 T  S  A  V  D  A  A  A  D  G  D  Y  E  P  P  P  R  R  R  A  R  H  Y  L  D  L  E  E  G  E  G  L  A  R  L  G  A  P  S  P  E
ACATCCGCGGTTGACGCGGCAGCAGATGGTGATTACGAACCCCCGCGGCGCCGGGCCCGGCACTACCTGGACTTGGAGGAGGGCGAGGGCCTGGCGCGGCTAGGAGCGCCCTCTCCTGAG
   11170     11180     11190     11200     11210     11220     11230     11240     11250     11260     11270     11280
TGTAGGCGCCAACTGCGCCGTCGTCTACCACTAATGCTTGGGGGCGCCGCGGCCCGGGCCGTGATGGACCTGAACCTCCTCCCGCTCCCGGACCGCGCCGATCCTCGCGGGAGAGGACTC


 R  Y  P  R  V  Q  L  K  R  D  T  R  E  A  Y  V  P  R  Q  N  L  F  R  D  R  E  G  E  E  P  E  E  M  R  D  R  K  F  H  A
CGGTACCCAAGGGTGCAGCTGAAGCGTGATACGCGTGAGGCGTACGTGCCGCGGCAGAACCTGTTTCGCGACCGCGAGGGAGAGGAGCCCGAGGAGATGCGGGATCGAAAGTTCCACGCA
   11290     11300     11310     11320     11330     11340     11350     11360     11370     11380     11390     11400
GCCATGGGTTCCCACGTCGACTTCGCACTATGCGCACTCCGCATGCACGGCGCCGTCTTGGACAAAGCGCTGGCGCTCCCTCTCCTCGGGCTCCTCTACGCCCTAGCTTTCAAGGTGCGT


 G  R  E  L  R  H  G  L  N  R  E  R  L  L  R  E  E  D  F  E  P  D  A  R  T  G  I  S  P  A  R  A  H  V  A  A  A  D  L  V
GGGCGCGAGCTGCGGCATGGCCTGAATCGCGAGCGGTTGCTGCGCGAGGAGGACTTTGAGCCCGACGCGCGAACCGGGATTAGTCCCGCGCGCGCACACGTGGCCGGCCGCCGACCTGGTA
   11410     11420     11430     11440     11450     11460     11470     11480     11490     11500     11510     11520
CCCGCGCTCGACGCCGTACCGGACTTAGCGCTCGCCAACGACGCGCTCCTCCTGAAACTCGGGCTGCGCGCTTGGCCCTAATCAGGGCGCGCGCGTGTGCACCGCCGGCGGCTGGACCAT


                            HindIII
 T  A  Y  E  Q  T  V  N  Q  E  I  N  F  Q  K  S
ACCGCATACGAGCAGACGGTGAACCAGGAGATTAACTTTCAAAAAAGCTT
   11530     11540     11550     11560     11570
TGGCGTATGCTCGTCTGCCACTTGGTCCTCTAATTGAAAGTTTTTTCGAA
```

Table 2.2. Landmarks in the Ad5 DNA sequence 0–31.7%

Strand, nucleotide		Sequence	Identity
r	l		
	G103		last nucleotide of ITR
	T468	TATTTAA	"TATA" box E1A
	A499		cap sites E1A mRNAs
	A560	ATG	start E1A proteins
	G637		splice donor E1A 9S mRNA
	A917	ATCGAT	unique *Cla*I in Ad5 (d'HALLUIN et al. 1983)
	G974		splice donor E1A 12S mRNA
T1067		TAA	stop ORF 23K
	G1112		splice donor E1A 13S mRNA
	G1229		splice acceptor E1A mRNAs
	T1316	TGA	stop E1A 6K protein
	T1339	TCTAGA	*Xba*I 3.7%
	T1543	TAA	stop E1A 32K, 28K proteins
	G1572	GTTAAC	*Hpa*I 4.3%
	A1611	AATAAA	3'-poly(A) signal E1A mRNAs
	T1632		3'-poly(A) attachment site E1A mRNAs
	T1672	TATATAA	"TATA" box E1B
	A1702		cap sites E1B mRNAs
	A1704		
	A1714	ATG	start E1B 21K protein
A1715		ATG	start ORF 23K
	A2019	ATG	start E1B 55K, 8.3K proteins
	G2048	GGTACC	*Kpn*I 5.6%
	T2242	TGA	stop E1B 21K protein
	G2255		splice donor E1B mRNA
	A2804	AAGCTT	*Hind*III 7.7%
	A3328	AGATCT	*Bgl*II 9.1%
	T3507	TGA	stop E1B 55K, 8.3K proteins
	G3510		splice donor E1B mRNA
	T3551	TATATAA	"TATA" box protein IX mRNA
	G3580		cap sites protein IX mRNA
	A3582		

Table 2.2 (Continued)

Strand, nucleotide		Sequence	Identity
r	l		
	C3595		splice acceptor E1B mRNAs
	A3610	ATG	start protein IX
	T3611	TGA	stop E1B 8.3 K protein
	C3940	CCCGGG	*Sma*I 10.8%
	T4029	TAA	stop protein IX
	A4038	AATAAA	3′-poly(A) signal E1B, protein IX mRNAs
C4060			3′-poly(A) attachment site IVa2, E2B
	C4070		3′-poly(A) attachment site E1B, protein IX
T4093		TAA	stop protein IVa2
A4095		AATAAA	3′-poly(A) signal IVa2, E2B
	C4120	CCCGGG	*Sma*I 11.3%
T5199		TAG	stop E2B 120 K DNA polymerase
T5339		TAG	stop ORF 12.2 K
G5429			splice acceptor IVa2 mRNA
A5684		ATG	start ORF 12.2 K
G5706			splice donor IVa2 mRNA
A5718		ATG	start IVa2 protein
	C5788	CTCGAG	*Xho*I 15.9%
A5836			cap sites IVa2 mRNA
T5838			
	T6018	TATAAAA	"TATA" box major late mRNAs
	A6049		cap site major late RNAs (1st leader)
	G6089		splice donor 1st leader late RNAs
	A6241	AAGCTT	*Hin*dIII 17.1%
	A6290	ATG	start ORF 11.7 K
T6454		TGA	stop ORF 12.8 K
	T6608	TAG	stop ORF 11.7 K
A6790		ATG	start ORF 12.8 K
	C7111		splice acceptor 2nd major late leader
	G7182		splice donor 2nd major late leader
	A7310	ATG	start ORF 9.4 K
	T7559	TAA	stop ORF 9.4 K
	G7952		splice acceptor late i leader
	A7978	ATG	start agnoprotein 16.6 K
	C8254	CTCGAG	*Xho*I 22.6%
A8367		ATG	start E2B 120 K DNA polymerase
	G8391		splice donor late i leader
G8481			splice acceptor E2B mRNA
T8464		TAG	stop ORF 20.8 K
	G8533		*Kpn*I 23.4%
T8585		TAG	stop E2B pTB 75 K
	A8914	AGATCT	*Bgl*II 24.4%
A9040		ATG	start ORF 20.8 K
	G9280	GTTAAC	*Hpa*I 25.4%
	A9304	ATG	start ORF 17.7 K
	G9462	GTCGAC	*Sal*I 25.9%
	G9644		splice acceptor 3rd major late leader
	T9665	TGA	stop agnoprotein 16.6 K
	C9699	CTCGAG	*Xho*I 26.6%
	G9733		splice donor 3rd major late leader
	T9808	TAA	stop ORF 17.7 K

Table 2.2 (Continued)

Strand, nucleotide		Sequence	Identity
r	1		
	G9841	GTCGAC	*Sal*I 27.0%
	G10236	GTTAAC	*Hpa*I 28.0%
	C10294	CTCGAG	*Xho*I 28.2%
	A10411	AGATCT	*Bgl*II 28.5%
	A10431	ATG	start ORF 14.4K
A10544		ATG	start E2B pTP 75K
	T10589	TCTAGA	*Xba*I 29.0%
	G10620		5′-end VA1 RNA
	T10776		heterogeneous 3′-end VA1 RNA
	to		
	T10779		
	T10842	TAA	stop ORF 14.4K
	G10876		5′-end VA2 RNA
	T11033		heterogeneous 3′-end VA2 RNA
	to		
	T11038		
	A11050		splice acceptor L1 RNA
	A11050	ATG	start L1 55,52K protein?
	G11282	GGTACC	*Kpn*I 30.9% (not in Tooze 1981)
	A11565	AAGCTT	*Hin*dIII 31.7%

Fig. 2.1. Schematic representation of identified and unidentified reading frames and RNA coordinates in Ad5 DNA between coordinates 0.0 and 31.7. The map scale in the *center* of the figure reflects a conversion factor of 365 bp, which corresponds to 1% of the viral genome. Immediately *above* and *below* the scale, the locations of the various transcription units are indicated. The *continuous lines* above the transcription unit designations represent the segments of rightward transcripts present in mature RNAs; *interrupted carets* connecting the lines denote RNA splices. The coordinates of the RNA 5′ caps and 3′-poly(A) attachment sites and of splice donor and acceptor sites are also given in this part of the figure. On the *next line above* a number of RNA expression signals have been drawn: "TATA" boxes and 3′-poly(A) signals (AATAAA). Lines 1, 2, and 3 in the *upper part* of the figure represent the three possible frames in which the DNA 1-strand can be read. Tracts open for translation are indicated as *solid bars* for known genes and as *hatched bars* for unidentified translatable regions. The open frames are flanked by the symbols ? and ?, denoting initiation (ATG) and termination (TAA, TAG, or TGA) codons respectively. The *numbers* next to the codons are their coordinates, and the *numbers in larger type* refer to the predicted MW of the translation products. *Interrupted lines* connecting solid bars show how open frames are linked due to RNA splicing.

In the *bottom* half of the figure are the open frames in the DNA r-strand for known genes (*solid bars*) and potential (unidentified) polypeptides (*hatched bars*) and *below* them the schematic representation of the mRNAs transcribed from the 1-strand (as far as they have been determined at the nucleotide level)

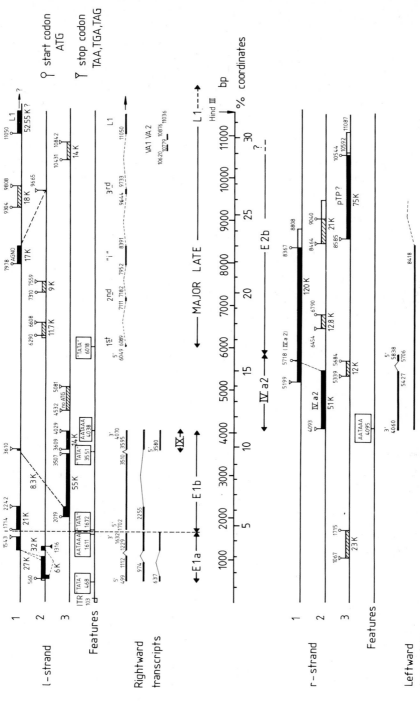

3 DNA Sequence of Human Ad2 (Subgroup C) Between Coordinates 43.4 and 44.9 (Gene for L2 Protein VII)

The sequence (Table 3.1) was determined by SUNG et al. (1983). It is given in double-stranded format with 120 nucleotides per line, the numbering starting at coordinate 43.37. Each number refers to the positions above and below its last zero. The features marked are the predicted initiation and termination codons and a potential splice acceptor site (Table 3.2) (G. AKUSJÄRVI, personal communication). Above the DNA sequence (sense strand) is given the predicted amino acid sequence (in one-letter code) for L2 protein VII. Apart from the gene for protein VII, a hitherto unidentified ORF was found in the opposite strand between TAA-667 and TAG-28; this frame does not contain an initiation triplet.

Table 3.1. Ad2 DNA sequence 43.4–44.9%

```
          potential splice acceptor L2 mRNA ┐     start L2 pro-VII
                                             M   S   I   L   I   S   P   S   N   N   T   G   W   G   L   R   F   P   S   K   M   F   G
CCTGGGCATAGTCTCGCCGCGCGTCCTATCGAGCCTCACTTTTTGAGCAAACATGTCCATCCTTATATCGCCCAGCAATAACACAGGCTGGGGTCTGCGCTTCCCAAGCAAGATGTTTGG
    10        20        30        40        50        60        70        80        90       100       110       120
GGACCCGTATCAGAGCGGCGCGCAGGATAGCTCGGAGTGAAAAACTCGTTTGTACAGGTAGGAATATAGCGGGTCGTTATTGTGTCCGACCCCAGACGCGAAGGGTTCGTTCTACAAACG


     ┌N terminus protein VII
 G   A   K   K   R   S   D   Q   H   P   V   R   V   R   G   H   Y   R   A   P   W   G   A   H   K   R   G   R   T   G   R   T   T   V   D   D   A   I   D   A
CGGGGCAAAGAAGCGCTCCGACCAACACCCAGTGCGCGTGCGCGGGCACTACCGCGCCCCCTGGGGCGGCACAAACGCGGCCGCACTGGGCGCACCACCGTCGATGACGCCATTGACGC
    130       140       150       160       170       180       190       200       210       220       230       240
GCCCCGTTTCTTCGCGAGGCTGGTTGTGGGTCACGCGCACGCGCCCGTGATGGCGCGGGGGACCCCGCGCGTGTTTGCGCCGGCGTGACCCGCTGGTGGCAGCTACTGCGGTAACTGCG


 V   V   E   E   A   R   N   Y   T   P   T   P   P   P   V   S   T   V   D   A   A   I   Q   T   V   V   R   G   A   R   R   Y   A   K   M   K   R   R   R   R
GGTGGTGGAGGAGGCGCGCAACTACACGCCCCACGCCGCCCACCAGTGTCCACAGTGGACGCGGCCATTCAGACCGTGGTGCGCGGAGCCCGGCGTTATGCTAAAATGAAGAGACGGCGGAG
    250       260       270       280       290       300       310       320       330       340       350       360
CCACCACCTCCTCCGCGCGTTGATGTGCGGGTGCGGCGGTGGTCACAGGTGTCACCTGCGCCGGTAAGTCTGGCACCACGCGCCTCGGGCCGCAATACGATTTTACTTCTCTGCCGCCTC


 R   V   A   R   R   H   R   R   P   G   T   A   A   Q   R   A   A   A   A   L   L   N   R   A   R   R   T   G   R   R   A   A   M   R   A   A   R   R   L   A
GCGCGTAGCACGTCGCCACCGCCGCCCCGGCACTGCCGCCCAACGCGCGGCGGCGGCCCTGCTTAACCGCGCACGTCGCACCGGCCGACGGGCGGCCATGCGGGCCGCTCGAAGGCTGGC
    370       380       390       400       410       420       430       440       450       460       470       480
CGCGCATCGTGCAGCGGTGGCGGCGGGGCCGTGACGGCGGGTTGCGCGCCGCCGCCGGGACGAATTGGCGCGTGCAGCGTGGCCGGCTGCCCGCCGGTACGCCCGGCGAGCTTCCGACCG


 A   G   I   V   T   V   P   P   R   S   R   R   R   A   A   A   A   A   A   A   A   A   I   S   A   M   T   Q   G   R   R   G   N   V   Y   W   V   R   D   S   V
CGCGGGTATTGTCACTGTGCCCCCCCAGGTCCAGGCGACGAGCGGCCGCCGCAGCAGCCGCGGCCATTAGTGCTATGACTCAGGGTCGCAGGGGCAACGTGTACTGGGTGCGCGACTCGGT
    490       500       510       520       530       540       550       560       570       580       590       600
GCGCCCATAACAGTGACACGGGGGGTCCAGGTCCGCTGCTCGCCGGCGGCGTCGTCGGCGCCGGTAATCACGATACTGAGTCCCAGCGTCCCGTTGCACATGACCCACGCGCTGAGCCA


                                                   stop L2 protein VII
 S   G   L   R   V   P   V   R   T   R   P   P   R   N   *
TAGCGGCCTGCGCGTGCCCGTGCGCACCCGCCCCCCGCGCAACTAGATTGCAAGAAAAAACTACTTAGACTC
    610       620       630       640       650       660       670
ATCGCCGGACGCGCACGGGCACGCGTGGGCGGGGGGCGCGTTGATCTAACGTTCTTTTTTGATGAATCTGAG
```

One-letter code for amin acids: A, ala; C, cys; D, asp; E, glu; F, phe; G, gly; H, his; I, ile; K, lys; L, leu; M, met; N, asn; P, pro; Q, gln; R, arg; S, ser; T, thr; V, val; W, trp; Y, tyr

Table 3.2. Landmarks in the Ad2 DNA sequence 43–45%

Strand nucleotide		Sequence	Identity
r	1		
T28		TAG	stop ORF in r-strand
	C49		potential splice acceptor L2 mRNA
	A53	ATG	start L2 protein VII precursor
	G125	GCA	codon for Ala: N-terminus of mature protein VII
	T644	TAG	stop L2 protein VII
T667		TAA	start ORF in r-strand (no ATG)

4 DNA Sequence of Human Ad2 (Subgroup C) Between Coordinates 48 and 66

The sequence (Table 4.1) was determined by AKUSJÄRVI and PETTERSSON (1978a, b; 1979a), JÖRNVALL et al. (1981), AKUSJÄRVI and PERSSON (1981a), P. ALE-STRÖM et al. (personal communication), AKUSJÄRVI et al. (1981), and KRUIJER et al. (1982). It is given in double-stranded format with 120 nucleotides per line, the numbering starting at the *Hpa*II site at coordinate 48. Each number refers to the positions above and below its last zero. The following features are marked: predicted or potential initiation and termination codons, 3'-poly(A) signals and attachment sites, and splice points (Table 4.2). Above or below the DNA sequence (sense strand) is given the predicted amino acid sequence (in one-letter code; see Footnote to Table 4.1) for L3 pVI, L3 hexon, L3 23K, the E2A DNA-binding protein (DBP), and the N-terminus of the L4 100K protein. Apart from the genes for these proteins, two hitherto unidentified ORFs have been found in the sequence; the amino acid sequences of their hypothetical translation products are also given.

Table 4.1 see page 90–93

Table 4.1. Ad2 DNA sequence 48–66%

```
                                                             3'-poly(A) L2 mRNA ⌐
CCGGAATTGCATCCGTGGCCTTGCAGGCGCAGAGACACTGATTAAAAACAAGTTGCATGTGGAAAAATCAAAATAAAAAGTCTGGAGTCTCACGCTCGCTTGGTCCTGTAACTATTTTGT
      10        20        30        40        50        60        70        80        90       100       110       120
GGCCTTAACGTAGGCACCGGAACGTCCGCGTCTCTGTGACTAATTTTTGTTCAACGTACACCTTTTTAGTTTTATTTTTCAGACCTCAGAGTGCGAGCGAACCAGGACATTGATAAAACA
```

```
  ⌐splice L3 mRNA
  │start L3 pVI
  │M  E  D  I  N  F  A  S  L  A  P  R  H  G  S  R  P  F  M  G  N  W  Q  D  I  G  T  S  N  M  S  G  G  A  F  S  W  G  S
AGAATGGAAGACATCAACTTTGCGTCTCTGGCCCCGCGACACGGCTCGCGCCCGTTCATGGGAAACTGGCAAGATATCGGCACCAGCAATATGAGCGGTGGCGCCTTCAGCTGGGGCTCG
     130       140       150       160       170       180       190       200       210       220       230       240
TCTTACCTTCTGTAGTTGAAACGCAGAGACCGGGGCGCTGTGCCGAGCGCGGGCAAGTACCCTTTGACGTTCTATAGCCGTGGTCGTTATACTCGCCACCGCGGAAGTCGACCCCGAGC
```

```
  L  W  S  G  I  K  N  F  G  S  T  I  K  N  Y  G  S  K  A  W  N  S  S  T  G  Q  M  L  R  D  K  L  K  E  Q  N  F  Q  Q  K
CTGTGGAGCGGCATTAAAAATTTCGGTTCCACCATTAAGAACTATGGCAGCAAGGCCTGGAACAGCAGCACAGGCCAGATGCTGAGGGACAAGTTGAAAGAGCAAAATTTCCAACAAAAG
     250       260       270       280       290       300       310       320       330       340       350       360
GACACCTCGCCGTAATTTTTAAAGCCAAGGTGGTAATTCTTGATACCGTCGTTCCGGACCTTGTCGTCGTATCCGGTCTACGACTCCCTGTTCAACTTTCTCGTTTTAAAGGTTGTTTTC
```

```
  V  V  D  G  L  A  S  G  I  S  G  V  V  D  L  A  N  Q  A  V  Q  N  K  I  N  S  K  L  D  P  R  P  P  V  E  E  P  P  P  A
GTGGTAGATGGCCTGGCCTCTGGCATTAGCGGGGTGGTGGACCTGGCCAACCAGGCAGTGCAAAATAAGATTAACAGTAAGCTTGATCCCCGCCCTCCCGTAGAGGAGGCCTCCACCGGCC
     370       380       390       400       410       420       430       440       450       460       470       480
CACCATCTACCGGACCGGAGACCGTAATCGCCCCACCACCTGGACCGGTTGGTCCGTCACGTTTTATTCTAATTGTCATTCGAACTAGGGCGGGAGGGCATCTCCTCGGAGGTGGCCGG
```

```
  V  E  T  V  S  P  E  G  R  G  E  K  R  P  R  P  D  R  E  E  T  L  V  T  Q  I  D  E  P  P  S  Y  E  E  A  L  K  Q  G  L
GTGGAGACAGTGTCTCCAGAGGGGCGTGGCGAAAAGCGTCCGCGGCCCGACAGGGAAGAAACTCTGGTGACGCAAATAGATGAGCCTCCCTCGTACGAGGAGGCACTAAAGCAAGGCCTG
     490       500       510       520       530       540       550       560       570       580       590       600
CACCTCTGTCACAGAGGTCTCCCCGCACCGCTTTTCGCAGGCGCCGGGCTGTCCCTTCTTTGAGACCACTGCGTTTATCTACTCGGAGGGAGCATGCTCCTCCGTGATTTCGTTCCGGAC
```

```
  P  T  T  R  P  I  A  P  M  A  T  G  V  L  G  Q  H  T  P  V  T  L  D  L  P  P  P  A  D  T  Q  Q  K  P  V  L  P  G  P  S
CCCACCACCCGTCCCATCGCGCCCATGGCTACCGGAGTGCTGGGCCAGCACACACCTGTAACGCTGGACCTGCCTCCCCCGCTGACACCCAGCAGAAACCTGTGCTGCCACGGGCCGTCC
     610       620       630       640       650       660       670       680       690       700       710       720
GGGTGGTGGGCAGGGTAGCGCGGGTACCGATGGCCTCACGACCCGGTCGTGTGTGGACATTGCGACCTGGACGGAGGGGGGCGACTGTGGGTCGTCTTTGGACACGACGGTCCCGGCAGG
```

```
  A  V  V  V  T  R  P  S  R  A  S  L  R  R  A  A  S  G  P  R  S  M  R  P  V  A  S  G  N  W  Q  S  T  L  N  S  I  V  G  L
GCCGTTGTTGTAACCCGCCCTAGCCGCGCGTCCCTGCGCCGTGCCGCCAGCGGTCCGCGATCGATGCGGCCCGTAGCCAGTGGCAACTGGCAAAGCACACTGAACAGCATCGTGGGTCTG
     730       740       750       760       770       780       790       800       810       820       830       840
CGGCAACAACATTGGGCGGGATCGGCGCGCAGGGACGCGGCACGGCGGTCGCCAGCGCGCTAGCTACGCCGGGCATCGGTCACCGTTGACCGTTTCGTGTGACTTGTCGTAGCACCCAGAC
```

```
  G  V  Q  S  L  K  R  R  R  C  F  *          stop L3 pVI                    splice L3 hexon mRNA ⌐
GGGGTGCAATCCCTGAAGCGCCGACGATGCTTCTAAATAGCTAACGTGTCGTATGTGTCATGTATGCGTCCATGTCGCCGCCAGAGGAGCTGCTGAGCCGCCGTGCGCCCGCTTTCCAAG
     850       860       870       880       890       900       910       920       930       940       950       960
CCCCACGTTAGGGACTTCGCGGCTGCTACGAAGATTTATCGATTGCACAGCATACACAGTACATACGCAGGTACAGCGGCGGTCTCCTCGACGACTCGGCGGCACGCGGGCGAAAGGTTC
```

```
start L3 hexon
  M  A  T  P  S  M  M  P  Q  W  S  Y  M  H  I  S  G  Q  D  A  S  E  Y  L  S  P  G  L  V  Q  F  A  R  A  T  E  T  Y  F  S
ATGGCTACCCCTTCGATGATGCCGCAGTGGTCTTACATGCACATCTCGGGCCAGGACGCCTCGGAGTACCTGAGCCCCGGGCTGGTGCAGTTTGCCCGCGCCACCGAGACGTACTTCAGC
     970       980       990      1000      1010      1020      1030      1040      1050      1060      1070      1080
TACCGATGGGGAAGCTACTACGGCGTCACCAGAATGTACGTGTAGAGCCCGGTCCTGCGGAGCCTCATGGACTCGGGGCCCGACCACGTCAAACGGGCGCGGTGGCTCTGCATGAAGTCG
                                            *  M  C  M  E  P  W  S  A  E  S  Y  R  L  G  P  S  T  C  N  A  R  A  V  S  V  Y  K  L  R
                                            stop ORF 10.2K
```

```
  L  N  N  K  F  R  N  P  T  V  A  P  T  H  D  V  T  T  D  R  S  Q  R  L  T  L  R  F  I  P  V  D  R  E  D  T  A  Y  S  Y
CTGAATAACAAGTTTAGAAACCCCACGGTGGCCACCTACGCACGACGTAACCACAGACCGGTCCCAGCGTTTGACGCTGCCGGTTCATCCCTGTGGACCGCGAGGATACCGCGTACTCGTAC
    1090      1100      1110      1120      1130      1140      1150      1160      1170      1180      1190      1200
GACTTATTGTTCAAATCTTTGGGGTGCCACCGGTGGATGCGTGCTGCATTGGTGTCTGGCCAGGGTCGCAAACTGCGACGCCAAGTAGGGACACCTGGCGCTCCTATGGCGCATGAGCATG
  F  L  L  N  L  F  G  V  T  A  G  V  C  S  T  V  V  S  R  D  W  R  K  V  S  R  N  M  G  T  S  R  S  S  V  A  Y  E  Y  L
```

```
  K  A  R  F  T  L  A  V  G  D  N  R  V  L  D  M  A  S  T  Y  F  D  I  R  G  V  L  D  R  G  P  T  F  K  P  Y  S  G  T  A
AAAGCGCGGTTCACCCTGGCTGTGGGTGACAACCGTGTGCTTGATATGGCTTCCACGTACTTTGACATCCGCGGCGTGCTGGACAGGGGGCCTACTTTTAAGCCCTACTCCGGCACTGCC
    1210      1220      1230      1240      1250      1260      1270      1280      1290      1300      1310      1320
TTTCGCGCCAAGTGGGACCGACACCCACTGTTGGCACACGAACTATACCGAAGGTGCATGAAACTGTAGGCGCGCACGACCTGTCCCCCGGATGAAAATTCGGGATGAGGCCGTGACGG
  A  R  N  V  R  A  T  P  S  L  R  T  S  S  I  A  E  V  Y  K  S  M
                                            start ORF 10.2K
```

```
  Y  N  A  L  A  P  K  G  A  P  N  S  C  E  W  E  Q  T  E  D  S  G  R  A  V  A  E  D  E  E  E  E  D  E  D  E  E  E  E
TACAACGCTCTAGCTCCCAAGGGCGCTCCTAACTCCTGTGAGTGGGAACAAACCGAAGATAGCGGCCGGGCAGTTGCCGAGGATGAAGAAGAGGAAGATGAAGATGAAGAAGAGGAAGAA
    1330      1340      1350      1360      1370      1380      1390      1400      1410      1420      1430      1440
ATGTTGCGAGATCGAGGGTTCCCGCGAGGATTGAGGACACTCACCCTTGTTTGGCTTCTATCGCCGGCCCGTCAACGGCTCCTACTTCTTCTCCTTCTACTTCTACTTCTTCTCCTTCTT
```

```
  E  E  Q  N  A  R  D  Q  A  T  K  K  T  H  V  Y  A  Q  A  P  L  S  G  E  T  I  T  K  S  G  L  Q  I  G  S  D  N  A  E  T
GAAGAGCAAAACGCTCGAGATCAGGCTACTAAGAAAACACATGTCTATGCCCAGGCTCCTTTGTCTGGAGAAACAATTACAAAAAGCGGGCTACAAATAGGATCAGACAATGCAGAAACA
    1450      1460      1470      1480      1490      1500      1510      1520      1530      1540      1550      1560
CTTCTCGTTTTGCGAGCTCTAGTCCGATGATTCTTTTGTGTACAGATACGGGTCCGAGGAAACAGACCTCTTTGTTAATGTTTTTCGCCCGATGTTTATCCTAGTCTGTTACGTCTTTGT
```

```
  Q  A  K  P  V  Y  A  D  P  S  Y  Q  P  E  P  Q  I  G  E  S  Q  W  N  E  A  D  A  N  A  A  G  G  R  V  L  K  K  T  T  P
CAAGCTAAACCTGTATACGCAGATCCTTCCTATCAACCAGAACCTCAAATTGGCGAATCTCAGTGGAACGAAGCTGATGCTAATGCGGCCAGGAGGGAGAGTGCTTAAAAAAACAACTCCC
    1570      1580      1590      1600      1610      1620      1630      1640      1650      1660      1670      1680
GTTCGATTTGGACATATGCGTCTAGGAAGGATAGTTGGTCTTGGAGTTTAACCGCTTAGAGTCACCTTGCTTCGACTACGATTACGCCGGTCCTCCCTCTCACGAATTTTTTGTTGGAGGG
```

```
  M  K  P  C  Y  G  S  Y  A  R  P  T  N  P  F  G  G  Q  S  V  L  V  P  D  E  K  G  V  P  L  P  K  V  D  L  Q  F  F  S  N
ATGAAACCATGCTATGGATCTTATGCCAGGCCTACAAATCCTTTTGGTGGTCAATCCGTTCTGGTTCCGGATGAAAAAGGGGTGCCTCTTCCCAAAGGTTGACTTGCAATTCTTCTCAAAT
    1690      1700      1710      1720      1730      1740      1750      1760      1770      1780      1790      1800
TACTTTGGTACGATACCTAGAATACGGTCCGGATGTTTAGGAAAACCACCAGTTAGGCAAGACCAAGGCCTACTTTTTCCCCACGGAGAAGGTTTCCAACTGAACGTTAAGAAGAGTTTA
```

One-letter code for amino acids: A, ala; C, cys; D, asp; E, glu; F, phe; G, gly; H, his; I, ile;
K, lys; L, leu; M, met; N, asn; P, pro; Q, gln; R, arg; S, ser; T, thr; V, val; W, trp; Y, tyr

Table 4.1 (Continued)

```
 T  T  S  L  N  D  R  Q  G  N  A  T  K  P  K  V  V  L  Y  S  E  D  V  N  M  E  T  P  D  T  H  L  S  Y  K  P  G  K  G  D
ACTACCTCTTTGAACGACCGGCAAGGCAATGCTACTAAACCAAAAGTGGTTTTGTACAGTGAAGATGTCAATATGGAAACCCCAGACACACATCTGTCTTACAAACCTGGAAAAGGTGAT
     1810      1820      1830      1840      1850      1860      1870      1880      1890      1900      1910      1920
TGATGGAGAAACTTGCTGGCCGTTCCGTTACGATGATTTGGTTTTCACCAAAACATGTCACTTCTACAGTTATACCTTTGGGGTCTGTGTGTAGACAGAATGTTTGGACCTTTCCACTA

 E  N  S  K  A  M  L  G  Q  Q  S  M  P  N  R  P  N  Y  I  A  F  R  D  N  F  I  G  L  M  Y  Y  N  S  T  G  N  M  G  V  L
GAAAATTCTAAAGCTATGTTGGGTCAACAATCTATGCCAAACAGACCCAATTACATTGCTTTCAGGGACAATTTTATTGGCCTAATGTATTATAACAGCACTGGCAACATGGGTGTTCTT
     1930      1940      1950      1960      1970      1980      1990      2000      2010      2020      2030      2040
CTTTTAAGATTTCGATACAACCCAGTTGTTAGATACGGTTTGTCTGGGTTAATGTAACGAAAGTCCCTGTTAAAATAACCGGATTACATAATATTGTCGTGACCGTTGTACCCACAAGAA

 A  G  Q  A  S  Q  L  N  A  V  V  D  L  Q  D  R  N  T  E  L  S  Y  Q  L  L  L  D  S  I  G  D  R  T  R  Y  F  S  M  W  N
GCTGGTCAGGCATCGCAGCTAAATGCCGTGGTAGATTTGCAAGACAGAAACACAGAGCTGTCCTATCAACTCTTGCTTGATTCCATAGGTGATAGAACCAGATATTTTTCTATGTGGAAT
     2050      2060      2070      2080      2090      2100      2110      2120      2130      2140      2150      2160
CGACCAGTCCGTAGCGTCGATTTACGGCACCATCTAAACGTTCTGTCTTTGTGTCTCGACAGGATAGTTGAGAACGAACTAAGGTATCCACTATCTTGGTCTATAAAAAGATACACCTTA

 Q  A  V  D  S  Y  D  P  D  V  R  I  I  E  N  H  G  T  E  D  E  L  P  N  Y  C  F  P  L  G  G  I  G  V  T  D  T  Y  Q  A
CAGGCTGTAGACAGCTATGATCCAGATGTTAGAATCATTGAAAACCATGGAACTGAGGATGAATTGCCAAATTATTGTTTTCCTCTTGGGGGTATTGGGGTAACTGACACCTATCAAGCT
     2170      2180      2190      2200      2210      2220      2230      2240      2250      2260      2270      2280
GTCCGACATCTGTCGATACTAGGTCTACAATCTTAGTAACTTTTGGTACCTTGACTCCTACTTAACGGTTTAATAACAAAAGGAGAACCCCCATAACCCCATTGACTGTGGATAGTTCGA

 I  K  A  N  G  N  G  S  G  D  N  G  D  T  T  W  T  K  D  E  T  F  A  T  R  N  E  I  G  V  G  N  N  F  A  M  E  I  N  L
ATTAAGGCTAATGGCAATGGCTCAGGCGATAATGGAGATACTACATGGACAAAAGATGAAACTTTTGCAACACGTAATGAAATAGGAGTGGGTAACAACTTTGCCATGGAAATTAACCTA
     2290      2300      2310      2320      2330      2340      2350      2360      2370      2380      2390      2400
TAATTCCGATTACCGTTACCGAGTCCGCTATTACCTCTATGATGTACCTGTTTTCTACTTTGAAAACGTTGTGCATTACTTTATCCTCACCCATTGTTGAAACGGTACCTTTAATTGGAT

 N  A  N  L  W  R  N  F  L  Y  S  N  I  A  L  Y  L  P  D  K  L  K  Y  N  P  T  N  V  E  I  S  D  N  P  N  T  Y  D  Y  M
AATGCCAACCTATGGAGAAATTTCCTTTACTCCAATATTGCGCTGTACCTGCCAGACAAGCTAAAATACAACCCCACCAATGTGGAAATATCTGACAACCCCAACACCTACGACTACATG
     2410      2420      2430      2440      2450      2460      2470      2480      2490      2500      2510      2520
TTACGGTTGGATACCTCTTTAAAGGAAATGAGGTTATAACGCGACATGGACGGTCGTTCGATTTTATGTTGGGGTGGTTACACCTTTATAGACTGTTGGGGGTTGTGGATGCTGATGTAC

                                                                                    start ORF 15.7K
 N  K  R  V  V  A  P  G  L  V  D  C  Y  I  N  L  G  A  R  W  S  L  D  Y  M  D  N  V  N  P  F  N  H  H  R  N  A  G  L  R
AACAAGCGAGTGGTGGCTCCCGGGCTTGTAGACTGCTACATTAACCTTGGGGCGCGCTGGTCTCTGGACTACATGGACAACGTTAATCCCTTTAACCACCACCGCAATGCGGGCCTCCGT
     2530      2540      2550      2560      2570      2580      2590      2600      2610      2620      2630      2640
TTGTTCGCTCACCACCGAGGGCCCGAACATCTGACGATGTAATTGGAACCCCGCGCGACCAGAGACCTGATGTACCTGTTGCAATTAGGGAAATTGGTGGTGGCGTTACGCCCGGAGGCA
                                                                                                   M  R  A  S  V

 Y  R  S  M  L  L  G  N  G  R  Y  V  V  P  F  H  I  Q  V  P  Q  K  F  F  A  I  K  N  L  L  L  L  P  G  S  Y  T  Y  E  W  N
 I  A  P  C  C  W  E  T  A  A  T  C  P  F  T  F  R  C  P  K  S  F  L  P  L  K  T  S  S  S  C  Q  A  H  I  H  M  N  G  T
TATCGCTCCATGTTGTTGGGAAACGGCCGCTACGTGCCCTTTCACATTCAGGTGCCCCAAAAGTTTTTTGCCATTAAAAACCTCCTCCTCCTGCCAGGCTCATATACATATGAATGGAAC
     2650      2660      2670      2680      2690      2700      2710      2720      2730      2740      2750      2760
ATAGCGAGGTACAACAACCCTTTGCCGGCGATGCACGGGAAAGTGTAAGTCCACGGGGTTTTCAAAAAACGGTAATTTTTGGAGGAGGAGGACGGTCCGAGTATATGTATACTTACCTTG

 F  R  K  D  V  N  M  V  L  Q  S  S  L  G  N  D  L  R  V  D  G  A  S  I  K  F  D  S  I  C  L  Y  A  T  F  P  M  A  H
 S  G  R  M  L  T  W  F  C  R  A  L  W  E  T  I  L  E  L  T  G  L  A  L  S  L  T  A  F  V  F  T  P  P  S  S  P  W  P  T
TTCAGGAAGGATGTTAACATGGTTCTGCAGAGCTCTCTGGGAAACGATCTTAGAGTTGACGGGGCTAGCATTAAGTTTGACAGCATTTGTCTTTACGCCACCTTCTTCCCCATGGCCCAC
     2770      2780      2790      2800      2810      2820      2830      2840      2850      2860      2870      2880
AAGTCCTTCCTACAATTGTACCAAGACGTCTCGAGAGACCCTTTGCTAGAATCTCAACTGCCCGATCGTAATTCAAACTGTCGTAAACAGAAATGCGGTGGAAGAAGGGGTACCGGGTG

 N  T  A  S  T  L  E  A  M  L  R  N  D  T  N  D  Q  S  F  N  D  Y  L  S  A  A  N  M  L  Y  P  I  P  A  N  A  T  N  V  P
 T  R  P  P  R  W  K  L  C  S  E  M  T  P  T  T  S  P  L  M  T  T  F  P  P  P  T  C  Y  T  P  Y  P  P  T  P  P  T  C  P
AACACGGCCTCCACGCTGGAAGCTATGCTCAGAAATGACACCAACGACCAGTCCTTTAATGACTACCTTTCCGCCGCCAACATGCTATACCCCATACCCGCCAACGCCAACGATGCCC
     2890      2900      2910      2920      2930      2940      2950      2960      2970      2980      2990      3000
TTGTGCCGGAGGTGCGACCTTCGATCAGAGTCTTTACTGTGGTTGCTGGTCAGGAAATTACTGATGGAAAGGCGGCGGTTGTACGATATGGGGTATGGGCGGTTGCGGTGGTTGCACGGG

                                   stop ORF 15.7K
 I  S  I  P  S  R  N  W  A  A  F  R  G  W  A  F  T  R  L  K  T  K  E  T  P  S  L  G  S  G  Y  D  P  Y  Y  T  Y  S  G  S
 S  P  S  H  R  A  T  G  Q  H  F  A  V  G  P  S  H  A  *
ATCTCCATCCCATCGCGCAACTGGGCAGCATTTCGCGGTTGGGCCTTCACACGCTTGAAGACAAAGGAAACCCCTTCCCTGGGATCAGGCTACGACCCTTACTACACCTACTCTGGCTCC
     3010      3020      3030      3040      3050      3060      3070      3080      3090      3100      3110      3120
TAGAGGTAGGGTAGCGCGTTGACCCGTCGTAAAGCGCCAACCCGGAAGTGTGCGAACTTCTGTTTCCTTTGGGGAAGGGACCCTAGTCCGATGCTGGGAATGATGTGGATGAGACCGAGG

 I  P  Y  L  D  G  T  F  Y  L  N  H  T  F  K  K  V  A  I  T  F  D  S  S  V  S  W  P  G  N  D  R  L  L  T  P  K  E  F  E
ATACCATACCTTGACGGAACCTTCTATCTTAATCACACCTTTAAGAAGGTGGCCATTACCTTTGACTCTTCTGTTAGCTGGCCGGGCAACGACCGCCTGCTTACTCCCAAGGAGTTTGAG
     3130      3140      3150      3160      3170      3180      3190      3200      3210      3220      3230      3240
TATGGTATGGAACTGCCTTGGAAGATAGAATTAGTGTGGAAATTCTTCCACCGGTAATGGAAACTGAGAAGACAATCGACCGGCCCGTTGCTGGCGGACGAATGAGGGTTCCTCAAACTC

 I  K  R  S  V  D  G  E  G  Y  N  V  A  Q  C  N  M  T  K  D  W  F  L  V  Q  M  L  A  N  Y  N  I  G  Y  Q  G  F  Y  I  P
ATTAAACGCTCAGTTGACGGGGAGGGCTACAACGTAGCTCAGTGCAACATGACCAAGGACTGGTTCCTGGTGCAGATGTTGGCCAACTACAATATTGGCTACCAGGGCTTCTACATTCCA
     3250      3260      3270      3280      3290      3300      3310      3320      3330      3340      3350      3360
TAATTTGCGAGTCAACTGCCCCTCCCGATGTTGCATCGAGTCACGTTGTACTGGTTCCTGACCAAGGACCACGTCTACAACCGGTTGATGTTATAACCGATGGTCCCGAAGATGTAAGGT

                                                                                           A<----EcoRI---->B
 E  S  Y  K  D  R  M  Y  S  F  F  R  N  F  Q  P  M  S  R  Q  V  V  D  D  T  K  Y  K  E  Y  Q  Q  V  G  I  L  H  Q  H  N
GAAAGCTACAAGGACCGGCATGTACTCCGTTCTTCAGAAACTTCCAGCCCATGAGCCGGCAAGTGGTTGACGATACTAAATACAAGGAGTATCAGCAGGTTGGAATTCTTCACCAGCATAAC
     3370      3380      3390      3400      3410      3420      3430      3440      3450      3460      3470      3480
CTTTCGATGTTCCTGGCCGTACATGAGCAAGAAGTCTTTGAAGGTCGGGTACTCGGCCGTTCACCAACTGCTATGATTTATGTTCCTCATAGTCGTCCAACCTTAAGAAGTGGTCGTATTG

 N  S  G  F  V  G  Y  L  A  P  T  M  R  E  G  Q  A  Y  P  A  N  V  P  Y  P  L  I  G  K  T  A  V  D  S  I  T  Q  K  K  F
AACTCAGGATTCGTAGGCTACCTCGCTCCCACCATGCGCGAGGGACAGGCTTACCCGCCAACGTGCCCTACCCACTAATAGGCAAAACCGCGGTTGACAGTATTACCCAGAAAAAGTTT
     3490      3500      3510      3520      3530      3540      3550      3560      3570      3580      3590      3600
```

Table 4.1 (Continued)

```
  L   C   D   R   T   L   W   R   I   P   F   S   S   N   F   M   S   M   G   A   L   T   D   L   G   Q   N   L   L   Y   A   N   S   A   H   A   L   D   M   T
CTTTGCGATCGCACCCTTTGGCGCATCCCATTCTCCAGTAACTTTATGTCCATGGGCGCACTCACAGACCTGGGCCAAAACCTTCTCTACGCCAACTCCGCCCACGCGCTAGACATGACT
      3610      3620      3630      3640      3650      3660      3670      3680      3690      3700      3710      3720
GAAACGCTAGCGTGGGAAACCGCGTAGGGTAAGAGGTCATTGAAATACAGGTACCCGCGTGAGTGTCTGGACCCGGTTTTGGAAGAGATGCGGTTGAGGCGGGTGCGCGATCGTGTACTGA
```

```
                                                          ┌─ splice L3 23K mRNA
  F   E   V   D   P   M   D   E   P   T   L   L   Y   V   L   F   E │ V   F   D   V   V   R   V   H   Q   P   H   R   G   V   I   E   T   V   Y   L   R   T   P
TTTGAGGTGGATCCCATGGACGAGCCCACCCTTCTTTATGTTTTGTTTGAAGTCTTTGACGTGGTCCGTGTGCACCAGCCGCACCGCGGCGTCATCGAGACCGTGTACCTGCGCACGCCC
      3730      3740      3750      3760      3770      3780      3790      3800      3810      3820      3830      3840
AAACTCCACCTAGGGTACCTGCTCGGGTGGGAAGAAATACAAAACAAACTTCAGAAACTGCACCAGGCACACGTGGTCGGCGTGGCGCCGCAGTAGCTCTGGCACATGGACGCGTGCGGG
```

```
                   stop L3 hexon                                                start L3 23K
  F   S   A   G   N   A   T   T   *                                      M   G   S   S   E   Q   E   L   K   A   I   V   K   D   L   G   C   G   P   Y
TTCTCGGCCGGCAACGCCACAACATAAAAGAAGCAAGCAACATCAACAACAGCTGCCGCCATGGGCTCCAGTGAGCAGGAACTGAAAGCCATTGTCAAAGATCTTGGTTGTGGGCCATAT
      3850      3860      3870      3880      3890      3900      3910      3920      3930      3940      3950      3960
AAGAGCCGGCCGTTGCGGTGTTGTATTTTCTTCGTTCGTTGTAGTTGTTGTCGACGGCGGTACCCGAGGTCACTCGTCCTTGACTTTCGGTAACAGTTTCTAGAACCAACACCCGGTATA
```

```
  F   L   G   T   Y   D   K   R   F   P   G   F   V   S   P   H   K   L   A   C   A   I   V   N   T   A   G   R   E   T   G   G   V   H   W   M   A   F   A   W
TTTTTGGGCACCTATGACAAGCGCTTTCCAGGCTTTGTTTCTCCACACAAGCTCGCCTGCGCCATAGTCAATACGGCCGGTCGCGAGACTGGGGGCGTACACTGGATGGCCTTTGCCTGG
      3970      3980      3990      4000      4010      4020      4030      4040      4050      4060      4070      4080
AAAAACCCGTGGATACTGTTCGCGAAAGGTCCGAAACAAAGAGGTGTGTTCGAGCGGACGCGGTATCAGTTATGCCGGCCAGCGCTCTGACCCCCGCATGTGACCTACCGGAAACGGACC
```

```
  N   P   R   S   K   T   C   Y   L   F   E   P   F   G   F   S   D   Q   R   L   K   Q   V   V   Y   Q   F   E   Y   E   S   L   L   R   R   S   A   I   A   S   S
AACCCGCGCTCAAAAACATGCTACCTCTTTGAGCCCTTTGGCTTTTCTGACCAACGACTCAAGCAGGTTTACCAGTTTGAGTACGAGTCACTCCTGCGCCGTAGCGCCATTGCTTCTTCC
      4090      4100      4110      4120      4130      4140      4150      4160      4170      4180      4190      4200
TTGGGCGCGAGTTTTTGTACGATGGAGAAACTCGGGAAACCGAAAAGACTGGTTGCTGAGTTCGTCCAAATGGTCAAACTCATGCTCAGTGAGGACGCGGCATCGCGGTAACGAAGAAGG
```

```
  P   D   R   C   I   T   L   E   K   S   T   Q   S   V   Q   G   P   N   S   A   A   C   G   L   F   C   C   M   F   L   H   A   F   A   N   W   P   Q   T   P
CCCGACCGCTGTATAACGCTGGAAAAGTCCACCCAAAGCGTGCAGGGGCCCAACTCGGCCGCCTGTGGACTATTCTGCTGCATGTTTCTCCACGCCTTTGCCAACTGGCCCCAAACTCCC
      4210      4220      4230      4240      4250      4260      4270      4280      4290      4300      4310      4320
GGGCTGGCGACATATTGCGACCTTTTCAGGTGGGTTTCGCACGTCCCCGGGTTGAGCCGGCGGACACCTGATAAGACGACGTACAAAGAGGTGCGGAAACGGTTGACCGGGTTTGAGGG
```

```
  M   D   H   N   P   T   M   N   L   I   T   G   V   P   N   S   M   L   N   S   P   Q   V   Q   P   T   L   R   R   N   Q   E   Q   L   Y   S   F   L   E   R
ATGGATCACAACCCCACCATGAACCTTATTACCGGGGTACCCAACTCCATGCTTAACAGTCCCCAGGTACAGCCCACCCTGCGTCGCAACCAGGAACAGCTCTACACGCTTCCTGGACCGC
      4330      4340      4350      4360      4370      4380      4390      4400      4410      4420      4430      4440
TACCTAGTGTTGGGGTGGTACTTGGAATAATGGCCCCATGGGTTGAGGTACGAATTGTCAGGGGTCCATGTCGGGTGGGACGCAGCGTTGGTCCTTGTCGAGATGTCGAAGGACCTCGCG
```

```
                                                                        stop L3 23K
  H   S   P   Y   F   R   S   H   S   A   Q   I   R   S   A   T   S   F   C   H   L   K   N   M   *
CACTCGCCCTACTTCCGCAGCCACAGTGCGCAGATTAGGAGCGCCACTTCTTTTTGTCACTTGAAAAACATGTAAAAATAATGTACTAGGAGACACTTTCAATAAAGGCAAATGTTTTTA
      4450      4460      4470      4480      4490      4500      4510      4520      4530      4540      4550      4560
GTGAGCGGGATGAAGGCGTCGGTGTCACGCGTCTAATCCTCGCGGTGAAGAAAAACAGTGAACTTTTTGTACATTTTATTACATGATCCTCTGTGAAAGTTATTTCCGTTTACAAAAT
                                                               3'-poly(A) E2a mRNA ─┘
```

```
┌─ 3'-poly(A) L3 mRNA
TTTGTACACTCTCGGGTGATTATTTACCCCCCACCCTTGCCGTCTGCGCCGTTTAAAAATCAAAGGGGTTCTGCCGCGCATCGCTATGCGCCACTGGCAGGGACACGTTGCGATACTGGT
      4570      4580      4590      4600      4610      4620      4630      4640      4650      4660      4670      4680
AAACATGTGAGAGCCCACTAATAAATGGGGGGTGGGAACGGCAGACGCGGCAAATTTTTAGTTTCCCCAAGACGGCGCGTAGCGATACGCGGTGACCGTCCCTGTGCAACGCTATGACCA
                                                                                *   F   D   F   P   N   Q   R   A   D   S   H   A   V   P   L   S   V   N   R   Y   Q   H
                                        stop E2a DBP
```

```
GTTTAGTGCTCCACTTAAACTCAGGCACAACCATCCGCGGCAGCTCGGTGAAGTTTTCACTCCACAGGCTGCGCACCATCACCAACGCGTTTAGCAGGTCGGGCGCCGATATCTTGAAGT
      4690      4700      4710      4720      4730      4740      4750      4760      4770      4780      4790      4800
CAAATCACGAGGTGAATTTGAGTCCGTGTTGGTAGGCGCCGTCGAGCCACTTCAAAAGTGAGGTGTCCGACGCGTGGTAGTGGTTGCGCAAATCGTCCAGCCCGCGGCTATAGAACTTCA
  K   T   S   W   K   F   E   P   V   V   M   R   P   L   E   T   F   N   E   S   W   L   S   R   V   M   V   L   A   N   L   L   D   P   A   S   I   K   F   D
```

```
CGCAGTTGGGGCCTCCGCCCTGCGCGCGCGAGTTGCGATACACAGGGTTGCAGCACTGGAACACTATCAGCGCCGGGTGGTGCACGCTGGCACACGCTCTTGTCGGAGATCAGATCCG
      4810      4820      4830      4840      4850      4860      4870      4880      4890      4900      4910      4920
GCGTCAACCCCGGAGGCGGGACGCGCGCGCTCAACGCTATGTGTCCCAACGTCGTGACCTTGTGATAGTCGCGGCCCACCACGTGCGACCGGTCGTGCGAGAACAGCCTCTAGTCTAGGC
  C   N   P   G   G   Q   A   R   S   N   R   Y   V   P   N   C   C   Q   F   V   I   L   A   P   H   H   V   S   A   L   V   S   K   D   S   I   L   D   A
```

```
CGTCCAGGTCCTCCGCGTTGCTCAGGGCGAACGGAGTCAACTTTGGTAGCTGCCTTCCCAAAAAGGGTGCATGCCCAGGCTTTGAGTTGCACTCGCACCGTAGTGGCATCAGAAGGTGAC
      4930      4940      4950      4960      4970      4980      4990      5000      5010      5020      5030      5040
GCAGGTCCAGGAGGCGCAACGAGTCCCGCTTGCCTCAGTTGAAACCATCGACGGAAGGGTTTTTCCCACGTACGGGTCCGAAACTCAACGTGAGCGTGGCATCACCGTAGTCTTCCACTG
  D   L   D   E   A   N   S   L   A   F   P   T   L   K   P   L   Q   R   G   L   F   P   A   H   G   P   K   S   N   C   E   C   R   L   P   M   L   L   H   G
```

```
CGTGCCCGGTCTGGGCGTTAGGATACAGCGCCTGCATGAAAGCCTTGATCTGCTTAAAAGCCACCTGAGCCTTTGCGCCTTCAGAGAAGAACATGCCGCAAGACTTGCCGGAAAACTGAT
      5050      5060      5070      5080      5090      5100      5110      5120      5130      5140      5150      5160
GCACGGGCCAGACCCGCAATCCTATGTCGCGGACGTACTTTCGGAACTAGACGAATTTTCGGTGGACTCGGAAACGCGGAAGTCTCTTCTTGTACGGCGTTCTGAACGGCCTTTTGACTA
  H   G   T   Q   A   N   P   Y   L   A   Q   M   F   A   K   I   Q   K   F   A   V   Q   A   K   A   G   E   S   F   F   M   G   C   S   K   G   S   F   Q   N
```

```
TGGCCGGACAGGCCGCGTCATGCACGCAGCACCTTGCGTCGGTGTTGGAGATCTGCACCACATTTCGGCCCCCACCGGTTCTTCACGATCTTGGCCTTGCTAGACTGCTCCTTCAGCGCGC
      5170      5180      5190      5200      5210      5220      5230      5240      5250      5260      5270      5280
ACCGGCCTGTCCGGCGCAGTACGTGCGTCGTGGAACGCAGCCACAACCTCTAGACGTGGTGTAAAGCCGGGGTGGCCAAGAAGTGCTAGAACCGGAACGATCTGACGAGGAAGTCGCGCG
  A   P   C   A   A   D   H   V   C   C   R   A   D   T   N   S   I   Q   V   V   N   R   G   W   R   N   K   V   I   K   A   K   S   S   Q   E   K   L   A   R
```

```
GCTGCCCGTTTCGCTCGTCACATCCATTTCAATCACGTGCTCCTTATTTATCATAATGCTCCCGTGTAGACACTTAAGCTCGCCTTCGATCTCAGCGCAGCGGTGCAGCCACAACGCGC
      5290      5300      5310      5320      5330      5340      5350      5360      5370      5380      5390      5400
CGACGGGCAAAAGCGAGCAGTGTAGGTAAAGTTAGTGCACGAGGAATAAATAGTATTACGAGGGCACATCTGTGAATTCGAGCGGAAGCTAGAGTCGCGTCGCCACGTCGGTGTTGCGCG
  Q   G   N   E   S   T   V   D   M   E   I   V   H   E   K   N   I   M   I   S   G   H   L   C   K   L   E   G   E   I   E   A   C   R   H   L   W   L   A   C
```

```
AGCCCGTGGGCTCGTGGTGCTTGTAGGTTACCTCTGCAAACGACTGCAGGTACGCCTGCAGGAATCGCCCCATCATCGTCACAAAGGTCTTGTTGCTGGTGAAGGTCAGCTGCAACCCGC
      5410      5420      5430      5440      5450      5460      5470      5480      5490      5500      5510      5520
TCGGGCACCCGAGCACCACGAACATCCAATGGAGACGTTTGCTGACGTCCATGCGACGTCCTTAGCGGGGTAGTAGCAGTGTTTCCAGAACAACGACCACTTCCAGTCGACGTTGGGCG
  G   T   P   E   H   H   K   Y   T   V   E   A   F   S   Q   L   Y   A   Q   L   F   R   G   M   M   T   V   F   T   K   N   S   T   F   T   L   Q   L   G   R
```

Table 4.1 (Continued)

```
GGTGCTCCTCGTTTAGCCAGGTCTTGCATACGGCCGCCAGAGCTTCCACTTGGTCAGGCAGTAGCTTGAAGTTTGCCTTTAGATCGTTATCCACGTGGTACTTGTCCATCAACGCGCGCG
    5530      5540      5550      5560      5570      5580      5590      5600      5610      5620      5630      5640
CCACGAGGAGCAAATCGGTCCAGAACGTATGCCGGCGGTCTCGAAGGTGAACCAGTCCGTCATCGAACTTCAAACGGAAATCTAGCAATAGGTGCACCATGAACAGGTAGTTGCGCGCGC
  H   E   E   N   L   W   T   K   C   V   A   A   L   A   E   V   Q   D   P   L   L   K   F   N   A   K   L   D   N   D   V   H   Y   K   D   M   L   A   R   A
```

```
CAGCCTCCATGCCCTTCTCCCACGCAGACACGATCGGCAGGCTCAGCGGGTTTATCACCGTGCTTTCACTTTCCGCTTCACTGGACTCTTCCTTTTCCTCTTGCGTCCGCATACCCCGCG
    5650      5660      5670      5680      5690      5700      5710      5720      5730      5740      5750      5760
GTCGGAGGTACGGGAAGAGGGTGCGTCTGTTGCTAGCCGTCCGAGTCGCCCAAATAGTGGCACGAAAGTGAAAGGCGAAGTGACCTGAGAAGGAAAAGGAGAACGCAGGCGTATGGGCCGC
  A   E   M   G   K   E   W   A   S   V   I   P   L   S   L   P   N   I   V   T   S   E   S   E   A   E   S   S   E   E   K   E   E   Q   T   R   M   G   R   A
```

```
CCACTGGGTCGTCTTCATTCAGCCGCCGCACCGTGCGCTTACCTCCCTTGCCGTGCTTGATTAGCACCGGTGGGTTGCTGAAACCCACCATTTGTAGCGCCACATCTTCTCTTTCTTCCT
    5770      5780      5790      5800      5810      5820      5830      5840      5850      5860      5870      5880
GGTGACCCAGCAGAAGTAAGTCGGCGGCGTGGCACGCGAATGGAGGGAACGGCACGAACTAATCGTGGCCACCCAACGACTTTGGGTGGTAAACATCGCGGTGTAGAAGAGAAAGAAGGA
  V   P   D   D   E   N   L   R   R   R   V   T   R   K   G   G   K   G   H   K   I   L   V   P   P   N   S   F   G   V   M   Q   L   A   V   D   E   R   E   E   E
```

```
CGCTGTCCACGATCACCTCTGGGGATGGCGGGCGCTCGGGCTTGGGAGAGGGGCGCTTCTTTTTCTTTTTGGACGCAATGGCCAAATCCGCCGTCGAGGTCGATGGCCGCGGGCTGGGTG
    5890      5900      5910      5920      5930      5940      5950      5960      5970      5980      5990      6000
GCGACAGGTGCTAGTGGAGACCCCTACCGCCCGCGAGCCCGAACCCTCTCCCCGCGAAGAAAAAGAAAAACCTGCGTTACCGGTTTAGGCGGCAGCTCCAGCTACCGGCGCCCGACCCAC
  S   D   V   I   V   E   P   S   P   P   R   E   P   K   P   S   P   R   K   K   K   K   K   S   A   I   A   L   D   A   T   S   T   S   P   R   P   S   P   T
```

```
TGCCGCGGCACCAGCGCATCTTGTGACGAGTCTTCTTCGTCCTCGGACTCGAGACGCCGCCTCAGCCGCTTTTTTGGGGGCGCGCGGGGAGGCGGCGGCGACGGCGACGGGGACGACACGT
    6010      6020      6030      6040      6050      6060      6070      6080      6090      6100      6110      6120
ACGGCGCCGTGGTCGCGTAGAACACTGCTCAGAAGAAGCAGGAGCCTGAGCTCTGCGGCGGAGTCGGCGAAAAAACCCCCGCGCGCCCTCCGCCGCCGCTGCCGCTGCCCCTGCTGTGCA
  R   P   V   L   A   D   Q   S   S   D   E   E   D   E   S   E   L   R   R   R   L   R   K   K   P   P   A   R   P   P   P   P   S   P   S   P   S   S   V   D
```

```
                                                                                                            ┌─── splice L4 mRNA
                                                                                                            │    L4 100K start
                                                                                                                          M   E   S   V
CCTCCATGGTTGGTGGACGTCGCGCCGCACCGCGTCCGCGCTCGGGGGTGGTTTCGCGCTGCTCCTCTTCCCGACTGGCCATTTCCTTCTCCTATAGGCAGAAAAAGATCATGGAGTCAG
    6130      6140      6150      6160      6170      6180      6190      6200      6210      6220      6230      6240
GGAGGTACCAACCACCTGCAGCGCGGCGTGGCGCAGGCGCGAGCCCCCACCAAAGCGCGACGAGGAGAAGGGCTGACCGGTAAAGGAAGAGGATATCCGTCTTTTTCTAGTACCTCAGTC
  E   M   T   P   P   R   R   A   A   G   R   G   R   E   P   T   T   E   R   Q   E   E   E   R   S   A   M
                                                                                                       start E2a DBP
                                                                                                       splice E2a mRNA┘
  E   K
TCGAGAAG

AGCTCTTC
```

Table 4.2. Landmarks in the Ad2 DNA sequence 48–66%

Strand nucleotide		Sequence	Identitiy
r	l		
	A72	AATAAA	3'-poly(A) signal L2 mRNA
	C91		3'-poly(A) attachment site L2 mRNA
	A123		acceptor L3 mRNA splice
	A124	ATG	start L3 protein VI
	T874	TAA	stop L3 protein VI
	A925		acceptor L3 hexon mRNA splice
	A961	ATG	start L3 hexon
T995		TAA	stop ORF 10.2 K
A1268		ATG	start ORF 10.2 K
	A2627	ATG	start ORF 15.7 K
	T3056	TGA	stop ORF 15.7 K
	G3461	GAATTC	*Eco*RI site 58.5% between fragments A and B
	G3729	GGATCC	*Bam*HI site 59.5% between fragments C and A
	T3773		acceptor L3 23 K mRNA splice
	T3865	TAA	stop L3 hexon
	A3901	ATG	start L3 23 K protein
	T4513	TAA	stop L3 23 K protein
	A4541	AATAAA	3'-poly(A) signal L3 mRNA
T4544			3'-poly(A) attachment site E2A mRNA
A4562		AATAAA	3'-poly(A) signal E2A mRNA
	T4565		3'-poly(A) attachment site L3 mRNA
T4615		TAA	stop E2A DBP
A6202		ATG	start E2A DBP
C6211			acceptor E2A mRNA splice
	G6218		acceptor L4 mRNA splice
	A6231	ATG	start L4 100 K protein

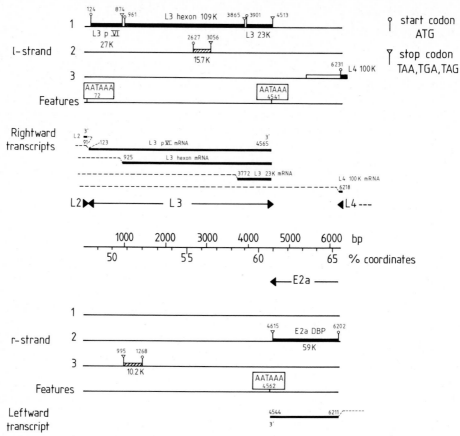

Fig. 4.1. Schematic representation of identified and unidentified reading frames and RNA coordinates in Ad2 DNA between coordinates 48 and 66. The map scale in the *center* of the figure reflects a conversion factor of 355 bp, which corresponds for the right end to 1% of the viral genome. Immediately *above* and *below* the scale, the locations of the various transcription units are indicated. The *continuous lines* above the transcription unit designations represent the segments of rightward transcripts present in mature RNAs; *interrupted lines* denote RNA splices. The coordinates of the 3'-poly(A) attachment sites, and of splice acceptor sites are also given in this part of the figure. On the *next line above* RNA expression signals have been drawn: in this case, 3'-poly(A) signals (AATAAA). Lines 1, 2, and 3 in the *upper part* of the figure represent the three possible frames in which the DNA l-strand can be read. Tracts open for translation are indicated as *solid bars* for known genes, and as *hatched bars* for unidentified translatable regions. The open frames are flanked by the symbols ⸸ and ⸸, denoting inititation (ATG) and termination (TAA, TAG or TGA) codons respectively. The *numbers* next to the codons are their coordinates, and the *numbers in larger type* refer to the predicted MW of the translation products. The *bottom* part of the figures represents the leftward transcripts

5 DNA Sequence of Human Ad5 (Subgroup C) Between Coordinates 60 and 72

The sequence (Table 5.1) was determined by KRUIJER et al. (1980, 1981). It is given in double-stranded format with 120 nucleotides per line, the numbering starting at the *Bgl*II site at coordinate 60 between fragments C and L. Each number refers to the positions above and below its last zero. The following features are marked: predicted or potential initiation and termination codons, 3′-poly(A) signals and attachment sites, and splice points (Table 5.2). Above or below the DNA sequence (sense strand) is given the predicted amino acid sequence (in one-letter code; see footnote to Table 5.1) for L3 23K, the E2A DBP and the N-terminal part of the L4 100K protein.

Table 5.1. Ad5 DNA sequence 60–72%

```
      start L3 23K
        M  G  S  S  E  Q  E  L  K  A  I  V  K  D  L  G  C  G  P  Y  F  L  G  T  Y  D  K  R  F  P  G  F  V  S  P  H  K  L
CTGCCGCCATGGGCTCCAGTGAGCAGGAACTGAAAGCCATTGTCAAAGATCTTGGTTGTGGGCCATATTTTTTGGGCACCTATGACAAGCGCTTTCCAGGCTTTGTTTCTCCACACAAGC
     10        20        30        40        50        60        70        80        90       100       110       120
GACGGCGGTACCCGAGGTCACTCGTCCTTGACTTTCGGTAACAGTTTCTAGAACCAACACCCGGTATAAAAAACCCGTGGATACTGTTCGCGAAAGGTCCGAAACAAAGAGGTGTGTTCG


        A  C  A  I  V  N  T  A  G  R  E  T  G  G  V  H  W  M  A  F  A  W  N  P  H  S  K  T  C  Y  L  F  E  P  F  G  F  S  D  Q
TCGCCTGCGCCATAGTCAATACGGCCGGTCGCGAGACTGGGGGCGTACACTGGATGGCCTTTGCCTGGAACCCGCACTCAAAAACATGCTACCTCTTTGAGCCCTTTGGCTTTTCTGACC
      130       140       150       160       170       180       190       200       210       220       230       240
AGCGGACGCGGTATCAGTTATGCCGGCCAGCGCTCTGACCCCCGCATGTGACCTACCGGAAACGGACCTTGGGCGTGAGTTTTTGTACGATGGAGAAACTCGGGAAACCGAAAAGACTGG


        R  L  K  Q  V  Y  Q  F  E  Y  E  S  L  L  R  R  S  A  I  A  S  S  P  D  R  C  I  T  L  E  K  S  T  Q  S  V  Q  G  P  N
AGCGACTCAAGCAGGTTTACCAGTTTGAGTACGAGTCACTCCTGCGCCGTAGCGCCATTGCTTCTTCCCCCGACCGCTGTATAACGCTGGAAAAGTCCACCCAAAGCGTACAGGGGCCCA
      250       260       270       280       290       300       310       320       330       340       350       360
TCGCTGAGTTCGTCCAAATGGTCAAACTCATGCTCAGTGAGGACGCGGCATCGCGGTAACGAAGAAGGGGGCTGGCGACATATTGCGACCTTTTCAGGTGGGTTTCGCATGTCCCCGGGT


        S  A  A  C  G  L  F  C  C  M  F  L  H  A  F  A  N  W  P  Q  T  P  M  D  H  N  P  T  M  N  L  I  T  G  V  P  N  S  M  L
ACTCGGCCGCCTGTGGACTATTCTGCTGCATGTTTCTCCACGCCTTTGCCAACTGGCCCCAAACTCCCATGGATCACAACCCCACCATGAACCTTATTACCGGGGTACCCAACTCCATGC
      370       380       390       400       410       420       430       440       450       460       470       480
TGAGCCGGCGGACACCTGATAAGACGACGTACAAAGAGGTGCGGAAACGGTTGACCGGGGTTTGAGGGTACCTAGTGTTGGGGTGGTACTTGGAATAATGGCCCCATGGGTTGAGGTACG


        N  S  P  Q  V  Q  P  T  L  R  R  N  Q  E  Q  L  Y  S  F  L  E  R  H  S  P  Y  F  R  S  H  S  A  Q  I  R  S  A  T  S  F
TCAACAGTCCCCAGGTACAGCCCACCCTGCGTCGCAACCAGGAACAGCTCTACAGCTTCCTGGAGCGCCACTCGCCCTACTTCCGCAGCCACAGTGCGCAGATTAGGAGCGCCACTTCTT
      490       500       510       520       530       540       550       560       570       580       590       600
AGTTGTCAGGGGTCCATGTCGGGTGGGACGCAGCGTTGGTCCTTGTCGAGATGTCGAAGGACCTCGCGGTGAGCGGGATGAAGGCGTCGGTGTCACGCGTCTAATCCTCGCGGTGAAGAA


                 stop L3 23K                                                                    ┌ 3'-poly(A) L3
      C  H  L  K  N  M  *                                                                       │
TTTGTCACTTGAAAAACATGTAAAAATAATGTACTAGAGACACTTTCAATAAAGGCAAATGCTTTTATTTGTACACTCTCGGGTGATTATTTACCCCCACCCTTGCCGTCTGCGCCGTTT
      610       620       630       640       650       660       670       680       690       700       710       720
AAACAGTGAACTTTTTGTACATTTTTATTACATGATCTCTGTGAAAGTTATTTCCGTTTACGAAAATAAACATGTGAGAGCCCACTAATAAATGGGGGTGGGAACGGCAGACGCGGCAAA
                    3'-poly(A) E2a ┘                                                                                    *


AAAAATCAAAGGGGTTCTGCCGCGCATCGCTATGCGCCACTGGCAGGGACACGTTGCGATACTGGTGTTTAGTGCTCCACTTAAACTCAGGCACAACCATCCGCGGCAGCTCGGTGAAGT
      730       740       750       760       770       780       790       800       810       820       830       840
TTTTTAGTTTCCCCAAGACGGCGCGTAGCGATACGCGGTGACCGTCCCTGTGCAACGCTATGACCACAAATCACGAGGTGAATTTGAGTCCGTGTTGGTAGGCGCCGTCGAGCCACTTCA
        F  D  F  P  N  Q  R  A  D  S  H  A  V  P  L  S  V  N  R  Y  Q  H  K  T  S  W  K  F  E  P  V  V  M  R  P  L  E  T  F  N
     stop E2a DBP


TTTCACTCCACAGGCTGCGCACCATCACCAACGCGTTTAGCAGGTCGGGCGCCGATATCTTGAAGTCGCAGTTGGGGCCTCCGCCCTGCGCGCGAGTTGCGATACACAGGGTTGCAGC
      850       860       870       880       890       900       910       920       930       940       950       960
AAAGTGAGGTGTCCGACGCGTGGTAGTGGTTGCGCAAATCGTCCAGCCCGCGGCTATAGAACTTCAGCGTCAACCCCGGAGGCGGGACGCGCGCGCTCAACGCTATGTGTCCCAACGTCG
        E  S  W  L  S  R  V  M  V  L  A  N  L  L  D  P  A  S  I  K  F  D  C  N  P  G  G  G  Q  A  R  S  N  R  Y  V  P  N  C  C


ACTGGAACACTATCAGCGCCGGGTGGTGCACGCTGGCCAGCACGCTCTTGTCGGAGATCAGATCCGCGTCCAGGTCCTCCGCGTTGCTCAGGGCGAACGGAGTCAACTTTGGTAGCTGCC
      970       980       990      1000      1010      1020      1030      1040      1050      1060      1070      1080
TGACCTGTGATAGTCGCGGCCCACCACGTGCGACCGGTCGTGCGAGAACAGCCTCTAGTCTAGGCGCAGGTCCAGGAGGCGCAACGAGTCCCGCTTGCCTCAGTTGAAACCATCGACGG
        Q  F  V  I  L  A  P  H  H  V  S  A  L  V  S  K  D  S  I  L  D  A  D  L  D  E  A  N  S  L  A  F  P  T  L  K  P  L  Q  R


TTCCCAAAAAGGGCGCGTGCCCAGGCTTTGAGTTGCACTCGCACCGTAGTGGCATCAAAAGGTGACCGTGCCCGGTCTGGGCGTTAGGATACAGCGCCTGCATAAAAGCCTTGATCTGCT
     1090      1100      1110      1120      1130      1140      1150      1160      1170      1180      1190      1200
AAGGGTTTTTCCCGCGCACGGGTCCGAAACTCAACGTGAGCGTGGCATCACCGTAGTTTTCCACTGGCACGGGCCAGACCCGCAATCCTATGTCGCGGACGTATTTTCGGAACTAGACGA
        G  L  F  P  A  H  G  P  K  S  N  C  E  C  R  L  P  M  L  L  H  G  H  G  T  Q  A  N  P  Y  L  A  Q  M  F  A  K  I  Q  K
```

One-letter code for amino acids: A, ala; C, cys; D, asp; E, glu; F, phe; G, gly; H, his; I, ile; K, lys; L, leu; M, met; N, asn; P, pro; Q, gln; R, arg; S, ser; T, thr; V, val; W, trp; Y, tyr

Table 5.1 (Continued)

```
TAAAAGCCACCTGAGCCTTTGCGCCTTCAGAGAAGAACATGCCGCAAGACTTGCCGGAAAACTGATTGGCCGGACAGGCCGCGTCGTGCACGCAGCACCTTGCGTCGGTGTTGGAGATCT
    1210      1220      1230      1240      1250      1260      1270      1280      1290      1300      1310      1320
ATTTTCGGTGGACTCGGAAACGCGGAAGTCTCTTCTTGTACGGCGTTCTGAACGGCCTTTTGACTAACCGGCCTGTCCGGCGCAGCACGTGCGTCGTGGAACGCAGCCACAACCTCTAGA
   F   A   V   Q   A   K   A   G   E   S   F   F   M   G   C   S   K   G   S   F   Q   N   A   P   C   A   A   A   D   H   V   C   C   R   A   D   T   N   S   I   Q

GCACCACATTTCGGCCCCACCGGTTCTTCACGATCTTGGCCTTGCTAGACTGCTCCTTCAGCGCGCGCTGCCCGTTTTCGCTCGTCACATCCATTTCAATCACGTGCTCCTTATTTATCA
    1330      1340      1350      1360      1370      1380      1390      1400      1410      1420      1430      1440
CGTGGTGTAAAGCCGGGGTGGCCAAGAAGTGCTAGAACCGGAACGATCTGACGAGGAAGTCGCGCGCGACGGGCAAAAGCGAGCAGTGTAGGTAAAGTTAGTGCACGAGGAATAAATAGT
   V   V   N   R   G   W   R   N   K   V   I   K   A   K   S   S   Q   E   K   L   A   R   Q   G   N   E   S   T   V   D   M   E   I   V   H   E   K   N   I   M

TAATGCTTCCGTGTAGACACTTAAGCTCGCCTTCGATCTCAGCGCAGCGGTGCAGCCACAACGCGCAGCCCGTGGGCTCGTGATGCTTGTAGGTCACCTCTGCAAACGACTGCAGGTACG
    1450      1460      1470      1480      1490      1500      1510      1520      1530      1540      1550      1560
ATTACGAAGGCACATCTGTGAATTCGAGCGGAAGCTAGAGTCGCGTCGCCACGTCGGTGTTGCGCGTCGGGCACCCGAGCACTACGAACATCCAGTGGAGACGTTTGCTGACGTCCATGC
   I   S   G   H   L   C   K   L   E   G   E   I   E   A   C   R   H   L   W   L   A   C   G   T   P   E   H   H   K   Y   T   V   E   A   F   S   Q   L   Y   A

CCTGCAGGAATCGCCCCATCATCGTCACAAAGGTCTTGTTGCTGGTGAAGGTCAGCTGCAACCCGCGGTGCTCCTCGTTCAGCCAGGTCTTGCATACGGCCGCCAGAGCTTCCACTTGGT
    1570      1580      1590      1600      1610      1620      1630      1640      1650      1660      1670      1680
GGACGTGCCTTAGCGGGGTAGTAGCAGTGTTTCCAGAACAACGACCCACTTCCAGTCGACGTTGGGCGCCACGAGGAGCAAGTCGGTCCAGAACGTATGCCGGCGGTCTCGAAGGTGAACCA
   Q   L   F   R   G   M   M   T   V   F   T   K   N   S   T   F   T   L   Q   L   G   R   H   E   E   N   L   W   T   K   C   V   A   A   L   A   E   V   Q   D

CAGGCAGTAGTTTGAAGTTCGCCTTTAGATCGTTATCCACGTGGTACTTGTCCATCAGCGCGCGCGCAGCCTCCATGCCCTTCTCCCACGCAGACACGATCGGCACACTCAGCGGGTTCA
    1690      1700      1710      1720      1730      1740      1750      1760      1770      1780      1790      1800
GTCCGTCATCAAACTTCAAGCGGAAATCTAGCAATAGGTGCACCATGAACAGGTAGTCGCGCGCGCGCGTCGGAGGTAGGGAAGAGGGTGCGTCTGTGCTAGCCGTGTGAGTCGCCCAAGT
   P   L   L   K   F   N   A   K   L   D   N   D   V   H   Y   K   D   M   L   A   R   A   A   E   M   G   K   E   W   A   S   V   I   P   V   S   L   P   N   M

TCACCGTAATTTCACTTTCCGCTTCGCTGGGCTCTTCCTCTTCCTCTTGCGTCCGCATACCACGCGCCACTGGGTCGTCTTCATTCAGCCGCCGCACTGTGCGCTTACCTCCTTTGCCAT
    1810      1820      1830      1840      1850      1860      1870      1880      1890      1900      1910      1920
AGTGGCATTAAAGTGAAAGGCGAAGCGACCCGAGAAGGAGAAGGAGAACGCAGGCGTATGGTGCGCGGTGACCCAGCAGAAGTAAGTCGGCGGCGTGACACGCGAATGGAGGAAACGGTA
   V   T   I   E   S   E   A   E   S   P   E   E   E   E   Q   T   R   M   G   R   A   V   P   D   D   E   N   L   R   R   V   T   R   K   G   G   K   H

GCTTGATTAGCACCGGTGGGTTGCTGAAACCCACCATTTGTAGCGCCACATCTTCTCTTTCTTCCTCGCTGTCCACGATTACCTCTGGTGATGGCGGGCGCTCGGGCTTGGGAGAAGGGC
    1930      1940      1950      1960      1970      1980      1990      2000      2010      2020      2030      2040
CGAACTAATCGTGGCCACCCAACGACTTTGGGTGGTAAACATCGCGGTGTAGAAGAGAAAGAAGGAGCGACAGGTGCTAATGGAGACCACTACCGCCCGCGAGCCCGAACCCTCTTCCCG
   K   I   L   V   P   P   N   S   F   G   V   M   Q   L   A   V   D   E   R   E   E   E   S   D   V   I   V   E   P   S   P   R   E   P   K   P   S   P   R

GCTTCTTTTTCTTCTTGGGCGCAATGGCCAAATCCGCCGCCGAGGTCGATGGCCGCGGGCTGGGTGTTGTGCCGGCACCAGCGCGTCTTGTGATGAGTCTTCCTCGTCCTCCGGACTCGATAC
    2050      2060      2070      2080      2090      2100      2110      2120      2130      2140      2150      2160
CGAAGAAAAAGAAGAACCCGCGTTACCGGTTTAGGCGGCGGCTCCAGCTACCGGCGCCGACCCACACGCGCCGTGGTCGCGCAGAACACTACTCAGAAGGAGCAGGAGCCTGAGCTATG
   K   K   K   K   P   A   I   A   L   D   A   A   S   T   S   P   R   P   S   P   T   R   P   V   L   A   D   Q   S   S   D   E   D   E   S   E   I   R

GCCGCCTCATCCGCTTTTTTGGGGGCGCCCGGGGAGGCGGCGGCGACGGGGACGGGGACGGGGACGACACGTCCTCCATGGTTGGGGGACGTCGCGCCGCCACCGCGTCCGCGCTCGGGGGTGGTTT
    2170      2180      2190      2200      2210      2220      2230      2240      2250      2260      2270      2280
CGGCGGAGTAGGCGAAAAAACCCCCGCGGGCCCCTCCGCCGCCGCTGCCCCTGCCCCTGCTGTGCAGGAGGTACCAACCCCCTGCAGCGCGGCGTGGCGCAGGCGCGAGCCCCCACCAAA
   R   R   M   R   K   K   P   P   A   R   P   P   P   P   S   P   S   P   S   S   V   D   E   M   T   P   P   R   R   A   A   G   R   G   R   E   P   T   T   E
```

```
                          splice L4 mRNA ⌐              start L4 100K
                                                        M   E   S   V   E   K   K   D   S   L   T   A   P   S   E   F   A   T   T   A   S   T
CGCGCTGCTCCTCTTCCCGACTGGCCATTTTCCTTCTCCTATAGGCAGAAAAAGATCATGGAGTCAGTCGAGAAGAAGGACAGCCTAACCGCCCCCTCTGAGTTCGCCACCACCGCCTCCA
    2290      2300      2310      2320      2330      2340      2350      2360      2370      2380      2390      2400
GCGCGACGAGGAGAAGGGCTGACCGGTAAAGGAAGAGGATATCCGTCTTTTTCTAGTACCTCAGTCAGCTCTTCTTCCTGTCGGATTGGCGGGGGAGACTCAAGCGGTGGTGGCCGGAGGT
   R   Q   E   E   E   R   S   A   M
            E2a DBP start         └─ splice E2a mRNA
```

```
   D   A   A   N   A   P   T   T   F   P   V   E   A   P   P   L   E   E   E   E   V   I   I   E   Q   D   P   G   F   V   S   E   D   D   E   D   R   S   V   P
CCGATGCCGCCAACGCGCGCCTACCACCTTCCCCGTCGAGGCACCCCCGCTTGAGGAGGAGGAAGTGATTATCGAGCAGGACCCAGGTTTTGTAAGCGAAGACGACGAGGACCGCTCAGTAC
    2410      2420      2430      2440      2450      2460      2470      2480      2490      2500      2510      2520
GGCTACGGCGGTTGCGCGGATGGTGGAAGGGGCAGCTCCGTGGGGGCGAACTCCTCCTCCTTCACTAATAGCTCGTCCTGGGTCCAAAACATTCGCTTCTGCTGCTCCTGGCAGTGATG
```

```
   T   E   D   K   K   Q   D   Q   D   N   A   E   A   N   E   E   Q   V   G   R   G   D   E   R   H   G   D   Y   L   D   V   G   D   D   V   L   L   K   H   L
CAACAGAGGATAAAAAGCAAGACCAGGACAACGCAGAGGCAAACGAGGAACAAGTCGGGCGGGGGGGGACGAAAGGCATGGCGACTACCTAGATGTGGGAGACGACGTGCTGTTGAAGCATC
    2530      2540      2550      2560      2570      2580      2590      2600      2610      2620      2630      2640
GTTGTCTCCTATTTTTCGTTCTGGTCCTGTTGCGTCTCCGTTTGCTCCTTGTTCAGCCCGCCCCCTGCTTTCCGTACCGCTGATGGATCTACACCCTCTGCTGCACGACAACTTCGTAG
```

```
   Q   R   Q   C   A   I   I   C   D   A   L   Q   E   R   S   D   V   P   L   A   I   A   D   V   S   L   A   Y   E   R   H   L   F   S   P   R   V   P   P   K
TGCAGCGCCAGTGCGCCATTATCTGCGACGCGTTGCAAGAGCGCAGCGATGTGCCCCTCGCCATAGCGGATGTCAGCCTTGCCTACGAACGCCACCTATTCTCACCGCGCGTACCCCCCA
    2650      2660      2670      2680      2690      2700      2710      2720      2730      2740      2750      2760
ACGTCGCGGTCACGCGGTAATAGACGCTGCGCAACGTTCTCGCGTCGCTACACGGGAGCGGTATCGCCTACAGTCGGAACGGATGCTTGCGGTGATAAGAGTGGCGCGCATGGGGGT
```

```
   R   Q   E   N   G   T   C   E   P   N   P   R   L   N   F   Y   P   V   F   A   V   P   E   V   L   A   T   Y   H   I   F   F   Q   N   C   K   I   P   L   S
AACGCCAAGAAAACGGCACATGCGAGCCCAACCCGCGCCTCAACTTCTACCCCGTATTTGCCGTGCCAGAGGTGCTTGCCACCTATCACATCTTTTTCCAAAACTGCAAGATACCCCTAT
    2770      2780      2790      2800      2810      2820      2830      2840      2850      2860      2870      2880
TTGCGGTTCTTTTGCCGTGTACGCTCGGGTTGGGCGCGGAGTTGAAGATGGGGCATAAACGGCACGGTCTCCACGAACGGTGGATAGTGTAGAAAAAGGTTTTGACGTTCTATGGGGATA
```

```
   C   R   A   N   R   S   R   A   D   K   Q   L   A   L   R   Q   G   A   V   I   P   D   I   A   S   L   N   E   V   P   K   I   F   E   G   L   G   R   D   E
CCTGCCGTGCCAACCGCAGCCGAGCGGACAAGCAGCTGGCCTTGCGGCAGGGCGCTGTCATACCTGATATCGCCTCGCTCAACGAAGTGCCAAAAATCTTTGAGGGTCTTGGACGCGACG
    2890      2900      2910      2920      2930      2940      2950      2960      2970      2980      2990      3000
GGACGGCACGGTTGGCGTCGGCTCGCCTGTTCGTCGACCGGAACGCCGTCCCGCGACAGTATGGACTATAGCGGAGCGAGTTGCTTCACGGTTTTAGAAACTCCCAGAACCTGCGCTAG
                                                           splice ─┴─ 3' 2nd E2a  leader
```

```
   K   R   A   A   N   A   L   Q   Q   Q   E   N   S   E   N   E   S   H   S   G   V   L   V   E   L   E   G   D   N   A   R   L   A   V   L   K   R   S   I   E   V
AGAAGCGCGGCAAACGCTCTGCAACAGGAAAACAGCGAAAATGAAAGTCACTCTGGAGTGTTGGTGGAACTCGAGGGTGACAACGCGCGCCTAGCCGTACTAAAACGCAGCATCGAGG
    3010      3020      3030      3040      3050      3060      3070      3080      3090      3100      3110      3120
TCTTCGCGCGCCGTTTGCGAGACGTTGTCCTTTTGTCGCTTTTACTTTCAGTGAGACCTCACAACCACCTTGAGCTCCCACTGTTGCGCGCGGATCGGCATGATTTTGCGTCGTAGCTCC
2nd E2a leader 5' ─┴─ splice
```

Table 5.1 (Continued)

```
      T  H  F  A  Y  P  A  L  N  L  P  P  K  V  M  S  T  V  M  S  E  L  I  V  R  R  A  Q  P  L  E  R  D  A  N  L  Q  E  Q  T
TCACCCACTTTGCCTACCCGGCACTTAACCTACCCCCCAAGGTCATGAGCACAGTCATGAGTGAGCTGATCGTGCGCCGTGCGCAGCCCCTGGAGAGGGATGCAAATTTGCAAGAACAAA
        3130      3140      3150      3160      3170      3180      3190      3200      3210      3220      3230      3240
AGTGGGTGAAACGGATGGGCCGTGAATTGGATGGGGGGGTTCCAGTACTCGTGTCAGTACTCACTCGACTAGCACGCGGCACGCGTCGGGGACCTCTCCCTACGTTTAAACGTTCTTGTTT


      E  E  G  L  P  A  V  G  D  E  Q  L  A  R  W  L  Q  T  R  E  P  A  D  L  E  E  R  R  K  L  M  M  A  A  V  L  V  T  V  E
CAGAGGAGGGCCTACCCGCAGTTGGCGACGAGCAGCTAGCGCGCTGGCTTCAAACGCGCGAGCCTGCCGACTTGGAGGAGCGACGCAAACTAATGATGGCCGCAGTGCTCGTTACCGTGG
        3250      3260      3270      3280      3290      3300      3310      3320      3330      3340      3350      3360
GTCTCCTCCCGGATGGGCGTCAACCGCTGCTCGTCGATCGCGCGACCGAAGTTGCGCGCTCGGACGGCTGAACCTCCTCGCTGCGTTTGATTACTACCGGCGTCACGAGCAATGGCACC


      L  E  C  M  Q  R  F  F  A  D  P  E  M  Q  R  K  L  E  E  T  L  H  Y  T  F  R  Q  G  Y  V  R  Q  A  C  K  I  S  N  V  E
AGCTTGAGTGCATGCAGCGGTTCTTTGCTGACCCGGAGATGCAGCGCAAGCTAGAGGAAACATTGCACTACACCTTTCGACAGGGCTACGTACGCCAGGCCTGCAAGATCTCCAACGTGG
        3370      3380      3390      3400      3410      3420      3430      3440      3450      3460      3470      3480
TCGAACTCACGTACGTCGCCAAGAAACGACTGGGCCTCTACGTCGCTTCGATCTCCTTTGTAACGTGATGTGGAAAGCTGTCCCGATGCATGCGGTCCGGACGTTCTAGAGGTTGCACC


      L  C  N  L  V  S  Y  L  G  I  L  H  E  N  R  L  G  Q  N  V  L  H  S  T  L  K  G  E  A  R  R  D  Y  V  R  D  C  V  Y  L
AGCTCTGCAACCTGGTCTCCTACCTTGGAATTTTGCACGAAAACCGCCTTGGGCAAAACGTGCTTCATTCCACGCTCAAGGGCGAGGCGCGCCGCGACTACGTCCGCGACTGCGTTTACT
        3490      3500      3510      3520      3530      3540      3550      3560      3570      3580      3590      3600
TCGAGACGTTGGACCAGAGGATGGAACCTTAAAACGTGCTTTGGCGGAACCCGTTTTGCACGAAGTAAGGTGCGAGTTCCGCTCGCGCGGCCGCTGATGCAGGCGCTGACGCAAATGA


      F  L  C  Y  T  W  Q  T  A  M  G  V  W  Q  Q  C  L  E  E  C  N  L  K  E  L  Q  K  L  L  K  Q  N  L  K  D  L  W  T  A  F
TATTTCTATGCTACACCTGGCAGACGGCCATGGGCGTTTGGCAGCAGTGCTTGGAGGAGTGCAACCTCAAGGAGCTGCAGAAACTGCTAAAGCAAAACTTGAAGGACCTATGGACGGCCT
        3610      3620      3630      3640      3650      3660      3670      3680      3690      3700      3710      3720
ATAAAGATACGATGTGGACCGTCTGCCGGTACCCGCAAACCGTCGTCACGAACCTCCTCACGTTGGAGTTCCTCGACGTCTTTGACGATTTCGTTTTGAACTTCCTGGATACCTGCCGGA


      N  E  R  S  V  A  A  H  L  A  D  I  I  F  P  E  R  L  L  L  K  T  L  Q  Q  Q  G  L  P  D  F  T  S  Q  S  M  L  Q  N  F  R  N
TCAACGAGCGCTCCGTGGCCGCGCACCTGGCGGACATCATTTTCCCCGAACGCCTGCTTAAAACCCTGCAACAGGGTCTGCCAGACTTCACCAGTCAAAGCATGTTGCAGAACTTTAGGA
        3730      3740      3750      3760      3770      3780      3790      3800      3810      3820      3830      3840
AGTTGCTCGCGAGGCACCGGCGCGTGGACCGCCTGTAGTAAAAGGGGCTTGCGGACGAATTTTGGGACGTTGTTCCCAGACGGTCTGAAGTGGTCAGTTTCGTACAACGTCTTGAAATCCT


          in Ad2 DNA:   gaattc (junction Ad2 EcoRI fragments B/F; beginning of Section 6)
      F  I  L  E  R  S  G  I  L  P  A  T  C  C  A  L  P  S  D  F  V  P  I  K  Y  R  E  C  P  P  P  L  W  G  H  C  Y  L  L  Q
ACTTTATCCTAGAGCGCTCAGGAATCTTGCCCGCCACCTGCTGTGCACTTCCTAGCGACTTTGTGCCCATTAAGTACCGCGAATGCCCTCCGCCGCTTTGGGGGCCACTGCTACCTTCTGC
        3850      3860      3870      3880      3890      3900      3910      3920      3930      3940      3950      3960
TGAAATAGGATCTCGCGAGTCCTTAGAACGGGCGGTGGACGACACGTGAAGGATCGCTGAAACACGGGTAATTCATGGCGCTTACGGGAGGCGGCGAAACCCCGGTGACGATGGAAGACG


      L  A  N  Y  L  A  Y  H  S  D  I  M  E  D  V  S  G  D  G  L  L  E  C  H  C  R  C  N  L  C  T  P  H  R  S  L  V  C  N  S
AGCTAGCCAACTACCTTGCCTACCACTCTGACATAATGGAAGACGTGAGCGGTGACGGTCTACTGGAGTGTCACTGTCGCTGCAACCTATGCACCCCGCACCGCTCCCTGGTTTGCAATT
        3970      3980      3990      4000      4010      4020      4030      4040      4050      4060      4070      4080
TCGATCGGTTGATGGAACGGATGGTGAGACTGTATTACCTTCTGCACTCGCCACTGCCAGATGACCTCACAGTGACAGCGACGTTGGATACGTGGGGCGTGGCGAGGGACCCAAACGTTAA


                        KpnI
      Q  L  L  N  E  S  Q  I  I  G  T
CGCAGCTGCTTAACGAAAGTCAAATTATCGGTACC
        4090      4100      4110
GCGTCGACGAATTGCTTTCAGTTTAATAGCCATGG
```

Table 5.2. Landmarks in the Ad5 DNA sequence 60–72%

Strands nucleotide		Sequence	Identity
r	l		
	A9	ATG	start L3 23K protein
	T621	TAA	stop L3 23K protein
	A648	AATAAA	3′-poly(A) signal L3 mRNA
T651			3′-poly(A) attachment site E2A DBP mRNA
A66g		AATAAA	3′-poly(A) signal E2A DBP mRNA
	T672		3′-poly(A) attachment site L3 mRNA
T721		TAA	stop E2A DBP
A2308		ATG	start E2A DBP
G2317			acceptor E2A mRNA splice
	G2324		acceptor L4 mRNA splice
	A2337	ATG	start L4 100K protein
G2944			donor 2nd E2A leader splice
A3020			acceptor 2nd E2A leader splice
	G4110	GGTACC	*Kpn*I site 72%

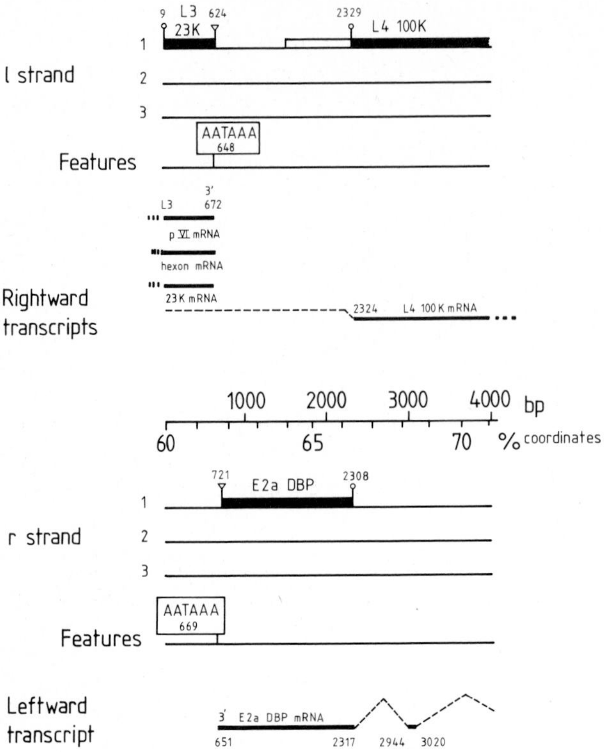

Fig. 5.1. Schematic representation of identified and unidentified reading frames and RNA coordinates in Ad5 DNA between coordinates 60 and 72. The map scale in the *center* of the figure reflects a conversion factor of 360 bp, which corresponds for this region to 1% of the viral genome. Immediately *above the sacle,* the locations of the various rightward transcripts are indicated; the *continuous lines* represent stretches of mature mRNA, the *interrupted line* symbolizes RNA splicing. On the *next line above* an RNA expression signal has been drawn: in this case, a 3′-poly(A) signal (AATAAA). Lines 1, 2, and 3 in the *upper part* of the figure represent the three possible frames in which the DNA l-strand can be read. Tracts open for translation are indicated as *solid bars.* The open frames are flanked by the symbols ⚲ and Y, denoting initiation (ATG) and termination (TAA, TAG or TGA) codons respectively. The *numbers* next to the codons are their coordinates, and the *numbers in larger type* refer to the predicted MW of the translation products. The *bottom* part of the figure represents the leftward transcripts

6 DNA Sequence of Human Ad2 (Subgroup C) Coordinates 70.7 and 100

The sequence (Table 6.1) was determined by GALIBERT et al. (1979), HÉRISSÉ et al. (1980, 1981a, b), and SHINAGAWA et al. (1980). It is given in double-stranded format with 120 nucleotides per line, the numbering starting at the *Eco*RI site at coordinate 70.7. Each number refers to the positions above and below its last zero. The following features are marked: the end of the ITR, RNA 5′ termini (cap sites), "TATA" boxes and 3′-poly(A) signals (AATAAA;

Table 6.1. Ad2 DNA sequence 70.7–100%

```
EcoRI fragment F---->
   I  L  P  A  T  C  C  A  L  P  S  D  F  V  P  I  K  Y  R  E  C  P  P  P  L  W  G  H  C  Y  L  L  Q  L  A  N  Y  L  A  Y
AATTCTGCCCGCCACCTGCTGTGCGCTTCCTAGCGACTTTGTGCCCATTAAGTACCGTGAATGCCCTCCGCCGCTTTGGGGTCACTGCTACCTTCTGCAGCTAGCCAACTACCTTGCCTA
        10        20        30        40        50        60        70        80        90       100       110       120
TTAAGACGGGCGGTGGACGACACGCGAAGGATCGCTGAAACACGGGTAATTCATGGCACTTACGGGAGGCGGCGAAACCCCAGTGACGATGGAAGACGTCGATCGGTTGATGGAACGGAT


   H  S  D  I  M  E  D  V  S  G  D  G  L  L  E  C  H  C  R  C  N  L  C  T  P  H  R  S  L  V  C  N  S  Q  L  L  S  E  S  Q
CCACTCCGACATCATGGAAGACGTGAGCGGTGACGGCCTACTGGAGTGTCACTGTCGCTGCAACCTATGCACCCCGCACCGCTCCCTGGTCTGCAATTCGCAACTGCTTAGCGAAAGTCA
       130       140       150       160       170       180       190       200       210       220       230       240
GGTGAGGCTGTAGTACCTTCTGCACTCGCCACTGCCGGATGACCTCACAGTGACAGCGACGTTGGATACGTGGGGCGTGGCGAGGGACCAGACGTTAAGCGTTGACGAATCGCTTTCAGT


        KpnI (end of Ad5 sequence,section D)
   I  I  G  T  F  E  L  Q  G  P  S  P  D  E  K  S  A  A  P  G  L  K  L  T  P  G  L  W  T  S  A  Y  L  R  K  F  V  P  E  D
AATTATCGGTACCTTTGAGCTGCAGGGTCCCTCGCCTGACGAAAAGTCCGCGGCTCCGGGGTTGAAACTCACTCCGGGGCTGTGGACGTCGGCTTACCTTCGCAAATTTGTACCTGAGGA
       250       260       270       280       290       300       310       320       330       340       350       360
TTAATAGCCATGGAAACTCGACGTCCCAGGGAGCGGACTGCTTTTCAGGCGCCGAGGCCCCAACTTTGAGTGAGGCCCCGACACCTGCAGCCGAATGGAAGCGTTTAAACATGGACTCCT
                                                         cap site E2a mRNA late ⌐┴┐              "TATA" E2a


        start L4 33K?
   Y  H  A  H  E  I  R  F  Y  E  D  Q  S  R  P  P  N  A  E  L  T  A  C  V  I  T  Q  G  H  I  L  G  Q  L  Q  A  I  N  K  A
CTACCACGCCCACGAGATTAGGTTCTACGAAGACCAATCCCGCCCGCCAAATGCGGAGCTTACCGCCTGCGTCATTACCCAGGGCCACATCCTTGGCCAATTGCAAGCCATCAACAAAGC
       370       380       390       400       410       420       430       440       450       460       470       480
GATGGTGCGGGTGCTCTAATCCAAGATGCTTCTGGTTAGGGCGGGCGGTTTACGCCTCGAATGGCGGACGCAGTAATGGGTCCCGGTGTAGGAACCGGTTAACGTTCGGTAGTTGTTTCG


   R  Q  E  F  L  L  R  K  G  R  G  V  Y  L  D  P  Q  S  G  E  E  L  N  P  I  P  P  P  P  P  Q  P  Y  Q  Q  P  R  A  L  A  S
CCGGCCAAGAGTTTCTGCTACGAAAGGGACGGGGGGTTTACCTGGACCCCCAGTCCGGCGAGGAGCTCAACCCAATCCCCCCGCCGCCGCAGCCCTATCAGCAGCCGCGGGCCCTTGCTTC
       490       500       510       520       530       540       550       560       570       580       590       600
GGCCGGTTCTCAAAGACGATGCTTTCCCTGCCCCCCAAATGGACCTGGGGGTCAGGCCGCTCCTCGAGTTGGGTTAGGGGGCGGCGGCGTCGGGATAGTCGTCGGCGCCCGGGAACGAAG


        start L4 33K (Oosterom-Dragon and Anderson, 1983)
   Q  D  G  T  Q  K  E  A  A  A  A  A  A  A  A  T  H  G  R  G  G  I  L  G  Q  S  G  R  G  G  F  G  R  G  G  G  D  D  G  R  L
        M  A  P  K  K  K  L  Q  L  P  P  P  P  P  T  D  E  E  E  Y  W  D  S  Q  A  E  E  V  L  D  E  E  E  E  M  M  E  D  W
CCAGGATGGCACCCAAAAAGAAGCTGCAGCTGCCGCCGCCGCCCACCCACGGACGAGGAGGAATACTGGGACAGTCAGGCAGGAGGAGGTTTTGGACGAGGAGGAGGAGATGATGGAAGACT
       610       620       630       640       650       660       670       680       690       700       710       720
GGTCCTACCGTGGGTTTTTCTTCGACGTCGACGGCGGCGGCGGTGGGTGCCTGCTCCTCCTTATGACCCTGTCAGTCCGTCTCCTCCAAAACCTGCTCCTCCTCCTCTACTACCTTCTGA


   G  Q  P  R  R  S  F  R  G  R  R  G  V  R  R  N  T  V  T  L  G  R  I  P  L  A  G  A  P  E  I  G  N  R  S  Q  H  R  Y  N
        D  S  L  D  E  A  S  E  A  E  E  V  S  D  E  T  P  S  P  S  V  A  F  P  S  P  A  P  Q  K  L  A  T  V  P  S  I  A  T  T
GGGACAGCCTAGACGAAGCTTCCGAGGCCGAAGAGGTGTCAGACGAAACACCGTCACCCTCGGTCGCATTCCCCTCGCCGGCGCCCCAGAAATTGGCAACCGTTCCCAGCATCGCTACAA
       730       740       750       760       770       780       790       800       810       820       830       840
CCCTGTCGGATCTGCTTCGAAGGCTCCGGCTTCTCCACAGTCTGCTTTGTGGCAGTGGGAGCCAGCGTAAGGGGAGCGGCCGCGGGGTCTTTAACCGTTGGCAAGGGTCGTAGCGATGTT


        stop L4 100K                        ⌐  splice L4 33K mRNA
   L  R  S  S  G  A  A  G  T  A  C  S  P  T  Q  P  *
        S  A  P  Q  A  P  P  A  L  P  V  R  R  P  N  R  R  W  D  T  T  G  T  R  A │
CCTCCGCTCCTCAGGCGCCCGGCCACTGCCTGTTCGCCGACCCAACCGTAGATGGGACACCACTGGAACCAGGGCCGGTAAGTCTAAGCAGCCGCCGCCGTTAGCCCAAGAGCAACAAC
       850       860       870       880       890       900       910       920       930       940       950       960
GGAGGCGAGGAGTCCGCGGCGGCCGTGACGGACAAGCGGCTGGGTTGGCATCTACCCTGTGGTGACCTTGGTCCCGGCCATTCAGATTCGTCGGCGGCGGCAATCGGGTTCTCGTTGTTG


AGCGCCAAGGCTACCGCTCGTGGCGCGGGCACAAGAACGCCATAGTTGCTTGCTTGCAAGACTGTGGGGGCAACATCTCCTTCGCCCGCCGCTTTCTTCTCTACCATCACGGCGTGGCCT
       970       980       990      1000      1010      1020      1030      1040      1050      1060      1070      1080
TCGCGGTTCCGATGGCGAGCACCGCGCCCGTGTTCTTGCGGTATCAACGAACGAACGTTCTGACACCCCCGTTGTAGAGGAAGCGGGCGGCGAAAGAAGAGATGGTAGTGCCGCACCGGA


        splice L4 33K mRNA ⌐                                      ┌A  P  T  A  P  A  A  A  A  A  A  A  A  T  A  A  V  T  Q  K  Q  R  R  P  D  S  K  T
TCCCCCGTAACATCCTGCATTACTACCGTCATCTCTACAGCCCCTACTGCACCGGCGGCAGCGGCAGCGGCAGCAACAGCAGCGGTCACACAGAAGCAAAGGCGACCGGATAGCAAGACT
      1090      1100      1110      1120      1130      1140      1150      1160      1170      1180      1190      1200
AGGGGGCATTGTAGGACGTAATGATGGCAGTAGAGATGTCGGGGATGACGTGGCCGCCGTCGCCGTCGCGTTGTCGTCGCCAGTGTGTCTTCGTTTCCGCTGGCCTATCGTTCTGA


   L  T  K  P  K  K  S  T  A  A  A  A  A  G  G  G  A  L  R  L  A  P  N  E  P  V  S  T  R  E  L  R  N  R  I  F  P  T  L  Y
CTGACAAAGCCCAAGAAATCCACAGCGGCGGCCAGCAGCAGGAGGAGGAGCGCTGCGTCTGGCGCCCAACGAACCCGTATCGACCCGCGAGCTTAGAAATAGGATTTTTCCCACTCTGTAT
      1210      1220      1230      1240      1250      1260      1270      1280      1290      1300      1310      1320
GACTGTTTCGGGTTCTTTAGGTGTCGCCGCCGTCGTCGTCCTCCTCCTCGCGACGCAGACCGCGGGTTGCTTGGGCATAGCTGGGCGCTCGAATCTTTATCCTAAAAAGGGTGAGACATA


   A  I  F  Q  Q  S  R  G  Q  E  Q  E  L  K  I  K  N  R  S  L  R  S  L  T  R  S  C  L  Y  H  K  S  E  D  Q  L  R  R  T  L
GCTATATTTCAACAAAGCAGGGGCCAAGAACAAGAGCTGAAAATAAAAAACAGGTCTCTGCGCTCCCTCACCCGCAGCTGCCTGTATCACAAAAGCGAAGATCAGCTTCGGCGCACGCTG
      1330      1340      1350      1360      1370      1380      1390      1400      1410      1420      1430      1440
CGATATAAAGTTGTTTCGTCCCCGGTTCTTGTTCTCGACTTTTATTTTTTGTCCAGAGACGCGAGGGAGTGGGCGTCGACGGACATAGTGTTTTCGCTTCTAGTCGAAGCCGCGTGCGAC
                                                                        splice E2a mRNA ─┘


                        stop L4 33K
   E  D  A  E  A  L  F  S  K  Y  C  A  L  T  L  K  D  *
GAAGACGCGGAGGCTCTCTTCAGCAAATACTGCGCGCTGACTCTTAAGGACTAGTTTCGCGCCCTTTCTCAAATTTAAGCGCGAAAACTACGTCATCTCCAGCGGCCACACCCGGCGCCA
      1450      1460      1470      1480      1490      1500      1510      1520      1530      1540      1550      1560
CTTCTGCGCCTCCGAGAGAAGTCGTTTATGACGCGCGACTGAGAATTCCTGATCAAAGCGCGGGAAAGAGTTTAAATTCGCGCTTTTGATGCAGTAGAGGTCGCCGGTGTGGGCCGCGGT
                                ↑↑ cap E2a mRNA


                        start L4 pVIII
                          M  S  K  E  I  P  T  P  Y  M  W  S  Y  Q  P  Q  M  G  L  A  A  G  A  A  Q  D  Y  S  T  R  I  N  Y
GCACCTGTCGTCAGCGCCATTATGAGCAAGGAAATTCCCACGCCCTACATGTGGAGTTACCAGCCACAAATGGGACTTGCGGCTGGAGCTGCCCAAGACTACTCAACCCGAATAAACTAC
      1570      1580      1590      1600      1610      1620      1630      1640      1650      1660      1670      1680
CGTGGACAGCAGTCGCGGTAATACTCGTTCCTTTAAGGGTGCGGGATTGTACACCTCAATGGTCGGTGTTTACCCTGAACGCCGACCTCGACGGGTTCTGATGAGTTGGGCTTATTTGATG
```

One-letter code for amino acids: A, ala; C, cys; D, asp; E, glu; F, phe; G, gly; H, his; I, ile; K, lys; L, leu; M, met; N, asn; P, pro; Q, gln; R, arg; S, ser; T, thr; V, val; W, trp; Y, tyr

Table 6.1 (Continued)

```
                                                          F <--- EcoRI ---> D
  M  S  A  G  P  H  M  I  S  R  V  N  G  I  R  A  H  R  N  R  I  L  L  E  Q  A  A  I  T  T  T  P  R  N  N  L  N  P  R  S
ATGAGCGCGGGACCCCACATGATATCCCGGGTCAACGGAATCCGCGCCCACCGAAACCGAATTCTCCTCGAACAGGCGGCTATTACCACCACACCTCGTAATAACCTTAATCCCCGTAGT
    1690      1700      1710      1720      1730      1740      1750      1760      1770      1780      1790      1800
TACTCGCGCCCTGGGGTGTACTATAGGGCCCAGTTGCCTTAGGCGCGGGTGGCTTTGGCTTAAGAGGAGCTTGTCCGCCGATAATGGTGGTGTGGAGCATTATTGGAATTAGGGGCATCA


  W  P  A  A  L  V  Y  Q  E  S  P  A  P  T  T  V  V  L  P  R  D  A  Q  A  E  V  Q  M  T  N  S  G  A  Q  L  A  G  G  F  R
TGGCCCGCTGCCCTGGTGTACCAGGAAAGTCCCGCTCCCACCACTGTGGTACTTCCCAGAGACGCCCAGGCCGAAGTTCAGATGACTAACTCAGGGGCGCAGCTTGCGGGCGGCTTTCGT
    1810      1820      1830      1840      1850      1860      1870      1880      1890      1900      1910      1920
ACCGGGCGACGGGACCACATGGTCCTTTCAGGGCGAGGGTGGTGACACCATGAAGGGTCTCTGCGGGTCCGGCTTCAAGTCTACTGATTGAGTCCCCGCGTCGAACGCCCGCCGAAAGCA


                     "TATA" E3        cap E3 mRNA┐
  H  R  V  R  S  P  G  Q  G  I  T  H  L  K  I  R  G  R G  I  Q  L  N  D  E  S  V  S  S  S  L  G  L  R  P  D  G  T  F  Q
CACAGGGTGCGGTCGCCCGGGCAGGGTATAACTCACCTGAAAATCAGAGGGCGAGGTATTCAGCTCAACGACGAGTCGGTGAGCTCCTCTTGGTCTCCGTCCGGACGGGACATTTCAG
    1930      1940      1950      1960      1970      1980      1990      2000      2010      2020      2030      2040
GTGTCCCACGCCAGCGGGCCCGTCCCATATTGAGTGGACTTTTAGTCTCCCGCTCCATAAGTCGAGTTGCTGCTCAGCCACTCGAGGAGGAGAACCAGAGGCAGGCCTGCCCTGTAAAGT


  I  G  G  A  G  R  S  S  F  T  P  R  Q  A  I  L  T  L  Q  T  S  S  S  E  P  R  S  G  G  I  G  T  L  Q  F  I  E  E  F  V
ATCGGCGGCGCTGGCCGCTCTTCATTTACGCCCCGTCAGGCGATCCTAACTCTGCAGACCTCGTCCTCGGAGCCGCGCTCCGGAGGCATTGGAACTCTACAATTTATTGAGGAGTTCGTG
    2050      2060      2070      2080      2090      2100      2110      2120      2130      2140      2150      2160
TAGCCGCCGCGACCGGCGAGAAGTAAATGCGGGGCAGTCCGCTAGGATTGAGACGTCTGGAGCAGGAGCCTCGGCGCGAGGCCTCCGTAACCTTGAGATGTTAAATAACTCCTCAAGCAC


                           splice───────5' late x leader                              stop L4 pVIII
                                                                                      start ORF 12.3K
  P  S  V  Y  F  N  P  F  S  G  P  P  G  H  Y  P  D  Q │F  I  P  N  F  D  A  V  K  D  S  A  D  G  Y  D ─* M  T  S  G  E
CCTTCGGTTTACTTCAACCCCTTTTCTGGACCTCCCGGCCACTACCCGGACCAGTTTATTCCCAACTTTGACGCGGTGAAAGACTCGGCGGACGGCTACGACTGAATGACCAGTGGAGAG
    2170      2180      2190      2200      2210      2220      2230      2240      2250      2260      2270      2280
GGAAGCCAAATGAAGTTGGGGAAAAGACCTGGAGGGCCGGTGATGGGCCTGGTCAAATAAGGGTTGAAACTGCGCCACTTTCTGAGCCGCCTGCCGATGCTGACTTACTGGTCACCTCTC


                                          3' late x leader;──also splice E3 mRNA
  A  E  R  L  R  L  T  H  L  D  H  C  R  R  H  K  C  F  A  R  G  S │G  E  F  C  Y  F  E  L  P  E  E  H  I  E  G  P  A  H
GCAGAGCGACTGCGCCTGACACACCTCGACCACTGCCGCCGCCACAAGTGCTTTGCCCGCGGCTCCGGTGAGTTTTGTTACTTTGAATTGCCCGAAGAGCATATCGAGGGCCCGGCGCAC
    2290      2300      2310      2320      2330      2340      2350      2360      2370      2380      2390      2400
CGTCTCGCTGACGCGGACTGTGTGGAGCTGGTGACGGCGGCGGTGTTCACGAAACGGGCGCCGAGGCCACTCAAAACAATGAAACTTAACGGGCTTCTCGTATAGCTCCCGGGCCGCGTG


  G  V  R  L  T  T  Q  V  E  L  T  R  S  L  I  R  E  F  T  K  R  P  L  L  V  E  R  E  R  G  P  C  V  L  T  V  V  C  N  C
GGCGTCCGGCTCACCACCCAGGTAGAGCTTACACGTAGCCTGATTCGGGAGTTTACCAAGCGCCCCTGCTAGTGGAGCGGGAGCGGGGTCCCTGTGTTCTGACCGTGGTTTGCAACTGT
    2410      2420      2430      2440      2450      2460      2470      2480      2490      2500      2510      2520
CCGCAGGCCGAGTGGTGGGTCCATCTCGAATGTGCATCGGACTAAGCCCTCAAATGGTTCGCGGGGGACGATCACCTCGCCCTCGCCCCAGGGACACAAGACTGGCACCAAACGTTGACA


                                poly(A) signal L4?    stop ORF 12.3K
  P  N  P  G  L  H  Q  D  L  C  C  H  L  C  A  E  Y  N  K  Y  R  N  *
CCTAACCCTGGATTACATCAAGATCTTTGTTGTCATCTCTGTGCTGAGTATAATAAATACAGAAATTAGAATCTACTGGGGCTCCTGTCGCCATCCTGTGAACGCCACCGTTTTTACCCA
    2530      2540      2550      2560      2570      2580      2590      2600      2610      2620      2630      2640
GGATTGGGACCTAATGTAGTTCTAGAAACAACAGTAGAGACACGACTCATATTATTTATGTCTTTAATCTTAGATGACCCCGAGGACAGCGGTAGGACACTTGCGGTGGCAAAAATGGGT


                                                              splice E3 mRNA─┐┌─5' late y leader
CCCAAAGCAGACCAAAGCAAACCTCACCTCCGGTTTGCACAAGCGGGCCAATAAGTACCTTACCTGGTACTTTAACGGCTCTTCATTTGTAATTTACAACAGTTTCCAGCGAGACGAAGT
    2650      2660      2670      2680      2690      2700      2710      2720      2730      2740      2750      2760
GGGTTTCGTCTGGTTTCGTTTGGAGTGGAGGCCAAACGTGTTCGCCCGGTTATTCATGGAATGGACCATGAAATTGCCGAGAAGTAAACATTAAATGTTGTCAAAGGTCGCTCTGCTTCA


AAGTTTGCCACACAACCTTCTCGGCTTCAACTACACCGTCAAGAAAAACACCACCACCACCACCACCTCCTCACCTGCCGGGAACGTACGAGTGCGTCACCGGTTGCTGCGCCCACACTAC
    2770      2780      2790      2800      2810      2820      2830      2840      2850      2860      2870      2880
TTCAAACGGTGTGTTGGAAGAGCCGAAGTTGATGTGGCAGTTCTTTTTGTGGTGGTGGTGGTGGTGGAGGAGTGGACGGCCCTTGCATGCTCACGCAGTGGCCAACGACGCGGGTGTGGATG


                    3' late y leader;──┬──also splice E3 mRNA
AGCCTGAGCGTAACCAGACATTACTCCCATTTTTCCAAAACAGGAGGTGAGCTCAACTCCCGGAACTCAGGTCAAAAAAGCATTTTGCGGGGTGCTGGGATTTTTTAATTAAGTATATGA
    2890      2900      2910      2920      2930      2940      2950      2960      2970      2980      2990      3000
TCGGACTCGCCATTGGTCTGTAATGAGGGTAAAAAGGTTTTGTCCTCCACTCGAGTTGAGGGCCTTGAGTCCAGTTTTTTCGTAAAACGCCCCACGACCCTAAAAAATTAATTCATATACT


GCAATTCAAGTAACTCTACAAGCTTGTCTAATTTTTCTGGAATTGGGGTCGGGGTTATCCTTACTCTTGTAATTCTGTTTATTCTTATACTAGCACTTCTGTGCCTTAGGGTTGCCGCCT
    3010      3020      3030      3040      3050      3060      3070      3080      3090      3100      3110      3120
CGTTAAGTTCATTGAGATGTTCGAACAGATTAAAAAGACCTTAACCCCAGCCCCAATAGGAATGAGAACATTAAGACAAATAAGAATATGATCGTGAAGACACGGAATCCCAACGGCAGA


                                                    start E3 19K glycoprotein
                                                    M  R  Y  M  I  L  G  L  L  A  L  A  A  V  C  S  A  A  K  K  V
GCTGCACGCACGTTTGTACCTATTGTCAGCTTTTTAAACGCTGGGGGCAACATCCAAGATGAGGTACATGATTTTAGGCTTGCTCGCCCTTGCGGCAGTCTGCAGCGCTGCCAAAAAGGT
    3130      3140      3150      3160      3170      3180      3190      3200      3210      3220      3230      3240
CGACGTGCGTGCAAACATGGATAACAGTCGAAAAATTTGCCGACCCCGTTGTAGGTTCTACTCCAGTCTACTAAAATCCGAACGACGGGAACGCCGTCAGACGTCGCGACGGTTTTTCCA


  E  F  K  E  P  A  C  N  V  T  F  K  S  E  A  N  E  C  T  T  L  I  K  C  T  T  E  H  E  K  L  I  I  R  H  K  D  K  I  G
TGAGTTTAAGGAACCAGCTTGCAATGTTACATTTAAATCAGAAGCTAATGAATGCACTACTCTTATAAAATGCACCACAGAACATGAAAAGCTTATTATTCGCCACAAAGACAAAATTGG
    3250      3260      3270      3280      3290      3300      3310      3320      3330      3340      3350      3360
ACTCAAATTCCTTGGTCGAACGTTACAATGTAAATTTAGTCTTCGATTACTTACGTGATGAGAATATTTTACGTGGTGTCTTGTACTTTTCGAATAATAAGCGGTGTTTCTGTTTTAACC


  K  Y  A  V  Y  A  I  W  Q  P  G  D  T  N  D  Y  N  V  T  V  F  Q  G  E  N  R  K  T  F  M  Y  K  F  P  F  Y  E  M  C  D
CAAGTATGCTGTATATGCTATTTGGCAGCCAGGTGACACTAACGACTATAATGTCACAGTCTTCCAAGGTGAAAATCGTAAAACTTTTATGTATAAATTTCCATTTTATGAAATGTGCGA
    3370      3380      3390      3400      3410      3420      3430      3440      3450      3460      3470      3480
GTTCATACGACATATACGATAAACCGTCGGTCCACTGTGATTGCTGATATTACAGTGTCAGAAGGTTCCACTTTTAGCATTTTGAAAATACATATTTAAAGGTAAAATACTTTACACGCT


  I  T  M  Y  M  S  K  Q  Y  K  L  W  P  Q  K  C  L  E  N  T  G  F  C  S  T  A  L  L  I  T  A  L  A  L  V  C  T  L
TATTACCATGTACATGAGCAAACAGTACAAGTTGTGGCCCCCACAAAAGTGTTTAGAGAACACTGGCACCTTTTGTTCCACCGCTCTGCTTATTACAGCGCTTGCTTTGGTATGTACCTT
    3490      3500      3510      3520      3530      3540      3550      3560      3570      3580      3590      3600
ATAATGGTACATGTACTCGTTTGTCATGTTCAACACCGGGGGTGTTTTCACAAATCTCTTGTGACCGTGGAAAAACAAGGTGGCGAGACGAATAATGTCGCGAACGAAACCATACATGGAA
```

Table 6.1 (Continued)

```
                          start ORF 11.4K
                                             stop E3 19K glycoprotein
  L  Y  L  K  Y  K  S  R  R  S  F  I  D  E  K  K  M  P  *
                          M  K  R  K  C  L  D  F  P  L  A  C  I  P  L  D  N  L  L  Y  V  G  Y  A  P  G  G  Q
ACTTTATCTCAAATACAAAAGCAGACGCAGTTTTATTGATGAAAAGAAAATGCCTTGATTTTCCGCTTGCTTGTATTCCCCTGGACAATTTACTCTATGTGGGATATGCTCCAGGCGGGC
   3610      3620      3630      3640      3650      3660      3670      3680      3690      3700      3710      3720
TGAAATAGAGTTTATGTTTTCGTCTGCGTCAAAATAACTACTTTTCTTTTACGGAACTAAAAGGCGAACGAACATAAGGGGACCTGTTAAATGAGATACACCCTATACGAGGTCCGCCCG
```

```
                                                                                        ORF 11.6K start
                                                                                                      M  T
  D  Y  T  H  N  L  Q  I  K  L  S  W  T  L  A  P  D  F  C  Q  R  L  H  C  K  F  D  Q  T  Q  L  Q  L  A  C  S  R  D  R
AAGATTATACCCACAACCTTCAAATCAAACTTTCCTGGACGTTAGCGCCTGATTTCTGCCAGCGCCTGCACTGCAAATTTGATCAAACCCAGCTTCAGCTTGCCTGCTCCAGAGATGACC
   3730      3740      3750      3760      3770      3780      3790      3800      3810      3820      3830      3840
TTCTAATATGGGTGTTGGAAGTTTAGTTTGAAAGGACCTGCAATCGCGGACTAAAGACGGTCGCGGACGTGACGTTTAAACTAGTTTGGGTCGAAGTCGAACGGACGAGGTCTCTACTGG
```

```
                                                                              stop ORF 11.4K
  G  S  T  I  A  P  T  T  D  Y  R  N  T  T  A  T  G  L  T  S  A  L  N  L  P  Q  V  H  A  F  V  N  D  W  A  S  L  D  M  W
     L  N  H  R  A  H  N  G  L  S  Q  H  H  C  Y  R  T  N  I  C  P  K  F  T  P  S  S  C  L  C  Q  *
GGCTCAACCATCGCGCCCACAACGGACTATCGCAACACCACTGCTACCGGACTAACATCTGCCCTAAATTTACCCCAAGTTCATGCCTTTGTCAATGACTGGGCGAGCTTGGACATGTGG
   3850      3860      3870      3880      3890      3900      3910      3920      3930      3940      3950      3960
CCGAGTTGGTAGCGCGGGTGTTGCCTGATAGCGTTGTGGTGACGATGGCCTGATTGTAGACGGGATTTAAATGGGGTTCAAGTACGGAAACAGTTACTGACCCGCTCGAACCTGTACACC
```

```
  W  F  S  I  A  L  M  F  V  C  L  I  I  M  W  L  I  C  C  L  K  R  R  R  A  R  P  P  I  Y  R  P  I  I  V  L  N  P  H  N
TGGTTTTCCATAGCGCTTATGTTTGTTTGCCTTATTATTATGTGGCTTATTTGTTGCCTAAAGCGCAAGCGCGCCAGACCCCCCATCTATAGGCCTATCATTGTGCTCAACCCACACAAT
   3970      3980      3990      4000      4010      4020      4030      4040      4050      4060      4070      4080
ACCAAAAGGTATCGCGAATACAAACAAACGGAATAATAATACACCGAATAAACAACGGATTTCGCGTCTGCGCGGTCTGGGGGGTAGATATCCGGATAGTAACACGAGTTGGGTGTGTTA
```

```
                                                        stop ORF 11.6K
                                                          start ORF 10.4K       3'-poly(A) E3 mRNA
  E  K  I  H  R  L  D  G  L  K  P  C  S  L  L  L  Q  Y  D  *
                                                              M  I  P  R  V  L  I  L  L  T  L  V  A  L  F  C  A  C
GAAAAAAATTCATAGATTGGACGGTCTGAAACCATGTTCTCTTCTTTTACAGTATGATTAAATGAGACATGATTCCTCGAGTTCTTATATTATTGACCCTTGTTGCGCTTTTCTGTGCGTG
   4090      4100      4110      4120      4130      4140      4150      4160      4170      4180      4190      4200
CTTTTTAAGTATCTAACCTGCCAGACTTTGGTACAAGAGAAGAAAATGTCATACTAATTTACTCTGTACTAAGGAGCTCAAGAATAATAACTGGGAACAACGCGAAAAGACACGCAC
```

```
  S  T  L  A  A  V  A  H  I  E  V  D  C  I  P  P  F  T  V  Y  L  L  Y  G  F  V  T  L  I  L  I  C  S  L  V  T  V  V  I  A
CTCTACATTGGCCGCGGTCGCTCACATCGAAGTAGATTGCATCCCACCTTTCACAGTTTACCTGCTTTACGGATTTGTCACCCTTATCCTCATCTGCAGCCTCGTCACTGTAGTCATCGC
   4210      4220      4230      4240      4250      4260      4270      4280      4290      4300      4310      4320
GAGATGTAACCGGCGCCAGCGAGTGTAGCTTCATCTAACGTAGGGTGGAAAGTGTCAAATGGACGAAATGCCTAAACAGTGGGAATAGGAGTAGACGTCGGAGCAGTGACATCAGTAGCG
```

```
                                                                                        stop ORF 10.4K
                                                                                          start E3 "14.5K"
                                                                          D  <--- EcoRI ---> E
                                                                                          M  K  R  S  V
  F  I  Q  F  I  D  W  V  C  V  R  I  A  Y  L  R  H  H  P  Q  Y  R  D  R  T  I  A  D  L  R  I  L  *
CTTCATTCAGTTCATTGACTGGGTTTGTGTGCGCATTGCGTACCTCAGGCACCATCCGCAATACAGAGACAGGACTATAGCTGATCTTCTCAGAATTCTTTAATTATGAAACGGAGTGTC
   4330      4340      4350      4360      4370      4380      4390      4400      4410      4420      4430      4440
GAAGTAAGTCAAGTAACTGACCCAAACACACGCGTAACGCATGGAGTCCGTGGTAGGCGTTATGTCTCTGTCCTGATATCGACTAGAAGAGTCTTAAGAAATTAATACTTTGCCTCACAG
```

```
  I  F  V  L  L  I  F  C  A  L  P  V  L  C  S  Q  T  S  A  P  P  K  R  H  I  S  C  R  F  T  Q  I  W  N  I  P  S  C  Y  N
ATTTTTGTTTTGCTGATTTTTTGCGCCCTACCTGTGCTTTGCTCCCAAACCTCAGCGCCTCCCAAAAGACATATTTCCTGCAGATTCACTCAAATATGGAACATTCCCAGCTGCTACAAC
   4450      4460      4470      4480      4490      4500      4510      4520      4530      4540      4550      4560
TAAAAACAAAACGACTAAAAAACGCGGGATGGACACGAAACGAGGGTTTGGAGTCGCGGAGGGTTTTCTGTATAAAGGACGTCTAAGTGAGTTTATACCTTGTAAGGGTCGACGATGTTG
```

```
  K  Q  S  D  L  S  E  A  W  L  Y  A  I  I  S  V  M  V  F  C  S  T  I  F  A  L  A  I  Y  P  Y  L  D  I  G  W  N  A  I  D
AAACAGAGCGATTTGTCAGAAGCCTGGTTATACGCCATCATCTCTGTCATGGTTTTTGCAGTACCATATATCCATACCTTGACATTGGCTGGAATGCCATAGAT
   4570      4580      4590      4600      4610      4620      4630      4640      4650      4660      4670      4680
TTTGTCTCGCTAAACAGTCTTCGGACCAATATGCGGTAGTAGAGACAGTACCAAAAAACGTCATGGTAAAAACGGGATCGGTATATAGGTATGGAACTGTAACCGACCTTACGGTATCTA
                                                                                          *  G  Y  I  W  V  K  V  N  A  P  I  G  Y  I
                                                                                          stop ORF 10.6K
```

```
  A  M  N  H  P  T  F  P  V  P  A  V  I  P  L  Q  Q  V  I  A  P  I  N  Q  P  R  P  P  S  P  T  P  T  E  I  S  Y  F  N  L
GCCATGAACCACCCTACTTTCCCAGTGCCCGCTGTCATACCACTGCAACAGGTTATTGCCCCAATCAATCAGCCTCGCCCCCCTTCTCCCACCCCCACTGAGATTAGCTACTTTAATTTG
   4690      4700      4710      4720      4730      4740      4750      4760      4770      4780      4790      4800
CGGTTACTTGGTGGGATGAAAGGGTCACGGGCGACAGTATGGTGACGTTGTCCAATAACGGGGTTAGTTAGTCGGAGCGGGGGGAAGAGGGTGGGGGTGACTCTAATCGATGAAATTAAAC
  G  H  V  V  R  S  E  W  H  G  S  D  Y  W  Q  L  L  N  N  G  W  D  I  L  R  A  G  R  R  G  G  G  S  L  N  A  V  K  I  Q
```

```
  ┌─5' late z leader; also splice E3 mRNA
  │    start E3 "14K"
  │         stop E3 "14.5K"
  T │  G  G  D  D  *
       M  T  E  S  L  D  L  E  L  D  G  I  N  T  E  Q  R  L  L  E  R  R  K  A  A  S  E  R  E  R  L  K  Q  E  V  E  D
ACAGGTGGAGATGACTGAATCTCTAGATCTAGAATTGGATGGAATTAACACCGAACAGCGCCTACTAGAAAGGCGCAAGGCGGCGTCCGAGCGAGAACGCCTAAAACAAGAAGTTGAAGA
   4810      4820      4830      4840      4850      4860      4870      4880      4890      4900      4910      4920
TGTCCACCTCTACTGACTTAGAGATCTAGATCTTAACCTACCTTAATTGTGGCTTGTCGCGGATGATCTTTCCGCGTTCCGCCGCAGGCTCGCTCTTGCGGATTTTGTTCTTCAACTTCT
  C  T  S  I  V  S  D  R  S  R  S  N  S  P  I  L  V  S  C  R  R  S  S  L  R  L  A  A  D  S  R  S  R  R  F  C  S  T  S  S
```

```
       3' late z leader;  ┌─also splice E3 mRNA
  M  V  N  L  H  Q  C  K  R │ G  I  F  C  V  V  K  Q  A  K  L  T  Y  E  K  T  T  T  G  N  R  L  S  Y  K  L  P  T  Q  R  Q
CATGGTTAACCTACACCAGTGTAAAAGAGGTATCTTTTGTGTGGTCAAGCAGGCCAAACTTACCTACGAAAAAACCACTACCGGCAACCGCCTCAGCTACAAGCTACCCACCCAGCGCCA
   4930      4940      4950      4960      4970      4980      4990      5000      5010      5020      5030      5040
GTACCAATTGGATGTGGTCACATTTCTCCATAGAAAACACACCAGTTCGTCCGGTTTGAATGGATGCTTTTTTGGTGATGGCCGTTGGCGGAGTCGATGTTCGATGGGTGGGTCGCGGT
GTACCAATTGGATGTGGTCACATTTCTCCATAGAAAACACACCAGTTCGTCCGGTTTGAATGGATGCTTTTTTGGTGATGGCCGTTGGCGGAGTCGATGTTCGATGGGTGGGTCGCGGT
  M
start ORF 10.6K
```

Table 6.1 (Continued)

```
     K L V L M V G E K P I T V T Q H S A E T E G C L H F P Y Q G P E D L C T L I K T
AAAACTGGTGCTTATGGTGGGAGAAAAACCTATCACCGTCACCCAGCACTCGGCAGAAACAGAGGGCTGCCTGCACTTCCCCTATCAGGGTCCAGAGGACCTCTGCACTCTTATTAAAAC
     5050      5060      5070      5080      5090      5100      5110      5120      5130      5140      5150      5160
TTTTGACCACGAATACCACCCTCTTTTTGGATAGTGGCAGTGGGTCGTGAGCCGTCTTTGTCTCCCGACGGACGTGAAGGGGATAGTCCCAGGTCTCCTGGAGACGTGAGAATAATTTTG


                                    stop E3 "14K"                          ┌─ 3'-poly(A) E3
      M C G I R D L I P F N *                                             ↓
CATGTGTGGTATTAGAGATCTTATTCCATTCAACTAACATAAACACAAATAAATTACTTACTTAAAATCAGTCAGCAAATCTTTGTCCAGCTTATTCAGCATCACCTCCTTTCCTTCCT
     5170      5180      5190      5200      5210      5220      5230      5240      5250      5260      5270      5280
GTACACACCATAATCTCTAGAATAAGGTAAGTTGATTGTATTTGTGTGTTATTTAATGAATGAATTTTAGTCAGTCGTTTAGAAACAGGTCGAATAAGTCGTAGTGGAGGAAAGGAAGGA
                                                                   * K F D T L L D K D L K N L M V E K G E E
                                                                     stop ORF 13.5K


                                                                                  splice L5 mRNA ┐
                                                                                  L5 fiber start │
                                                                                                 │M K
CCCAACTCTGGTATCTCAGCCGCCTTTTAGCTGCAAACTTTCTCCAAAGTTTAAATGGGATGTCAAATTCCTCATGTTCTTGTCCCTCCGCACCCACTATCTTCATATTGTTGCAGATGA
     5290      5300      5310      5320      5330      5340      5350      5360      5370      5380      5390      5400
GGGTTGAGACCATAGAGTCGGCGGAAAATCGACGTTTGAAAGAGGTTTCAAATTTACCCTACAGTTTAAGGAGTACAAGAACAGGGAGGCGTGGGTGATAGAAGTATAACAACGTCTACT
     W S Q Y R L R R K A A F K R W L K F P I D F E E H E Q G E A G V I K M N N C I F


      R A R P S E D T F N P V Y P Y D T E T G P P T V P F L T P P F V S P N G F Q E S
AACGCGCCAGACCGTCTGAAGACACCTTCAACCCCGTGTATCCATATGACACAGAAACCGGGCCTCCAACTGTGCCCTTTCTTACCCCTCCATTTGTTTCACCCAATGGTTTCCAAGAAA
     5410      5420      5430      5440      5450      5460      5470      5480      5490      5500      5510      5520
TTGCGCGGTCTGGCAGACTTCTGTGGAAGTTGGGGCACATAGGTATACTGTGTCGTTTGGCCCGGAGGTTGACACGGGAAAGAATGGGGAGGTAAACAAAGTGGGTTACCAAAGGTTCTTT
     R A L G D S S V K L G T Y G Y S V S V P G G V T G K R V G G N T E G L P K W S L


      P P G V L S L R V S E P L D T S H G M L A L K M G S G L T L D K A G N L T S Q N
GTCCCCCTGGAGTTCTCTCTCTACGCGTCTCCGAACCTTTGGACACCTCCCACGGCATGCTTGGCGCTTAAAATGGGCAGCGGTCTTACCCTAGACAAGGCCGGAAACCTCACCTCCCAA
     5530      5540      5550      5560      5570      5580      5590      5600      5610      5620      5630      5640
CAGGGGGGACCTCAAGAGAGAGATGCGCAGAGGCTTGGAAACCTGTGGAGGGTGCCGTACGAACGCGAATTTTACCCGTCGCCAGAATGGGATCTGTTCCGGCCTTTGGAGTGGAGGGTTT
     G G P T R E R R T E S G K S V E W P M
                            start ORF 13.5K


      V T T V T Q P L K K T K S N I S L D T S A P L T I T S G A L T V A T T A P L I V
ATGTAACCACTGTTACTCAGCCACTTAAAAAAACAAAGTCAAACATAAGTTTGGACACCTCCGCACCACTTACAATTACCTCAGGCGCCCTAACAGTGGCAACCACCGCTCCTCTGATAG
     5650      5660      5670      5680      5690      5700      5710      5720      5730      5740      5750      5760
TACATTGGTGACAATGAGTCGGTGAATTTTTTTGTTTCAGTTTGTATTCAAACCTGTGGAGGCGTGGTGAATGTTAATGGAGTCCGCGGGATTGTCACCGTTGGTGGCGAGGAGACTATC
     * G S L F V F D F M L K S V E A G S V I V E P A R V T A V V A G R I T
     stop ORF 10.7K


      T S G A L S V Q S Q A P L T V Q D S K L S I A T K G P I T V S D G K L A L Q T S
TTACTAGCGGCGCTCTTAGCGTACAGTCACAAGCCCCACTGACCGTGCAAGACTCCAAACTAAGCATTGCTACTAAAGGGCCCATTACAGTGTCAGATGGAAAGCTAGCCCTGCAAACAT
     5770      5780      5790      5800      5810      5820      5830      5840      5850      5860      5870      5880
AATGATCGCCGCGAGAATCGCATGTCAGTGTTCGGGGTGACTGGCACGTTCTGAGGTTTGATTCGTAACGATGATTTCCCGGGTAATGTCACAGTCTACCTTTCGATCGGGACGTTTGTA
     V L P A R L T C D C A G S V T C S E L S L M A V L P G M V T D S P F S A R C V D


      A P L S G S D S D T L T V T A S P P L T T A T G S L G I N M E D P I Y V N N G K
CAGCCCCCCTCTCTGGCAGTGACAGCGACCACCCTTACTGTAACTGCATCACCCCCGCTAACTACTGCCACGGGTAGCTTGGGCATTAACATGGAAGATCCTATTTATGTAAATAATGGAA
     5890      5900      5910      5920      5930      5940      5950      5960      5970      5980      5990      6000
GTCGGGGGGAGAGACCGTCACTGTCGCTGTGGGAATGACATTGACGTAGTGGGGGCGATTGATGACGGTGCCCATCGAACCCGTAATGTACCTTCTAGGATAAATACATTTATTACCTT
     A G R E P L S L S V R V T V A D G G S V V A V P L K P M L M
                                       start ORF 10.7K


      I G I K I S G P L Q V A Q N S D T L T V V T G P G V T V E Q N S L R T K V A G A
AAATAGGAATTAAAATAAGCGGTCCTTTGCAAGTAGCACAAAACTCCGATACACTAACAGTAGTTACTGGACCAGGTGTCACCGTTGAACAAAACTCCCTTAGAACCAAAGTTGCAGGAG
     6010      6020      6030      6040      6050      6060      6070      6080      6090      6100      6110      6120
TTTATCCTTAATTTTATTCGCCAGGAAACGTTCATCGTGTTTGAGGCTATGTGATTGTCATCAATGACCTGGTCCACAGTGGCAACTTGTTTTGAGGGAATCTTGGTTTCAACGTCCTC


      I G Y D S S N N M E I K T G G G M R I N N N L L I L D V D Y P F D A Q T K L R L
CTATTGGTTATGATTCATCAAACAACATGGAAATTAAAACGGGCGGTGGCATGCGTATAAATAACAACTTGTTAATTCTAGATGTGGATTACCCATTTGATGCTCAAACAAAACTACGTC
     6130      6140      6150      6160      6170      6180      6190      6200      6210      6220      6230      6240
GATAACCAATACTAAGTAGTTTGTTGTACCTTTAATTTTGCCCGCCACCGTACGCATATTTATTGTTGAACAATTAAGATCTACACCTAATGGGTAAACTACGAGTTTGTTTTGATGCAG


      K L G Q G P L Y I N A S H N L D I N Y N R G L Y L F N A S N N T K K L E V S I K
TTAAACTGGGGCAGGGACCCCTGTATATTAATGCATCTCATAACTTGGACATAAACTATAACAGAGGCCTATACCTTTTTAATGCATCAAACAATACTAAAAAACTGGAAGTTAGCATAA
     6250      6260      6270      6280      6290      6300      6310      6320      6330      6340      6350      6360
AATTTGACCCCGTCCCTGGGGACATATAATTACGTAGAGTATTGAACCTGTATTTGATATTGTCTCCGGATATGGAAAAATTACGTAGTTTGTTATGATTTTTTGACCTTCAATCGTATT


      K S S G L N F D N T A I A I N A G K G L E F D T N T S E S P D I N P I K T K I G
AAAAATCCAGTGGACTAAACTTTGATAATACTGCCATAGCTATAAATGCAGGAAAGGGTCTGGAGTTTGATACAAACACATCTGAGTCTCCAGATATCAACCCAATAAAAACTAAAATTG
     6370      6380      6390      6400      6410      6420      6430      6440      6450      6460      6470      6480
TTTTTAGGTCACCTGATTTGAAACTATTATGACGGTATCGATATTTACGTCCTTTCCCAGACCTCAAACTATGTTTGTGTAGACTCAGAGGTCTATAGTTGGGTTATTTTTGATTTTAAC


      S G I D Y N E N G A M I T K L G A G L S F D N S G A I T I G N K N D D K L T L W
GCTCTGGCATTGATTACAATGAAAACGGTGCCATGATTACTAAACTTGGAGCGGGTTTAAGCTTTGACAACTCAGGGGCCATTACAATAGGAAACAAAAATGATGACAAACTTACCCTGT
     6490      6500      6510      6520      6530      6540      6550      6560      6570      6580      6590      6600
CGAGACCGTAACTAATGTTACTTTTGCCACGGTACTAATGATTTGAACCTCGCCCAAATTCGAAACTGTTGAGTCCCCGGTAATGTTATCCTTTGTTTTTACTACTGTTTGAATGGGACA


                      E <---- EcoRI ----> C
      T T P D P S P N C R I H S D N D C K F T L V L T K C G S Q V L A T V A A L A V S
GGACAACCCCAGACCCATCTCCTAACTGCAGAATTCATTCAGTAATAATGACTGCAAATTTACTTTGGTTCTTACAAAATGTGGGAGTCAAGTACTACTGTAGCTGCTTTTGGCTGTAT
     6610      6620      6630      6640      6650      6660      6670      6680      6690      6700      6710      6720
CCTGTTGGGGTCTGGGTAGAGGATTGACGTCTTAAGTAAGTCTATTACTGACGTTTAAATGAAACCAAGAATGTTTTACACCCTCAGTTCATGATCGATGACATCGACGAAACCGACATA
```

Table 6.1 (Continued)

```
       G  D  L  S  S  M  T  G  T  V  A  S  V  S  I  F  L  R  F  D  Q  N  G  V  L  M  E  N  S  S  L  K  K  H  Y  W  N  F  R  N
CTGGAGATCTTTCATCCATGACACCGTTGCAAGTGTTAGTATATTCCTTAGATTTGACCAAAACGGTGTTCTAATGGAGAACTCCTCACTTAAAAAACATTACTGGAACTTTAGAA
    6730      6740      6750      6760      6770      6780      6790      6800      6810      6820      6830      6840
GACCTCTAGAAAGTAGGTACTGTCCGTGGCAACGTTCACAATCATATAAGGAATCTAAACTGGTTTTGCCACAAGATTACCTCTTGAGGAGTGAATTTTTTGTAATGACCTTGAAATCTT
```

```
       G  N  S  T  N  A  N  P  Y  T  N  A  V  G  F  M  P  N  L  L  A  Y  P  K  T  Q  S  Q  T  A  K  N  N  I  V  S  Q  V  Y  L
ATGGGAACTCAACTAATGCAAATCCATACACAAATGCAGTTGGATTTATGCCTAACCTTCTAGCCTATCCAAAAACCCAAAGTCAAACTGCTAAAAATAACATTGTCAGTCAAGTTTACT
    6850      6860      6870      6880      6890      6900      6910      6920      6930      6940      6950      6960
TACCCTTGAGTTGATTACGTTTAGGTATGTGTTTACGTCAACCTAAATACGGATTGGAAGATCGGATAGGTTTTTGGGTTTCAGTTTGACGATTTTTATTGTAACAGTCAGTTCAAATGA
                                                                      * G  I  W  F  G  L  T  L  S  S  F  I  V  N  D  T  L  N  V  Q
                                                                   stop ORF 9.7K
```

```
       H  G  D  K  T  K  P  M  I  L  T  I  T  L  N  G  T  S  E  S  T  E  T  S  E  V  S  T  Y  S  M  S  F  T  W  S  W  E  S  G
TGCATGGTGATAAAACTAAACCTATGATACTTACCATTACACTTAATGGCACTAGTGAATCCACAGAAACTAGCGAGGTAAGCACTTACTCTATGTCTTTTACATGGTCCTGGGAAAGTG
    6970      6980      6990      7000      7010      7020      7030      7040      7050      7060      7070      7080
ACGTACCACTATTTTGATTGGATACTATGAATGGTAATGTGAATTACCGTGATCACTTAGGTGTCTTTGATCGCTCCATTCGTGAATGAGATACAGAAATGTACCAGGACCCTTTCAC
    M  T  I  F  S  F  R  H  Y  K  G  N  C  K  I  A  S  T  F  G  C  F  S  A  L  Y  A  S  V  R  H  R  K  C  P  G  P  F  T  S
```

```
                                                                 3'-poly(A) signal L5  mRNA
                                                                 stop L5 fiber
       K  Y  T  T  E  T  F  A  T  N  S  Y  T  F  S  Y  I  A  Q  E  *
GAAAATACACCACTGAAACTTTTGCTACCAACTCTTACACCTTCTCCTACATTGCCCAGGAATAAAGAATCGTGAACCTGTTGCATGTTATGTTTCAACGTGTTTATTTTTCAATTGCAG
    7090      7100      7110      7120      7130      7140      7150      7160      7170      7180      7190      7200
CTTTTATGTGGTGACTTTGAAAACGATGGTTGAGAATGTGGAAGAGGATGTAACGGGTCCTTATTTCTTAGCACTTGGACAACGTACAATACAAAGTTGCACAAATAAAAAGTTAACGTC
    F  V  G  S  F  S  K  S  G  V  R  V  G  E  G  V  N  G  L  F  L  S  D  H  V  Q  Q  M
                                                                 start ORF 9.7K        3'-poly(A) E4?
```

```
AAAATTTCAAGTCATTTTTCATTCAGTAGTATAGCCCCACCACCACACATAGCTTATATTGATCACCGTACCTTAATCAAACTCACAGAACCCTAGTATTCAACCTGCCACCTCCCTCCCAA
    7210      7220      7230      7240      7250      7260      7270      7280      7290      7300      7310      7320
TTTTAAAGTTCAGTAAAAAGTAAGTCATCATATCGGGGTGGTGGTATCGAATATAACTAGTGGCATGGAATTAGTTTGAGTGTCTTGGGATCATAAGTTGGACGGTGGAGGGGAGGGTT
                                                             L  V  R  T  N  L  R  G  G  G  E  W  C
                                                             stop E4 region 7
```

```
CACACAGAGTACACAGTCCTTTCTCCCCGGCTGGCCTTAAAAAGCATCATATCATGGGTAACAGACATATTCTTAGGTGTTATATTCCACACGGTTTCCTGTCGAGCCAAACGCTCATCA
    7330      7340      7350      7360      7370      7380      7390      7400      7410      7420      7430      7440
GTGTGTCTCATGTGTCAGGAAAGAGGGGCCGACCGGAATTTTTCGTAGTATAGTACCCATTGTCTGTATAAGAATCCACAATATAAGGTGTGCCAAAGGACAGCTCGGTTTGCGAGTAGT
    V  S  Y  V  T  R  E  G  R  S  A  K  F  L  M  M  D  H  T  V  S  M  N  K  P  T  I  N  W  V  T  E  Q  R  A  L  R  E  D  T
```

```
GTGATATTAATAAACTCCCCGGGCAGCTCGCTTAAGTTCATGTCGCTGTCCAGCTGCTGAGCCACAGGCTGCTGTCCAACTTGCGGTTGCTCAACGGGCGGCGAAGGGGAAGTCCACGCC
    7450      7460      7470      7480      7490      7500      7510      7520      7530      7540      7550      7560
CACTATAATTATTTGAGGGGCCCGTCGAGCGAATTCAAGTACAGCGACAGGTCGACGACTCGGTGTCCGACGACAGGTTGAACGCCAACGAGTTGCCCGCCGCTTCCCCTTCAGGTGCGG
    I  N  I  F  E  G  P  L  E  S  L  N  M  D  S  D  L  Q  Q  A  V  P  Q  Q  Q  G  V  Q  P  Q ⌐
                                                                                      └ splice E4 region 7
```

```
TACATGGGGGTAGAGTCATAATCGTGCATCAGGATAGGGCGGTGGTGCTGCAGCAGCGCGCGAATAAAACTGCTGCCGCCGCCGCTCCGTCCTGCAGGAATACAACATGGCAGTGGTCTCC
    7570      7580      7590      7600      7610      7620      7630      7640      7650      7660      7670      7680
ATGTACCCCATCTCAGTATTAGCACGTAGTCCTATCCCGCCCACCACGACGTCGTCGCGCGCTTATTTGACGACGGCGGCGGCGAGGCAGGACGTCCTTATGTTGTACGTCACCAGAGG
    * M  P  T  S  D  Y  D  H  M  L  I  P  R  H  H  Q  L  L  A  R  I  F  Q  Q  R  R  R  E  T  R  C  S  Y  L  M  A  T  T  E  E
stop ORF starting at 8444 (region 6)
```

```
TCAGCGATGATTCGCACCGCCCGCAGCATGAGACGCCTTGTCCTCCGGGCACAGCAGCGCACCCTGATCTCACTTAAATCAGCACAGTAACTGCAGCACAGCACCACAATATTGTTCAAA
    7690      7700      7710      7720      7730      7740      7750      7760      7770      7780      7790      7800
AGTCGCTACTAAGCGTGGCGGGCGTCGTACTCTGCGGAACAGGAGGCCCGTGTCGTCGCGTGGGACTAGAGTGAATTTAGTCGTGTCATTGACGTCGTGTCGTGGTGTTATAACAAGTTT
    A  I  I  R  V  A  R  L  M  L  R  R  T  R  R  A  C  C  R  V  R  I  E  S  L  D  A  C  Y  S  C  C  L  V  V  I  N  N  L  I
```

```
ATCCCACAGTGCAAGGCGCTGTATCCAAAGCTCATGGCGGGGACCACAGAACCCACGTGGCCATCATACCAACAAGCGCAGGTAGATTAAGTGGCGACCCCTCATAAACACGCTGGACATA
    7810      7820      7830      7840      7850      7860      7870      7880      7890      7900      7910      7920
TAGGGTGTCACGTTCCGCGACATAGGTTTCGAGTACCGCCCCTGGTGTCTGGGTGCACCGGTAGTATGGTGTTCGCGTCCATCTAATTCACCGCTGGGGAGTATTTGTGCGACCTGTAT
    G  C  H  L  A  S  Y  G  F  S  M  A  P  V  V  S  G  V  H  G  D  Y  W  L  R  L  Y  I  L  H  R  G  R  M  F  V  S  S  M  F
```

```
AACATTACCTCTTTTGGCATGTTGTAATTCACCACCTCCCGGTACCATATAAACCTCTGATTAAACATGGCGCCATCCACCACCATCCTAAACCAGCTGGCCAAAACCTGCCCGCCGGCT
    7930      7940      7950      7960      7970      7980      7990      8000      8010      8020      8030      8040
TTGTAATGGAGAAAACCGTACAACATTAAGTGGTGGAGGGCCATGGTATATTTGGAGACTAATTTGTACCGCGGTAGGTGGTGGTAGGATTTGGTCGACCGGTTTTGGACGGGCGGCCGA
    M  V  E  K  P  M  N  Y  N  V  V  E  R  Y  W  I  F  R  Q  N  F  M  A  G  D  V  V  M  R  F  W  S  A  L  V  Q  G  G  A  I
```

```
                                        start ORF 10.7K
                                        M  T  V  E  S  P  G  L  V  T  M  D  H  H  A  R  H  D  I  N  V  G  T  T  Q  A  H  V  H  T  L
ATGCACTGCAGGGAACCGGGACTGGAACAATGACAGTGGAGAGCCCAGGACTCGTAACCATGGATCATCATGCTCGTCATGATATCAATGTTGGCACAACACAGGCACACGTGCATACAC
    8050      8060      8070      8080      8090      8100      8110      8120      8130      8140      8150      8160
TACGTGACGTCCCTTGGCCCTGACCTTGTTACTGTCACCTCTCGGGTCCTGAGCATTGGTACCTAGTAGTACGAGCAGTACTATAGTTACAACCGTGTTGTGTCCGTGTGCACGTATGTG
    C  Q  L  S  G  P  S  S  C  H  C  H  L  A  W  S  E  Y  G  H  I  M  M  S  T  M  I  D  I  N  A  C  C  L  C  V  H  M  C  K
```

```
       P  Q  D  Y  K  L  L  P  R  Q  N  H  I  P  G  N  N  P  F  L  N  Q  R  K  S  H  T  A  G  K  T  S  H  V  T  H  V  V  H  C
TTCCTCAGGATTACAAGCTCCTCCCGCGTCAGAACCATATCCCAGGGAACAACCCATTCCTGAATCAGCGTAAATCCCACACTGCAGGGAGACCTCGCACGTAACTCACGTTGTGCATT
    8170      8180      8190      8200      8210      8220      8230      8240      8250      8260      8270      8280
AAGGAGTCCTAATGTTCGAGGAGGGCGCAGTCTTGGTATAGGGTCCCTTGTTGGGTAAGGACTTAGTCGCATTTAGGGTGTGACGTCCCTTCTGGAGCGTGCATTGAGTGCAACACGTAA
    R  L  I  V  L  E  E  R  T  L  V  M  D  W  P  V  V  W  E  Q  I  L  T  F  G  V  S  C  P  L  G  R  V  S  V↑N  H  M  T
                                                                                          splice E4 mRNA ┘
```

```
                                start ORF 16.6K            stop ORF 10.7K
                                M  V  A  R  V  S  V  S  K  G  G  R  R  S  L  L  Y  G  V  R  R  D  N  R  D  R
       Q  S  V  T  F  G  Q  Q  R  M  I  L  Q  Y  S  A  G  L  C  L  K  R  R  *
GTCAAAGTGTTACATTCGGGCAGCAGCGGATGATCCTCCAGTATGGTAGCGCGGGTCTCTGTCTCAAAAGGAGGTAGGCGATCCCTACTGTACGGAGTGCGCCGAGACAACCGAGATCGT
    8290      8300      8310      8320      8330      8340      8350      8360      8370      8380      8390      8400
CAGTTTCACAATGTAAGCCCGTCGTCGCCTACTAGGAGGTCATACCATCGCGCCCAGAGACAGAGTTTTCCTCCATCCGCTAGGGATGACATGCCTCACGCGGCTCTGTTGGCTCTAGCA
    L  T  N  C  E  P  L  L  P  H  D  E  L  I  T  A  R  T  E  T  E  F  P  P  L  R  D  R  S  Y  P  T  R  R  S  L  R  S  R  T
                                                                 * Q  V  S  H  A  S  V  V  S  I  T
                                                                 stop E4 region 4
```

Table 6.1 (Continued)

```
  V G R S V M P N G T P D V V I F P E A K P G A G V T N R S A S P V S S L S S L C
GTTGGTCGTAGTGTCATGCCAAATGGAACGCCGGACGTAGTCATATTTCCTGAAGCAAAACCAGGTGCGGGCGTGACAAACAGATCTGCGTCTCCGGTCTCGTCGCTTAGCTCGCTCTGT
    8410      8420      8430      8440      8450      8460      8470      8480      8490      8500      8510      8520
CAACCAGCATCACAGTACGGTTTACCTTGCGGCCTGCATCAGTATAAAGGACTTCGTTTTGGTCCACGCCCGCACTGTTTGTCTAGACGCAGAGGCCAGAGCAGCGAATCGAGCGAGACA
  N T T T D H W I S R R V Y D Y K R F C F W T R A H C V S R R R R R D R R K A R E T
  P R L T M G F P V G S T T M
                    E4 region 6 start     └ splice E4 mRNA


  V V V V V V Y P L S Q S I Q A P P G F G F Y V N S F M R R C P D N I H H R R I S H
GTAGTAGTTGTAGTATATCCACTCTCTCAAAGCATCCAGGCGCCCCCTGGCTTCGGGTTCTATGTAAACTCCTTCATGCGCCGCTGCCCTGATAACATCCACCACCGCAGAATAAGCCAC
    8530      8540      8550      8560      8570      8580      8590      8600      8610      8620      8630      8640
CATCATCAACATCATATAGGTGAGAGAGTTTCGTAGGTCCGCGGGGGACCGAAGCCCAAGATACATTTGAGGAAGTACGCGGCGACGGGACTATTGTAGGTGGTGGCGTCTTATTCGGTG
  Y Y N Y Y I W E R L A D L R G R A E P E I Y V G E H A A A R I V D V V A S Y A V


  T Q P T Y T F V L R V T H G R S G K S W K N H V F F F L F Q K I I Q N L K M K I
ACCCAGCCAACCTACACATTCGTTCTGCGAGTCACACACGGGAGGAGCGGGAAGAGCTGGAAGAACCATGTTTTTTTTTTTTTATTCCAAAAGATTATCCAAAACCTCAAATGAAGATC
    8650      8660      8670      8680      8690      8700      8710      8720      8730      8740      8750      8760
TGGGTCGGTTGGATGTGTAAGCAAGACGCTCAGTGTGTGCCCTCCTCGCCCTTCTCGACCTTCTTGGTACAAAAAAAAAAAAATAAGGTTTTCTAATAGGTTTTGGAGTTTTACTTCTAG
  G L W G V C E N Q S D C V P P A P L A P L V M     *   E L L N D L V E F H L D
                              E4 region 4 start        stop E4 region 3


        stop ORF 16.6K                                        start ORF 12.7K
        Y  *                                                  M L H N G F Q K A N C P H V Q
TATTAAGTGAACGCGCTCCCCTCCGGTGGCGTGGTCAAACTCTACAGCCAAAGAACAGATAATGGCATTTGTAAGATGTTGCACAATGGCTTCCAAAAGGCAAACTGCCCTCACGTCCAA
    8770      8780      8790      8800      8810      8820      8830      8840      8850      8860      8870      8880
ATAATTCACTTGCGCGAGGGGAGGCCACCGCACCAGTTTGAGATGTCGGTTTCTTGTCTATTACCGTAAACATTCTACAACGTGTTACCGAAGGTTTTCCGTTTGACGGGAGTGCAGGTT
  I L H V R E G G T A H D F E V A L S C I I A N T L H Q V I A E L L C V A R V D L


  V D V K A K P F R V N L L L Y K H S S T F N H A Q I I F I S P P Y Q Y V S K Q I P
GTGGACGTAAAGGCTAAACCCTTCAGGGTGAATCTCCTCTATAAACATTCCAGCACCTTCAACCATGCCCAAATAATTTTCATCTCGCCACCTTATCAATATGTCTCTAAGCAAATCCCG
    8890      8900      8910      8920      8930      8940      8950      8960      8970      8980      8990      9000
CACCTGCATTTCCGATTTGGGAAGTCCCACTTAGAGGAGTATATTTGTAAGGTCGTGGAAGTTGGTACGGGTTTATTAAAAGTAGAGCGGTGGAATAGTTATACAGAGATTCGTTTAGGGC
  H V Y L S F G E P H I E E I F M G A G E V M G L Y N E D R W R I L I D R L L D R


  N I K S G H C K N L L Q S A L H L Q P P Q A A N H D C K N S G S S Q T C I R F K S
AATATTAAGTCCGGCCATTGTAAAAATCTGCTCCAGAGCGCCCTCCACCTTCAGCCTCAAGCAGCGAATCATGATTGCAAAAATTCAGGTTCCTCACAGACCTGTATAAGATTCAAAAGC
    9010      9020      9030      9040      9050      9060      9070      9080      9090      9100      9110      9120
TTATAATTCAGGCCGGTAACATTTTTAGACGAGGTCTCGCGGGAGGTGGAAGTCGGAGTTCGTCGCTTAGTACTAACGTTTTTAAGTCCAAGGAGTGTCTGGACATATTCTAAGTTTTCG
  I N L G A M T F I Q E L A G E V K L R L C R I M                *   S Q L F E P E E C V Q I L N L L P
                                            start E4 region 3
                                            stop E4 region 2                           └ splice E4 mRNA


                            stop ORF 12.7K
  G T L T K I P R S R R S L R R A S  *
GGAACATTAACAAAAATACCGCGATCCCGTAGGTCCCTTCGCAGGGCCAGCTGAACATAATCGTGCAGGTCTGCACGGACCAGCGCGGCCACTTCCCCGCCAGGAACCATGACAAAAGAA
    9130      9140      9150      9160      9170      9180      9190      9200      9210      9220      9230      9240
CCTTGTAATTGTTTTTATGGCGCTAGGGCATCCAGGGAAGCGTCCCGGTCGACTTGTATTAGCACGTCCAGACGTGCCTGGTCGCGCCGGTGAAGGGCGGTCCTTGGTACTGTTTTCTT
  V N V F I G R D R L D R R L A L Q V Y D H L D A R V L A A V E G G P V M V F S G


CCCACACTGATTATGCACGCGCATACTCGGAGCTATGCTAACCAGCGTAGCCCCTATGTAAGCTTGTTGCATGGGCGGCGATATAAAATGCAAGGTGCTGCTCAAAAAAATCAGGCAAAGCC
    9250      9260      9270      9280      9290      9300      9310      9320      9330      9340      9350      9360
GGGTGTGACTAATACTGTGCGTATGAGCCTCGATACGATTGGTCGCATCGGGGATACATTCGAACAACGCTCCCGCCGCTATATTTTACGTTCCACGACGAGTTTTTTAGTCCGTTTCGG
  V S I I V R M S P A I S V L T A G I Y A Q Q M P P S I F H L T S S L F D P L A E


TCGCGCAAAAAAGCAAGCACATCGTAGTCATGCTCATGCAGATAAAGGCAGGTAAGTTCCGGAACCACCACAGAAAAAGACACCATTTTTCTCTCAAACATGTCTGCGGGTTCCTGCATT
    9370      9380      9390      9400      9410      9420      9430      9440      9450      9460      9470      9480
AGCGCGTTTTTTCGTTCGTGTAGCATCAGTACGAGTACGTCTATTTCCGTCCATTCAAGGCCTTGGTGGTGTCTTTTTCTGTGGTAAAAAGAGAGTTTGTACAGACGCCCAAGGACGTAA
  R L F A L V D Y D H E H L Y L C T L E P V V V S F S V M K R E F M D A P E Q M
                                                                         E4 region 2 start
                                                                         splice E4 mRNA


AAACACAAAATAAAATAACAAAAAAAAAAACATTTAAACATTAGAAGCCTGTCTTACAACAGGAAAAACAACCCTTATAAGCATAAGACGGACTACGGCCATGCCGGCGTGACCGTAAAAA
    9490      9500      9510      9520      9530      9540      9550      9560      9570      9580      9590      9600
TTTGTGTTTTATTTTATTGTTTTTTTTTTGTAAATTTGTAATCTTCGGACAGAATGTTGTCCTTTTTGTTGGGAATATTCGTATTCTGCCTGATGCCGGTACGGCCGCACTGGCATTTTT
       *   V N S A Q R V V P F V V R I L M L R V V A M G A H G Y F F
       stop E4 region 1           └ splice E4 region 1--->2


AACTGGTCACCGTGATTAAAAAGCACCACCGACAGTTCCTCGGTCATGTCCGGAGTCATAATGTAAGACTCGGTAAACACATCAGGTTGGTTAACATCGGTCAGTGCTAAAAAGCGACCG
    9610      9620      9630      9640      9650      9660      9670      9680      9690      9700      9710      9720
TTGACCAGTGGCACTAATTTTTCGTGGTGGCTGTCAAGGAGCCAGTACAGGCCTCAGTATTACATTCTGAGCCATTTGTGTAGTCCAACCAATTGTAGCCAGTCACGATTTTTCGCTGGC
  Q D G H N F L V V S L E E T M D P T M I Y S E T F V D P Q N V D T L A L F R G F


AAATAGCCCGGGGGAATACATACCCGCAGGCGTAGAGACAACATTACAGCCCCCATAGGAGGTATAACAAAATTAATAGGAGAGAAAAACACATAAACACCTGAAAAACCCTCCTGCCTA
    9730      9740      9750      9760      9770      9780      9790      9800      9810      9820      9830      9840
TTTATCGGGCCCCCTTATGTATGGGCGTCCGCATCTCTGTTGTAATGTCGGGGGTATCCTCCATATTGTTTTAATTATCCTCTCTTTTTGTGTATTTGTGGACTTTTTGGGAGGACGGAT
  Y G P F I C V R L R L S L M V A G M P V N F N I P S F F V Y V G S F G R P


GGCAAAATAGCACCCTCCCGCTCCAGAACAACATACAGCGCTTCCACAGCGGCAGCCATAACAGTCAGCCTTACCAGTAAAAAAACCTATTAAAAAAACACCACTCGACACGGCACCAGCT
    9850      9860      9870      9880      9890      9900      9910      9920      9930      9940      9950      9960
CCGTTTTATCGTGGGAGGGCGAGGTCTTGTTGTATGTCGCGAAGGTGTCGCCGTCGGTATTGTCAGTCGGAATGGTCATTTTTTGGATAATTTTTTGTGGTGAGCTGTGCCGGTGGTCGA
  L I A G E R E L V V Y L A E V A A A M
               E4 region 1 start        └ splice E4 mRNA
```

Table 6.1 (Continued)

```
CAATCAGTCACAGTGTAAAAAGGGCCAAGTACAGAGCGAGTATATATAGGACTAAAAAATGACGTAACGGTTAAAGTCCACAAAAAACACCCAGAAAACCGCACGCGAACCTACGCCCAG
    9970      9980      9990     10000     10010     10020     10030     10040     10050     10060     10070     10080
GTTAGTCAGTGTCACATTTTTCCCGGTTCATGTCTCGCTCATATATATCCTGATTTTTTACTGCATTGCCAATTTCAGGTGTTTTTTGTGGGTCTTTTGGCGTGCGCTTGGATGCGGGTC
    cap E4 mRNA  ᴸ⊔⊔⊔⊔                                   "TATA" E4
```

```
AAACGAAAGCCAAAAAACCCACAACTTCCTCAAATCTTCACTTCCGTTTTCCCACGATACGTCACTTCCCATTTTAAAAAAACTACAATTCCCAATACATGCAAGTTACTCCGCCCTAAA
    10090     10100     10110     10120     10130     10140     10150     10160     10170     10180     10190     10200
TTTGCTTTCGGTTTTTTGGGTGTTGAAGGAGTTTAGAAGTGAAGGCAAAAGGGTGCTATGCAGTGAAGGGTAAAATTTTTTTGATGTTAAGGGTTATGTACGTTCAATGAGGCGGGATTT
```

```
ACCTACGTCACCCGCCCCGTTCCCACGCCCCGCGCCACGTCACAAACTCCCACCCCCTCATTATCATATTGGCTTCAATCCAAAATAAGGTATATTATTGATGATG
    10210     10220     10230     10240     10250     10260     10270     10280     10290     10300
TGGATGCAGTGGGCGGGGCAAGGGTGCGGGGCGCGGTGCAGTGTTTGAGGTGGGGGAGTAATAGTATAACCGAAGTTAGGTTTTATTCCATATAATAACTACTAC
    ᴸ end ITR
```

underlined), predicted or potential initiation and termination codons (under-lined), and predicted or defined splice points (Table 6.2) (BAKER et al. 1979; AHMED et al. 1982a, b; STÅLHANDSKE et al. (1983); HÉRISSÉ et al. 1981b; M. Rigolet et al., personal communication; PERSSON et al. 1980; FRASER and ZIFF 1978; ZAIN and ROBERTS 1979; ZAIN et al. 1979; BAKER and ZIFF 1981; OOS-TEROM-DRAGON and ANDERSON 1983; CHOW et al. 1979; BERK and SHARP 1978). Above or below the DNA sequence (sense strand) is given the predicted amino acid sequence (in one-letter code; see footnote to Table 6.1) for the C-terminal part of the L4 100K protein, L4 33K, L4 pVIII, the E3 19K glycoprotein, E3 14.5K, E3 14K, the L5 fiber and the presumed E4 proteins. Apart from the genes for these proteins, a number of hitherto unidentified ORFs have been found in the sequence; the amino acid sequences of their hypothetical translation products are also given.

Recently, a sequence comparison between coordinates 89 and 100 has been derived by GINGERAS et al. (1982) using viral Ad2 DNA instead of *E. coli*-cloned Ad2 DNA fragments. Their sequence agrees with the previously published data. It shows a sequence heterogeneity at nucleotide 8711, where the number of T residues in the l-strand is variable, with an average value of 14.

Table 6.2. Landmarks in the Ad2 DNA sequence 70.7–100%

Strand nucleotide		Sequence	Identity
r	l		
	A1	AATTC	*Eco*RI site 70.7% between fragments B and F
	G248	GGTACC	*Kpn*I 72% (end of Sect. 5)
A321			cap sites E2A mRNA (late)
A323			
T352		TACAAA	"TATA" box E2A (late)
	A411	ATG	start L4 33K?
	A606	ATG	start L4 33K?
	T890	TAG	stop L4 100K
	G918		donor L4 33K mRNA splice
	C1121		acceptor L4 33K mRNA splice
	A1362	AATAAA	3′-poly(A) signal?
G1392			donor E2A mRNA splice (early)
G1458			cap sites E2A mRNA (early)

Table 6.2 (Continued)

Strand, nucleotide		Sequence	Identity
r	l		
A1459			
	T1492	TAG	stop L4 33K protein
	A1582	ATG	start L4 protein VIII?
	A1671	AATAAA	3′-poly(A) signal?
	G1739	GAATTC	*Eco*RI site 75.9% between fragments F and D
	T1947	TATAA	"TATA" box E3
	G1976		cap sites E3 mRNA
	A1978		
	T2215		5′-end late x leader
	T2263	TGA	stop L4 protein VIII
	A2266	ATG	start ORF 12.3K
	G2347		3′-end late x leader and donor E3 mRNA splice
	A2572	AATAAA	3′-poly(A) signal L4 mRNA?
	T2587	TAG	stop ORF 12.3K
	T2743		5′-end late y leader and acceptor E3 mRNA splice
	G2926		3′-end late y leader and donor E3 mRNA splice
	A3179	ATG	start E3 19K glycoprotein
A3637		AATAAA	3′-poly(A) signal?
	A3639	ATG	start ORF 11.4K
	T3656	TGA	stop E3 19K glycoprotein
	A3835	ATG	start ORF 11.6K
	T3936	TGA	stop ORF 11.4K
	A4136	ATTAAA	3′-poly(A) signal E3 mRNA
	T4138	TAA	stop ORF 11.6K
	A4148	ATG	start ORF 10.4K
	G4158		3′-poly(A) attachment sites E3 mRNA
	T4165		
	G4413	GAATTC	*Eco*RI site 83.4% between fragments D and E
	T4421	TAA	stop ORF 10.4K
	A4426	ATG	start E3 14.5K
A4638		TAG	stop ORF 10.6K
	G4805		5′-end late z leader and acceptor E3 mRNA splice
	A4811	ATG	start E3 14K
	T4816	TGA	stop E3 14.5K
A4923		ATG	start ORF 10.6K
	G4949		3′-end late z leader and donor E3 mRNA splice
	T5195	TAA	stop E3 14K
	A5209	AATAAA	3′-poly(A) signal E3 mRNA
T5221		TAA	stop ORF 13.5K
	C5230		3′-poly(A) attachment site E3 mRNA
	A5397		acceptor L5 mRNA splice
	A5397	ATG	start L5 fiber
A5578		ATG	start ORF 13.5K
T5659		TGA	stop ORF 10.7K
A5971		ATG	start ORF 10.7K
A6323		ATTAAA	3′-poly(A) signal?
	G6631	GAATTC	*Eco*RI site 89.7% between fragments E and C
T6902		TAG	stop ORF 9.7K
	A7141	AATAAA	3′-poly(A) signal L5 mRNA
	T7143	TAA	stop L5 fiber
A7166		ATG	start ORF 9.7K

Table 6.2 (Continued)

Strand, nucleotide		Sequence	Identity
r	l		
A7188		AATAAA	3'-poly(A) signal E4 mRNA
T7283		TGA	stop E4 region 7
C7559			acceptor E4 region 7 splice
T7562		TAG	stop E4 region 6
	A8070	ATG	start ORF 10.7K
C8271			donor E4 mRNA splice?
	A8323	ATG	start ORF 16.6K
	T8355	TAG	stop ORF 10.7K
T8367		TAG	stop E4 region 4
A8444		ATG	start E4 region 5
G8450			donor E4 mRNA splice?
A8709		ATG	start E4 region 4
T8724		TAA	stop E4 region 3
	T8764	TAA	stop ORF 16.6K
	A8836	ATG	start ORF 16.6K
T9071		TGA	stop E4 region 2
A9072		ATG	start E4 region 3
T9098			donor E4 mRNA splice?
	T9172	TGA	stop ORF 12.7K
G9473			acceptor E4 mRNA splice
A9479		ATG	start E4 region 2
	A9489	AATAAA	3'-poly(A) signal
T9515		TAA	stop E4 region 1
T9537			donor E4 mRNA splice?
A9899		ATG	start E4 region 1
G9914			donor E4 mRNA splice?
A9976			major cap site E4 mRNA
T9977			minor cap sites E4 mRNA
to			
T9981			
T10008		TATATATA	"TATA" box E4
G10203			end ITR

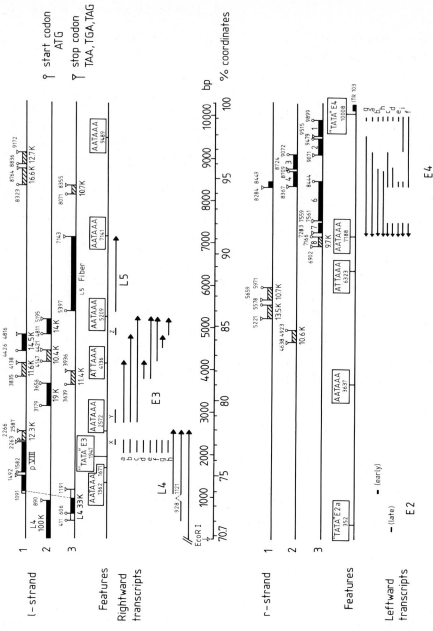

Fig. 6.1. Schematic representation of identified and unidentified reading frames and RNA coordinates in Ad2 DNA between coordinates 70.7 and 100. The map scale in the *center* of the figure reflects a conversion factor of 355 bp, which corresponds for the right end to 1% of the viral genome. Immediately *above* and *below* the scale, the locations of the various rightward transcripts are indicated. On the *next line above* a number of RNA expression signals have been drawn: "TATA" boxes and 3'-poly(A) signals (AATAAA). Lines 1, 2, and 3 in the *upper part* of the figure represent the three possible frames in which the DNA 1-strand can be read. Tracts open for translation are indicated as *solid bars* for known genes and as *hatched bars* for unidentified translatable regions. The open frames are flanked by the symbols ⸮ and Ⴤ, denoting initiation (ATG) and termination (TAA, TAG or TGA) codons respectively. The *numbers* next to the codons are their coordinates, and the *numbers in larger type* refer to the predicted MW of the translation products. *Interrupted lines* connecting solid bars show how open frames are linked due to RNA splicing. The *bottom part* of the figure corresponds to the leftward transcripts

7 DNA Sequence of Human Ad7 (Subgroup B) Between Coordinates 0.0 and 30.2

The sequence (Table 7.1) was determined by DIJKEMA and DEKKER (1979), DIJKEMA et al. (1982), ENGLER and VAN BREE (1982), and ENGLER et al. (1983). It is given in double-stranded format with 120 nucleotides per line, with the numbering (starting at the left terminus of Ad7 DNA) between the two strand sequences. Each number refers to the position above and below its last zero. The following features are marked: the end of the ITR, RNA 5′ termini (cap sites), splice donor and acceptor nucleotides, 3′-poly(A) addition sites, "TATA" boxes and 3′-poly(A) signals (AATAAA; underlined), and predicted or potential initiation and termination codons (underlined) (Table 7.2). For the region between coordinates 0 and 11, the RNA mapping data were described by DIJKEMA et al. (1982), for the remainder of the sequence they were inferred from those of Ad2/Ad5 on the basis of sequence homology. Above or below the DNA sequence (sense strand) are given the predicted amino acid sequences (in one-letter code; see footnote to Table 7.1) for the E1A proteins, the E1B proteins, protein IX (all from DIJKEMA et al. 1982), protein IVa2 (ENGLER and VAN BREE 1982), the 129K DNA polymerase, pTP, the Ad7 "agnoprotein", and the N-terminal residues of the L1 52K, 55K polypeptide (ENGLER et al. 1983). Apart from these identified proteins, a number of hitherto unidentified ORFs have been found in the sequence; the amino acid sequences of their hypothetical translation products are also given.

Table 7.1. Ad7 DNA sequence 0–30.2%

```
CTCTCTATATAATACCTTATAGATGGAATGGTGCCAACATGTAAATGAGGTAATTTAAAAAAGTGCGCGCTGTGTGGTGATTGGCTGTGGGGTGAATGACTAACATGGGCGGGCGGC
        10        20        30        40        50        60        70        80        90       100       110       120
GAGAGATATATTATATGGAATATCTACCTTACCACGGTTGTACATTTACTCCATTAAATTTTTTCACGCGCGACACACCACTAACCGACACCCCACTTACTGATTGTACCCGCCCCGCCG
```

```
                   ┌end ITR
CGTGGGAAAATGACGTGACTTATGTGGGAGGAGTTATGTTGCAAGTTATTGCGGTAAATGTGACGTAAAAGGAGGTGTGGTTTGAACACGGAAGTAGACAGTTTTCCCACGCTTACTGAT
        130       140       150       160       170       180       190       200       210       220       230       240
GCACCCTTTTACTGCACTGAATACACCCTCCTCAATACAACGTTCAATAACGCCATTTACACTGCATTTTCCTCCACACCAAACTTGTGCCTTCATCTGTCAAAAGGGTGCGAATGACTA
```

```
AGGATATGAGGTAGTTTTGGGCGGATGCAAGTGAAAATTCTCCATTTTCGCGCGAAAACTGAATGAGGAAGTGAATTTCTGAGTCATTTCGCGGTTATGACAGGGTGGAGTATTTGCCGA
        250       260       270       280       290       300       310       320       330       340       350       360
TCCTATACTCCATCAAAACCCGCCTACGTTCACTTTTAAGAGGTAAAAGCGCGCTTTTGACTTACTCCTTCACTTAAAGACTCAGTAAAGCGCCAATACTGTCCCACCTCATAAACGGCT
```

```
GGGCCGAGTAGACTTTGACCGTTTACGTGGAGGTTTCGATTACCGTGTTTTTCACCTAAATTTCCGCGTACGGTGTCAAAGTCCTGTGTTTTTACGTAGGTGTCAGCTGATCGCTAGGGT
        370       380       390       400       410       420       430       440       450       460       470       480
CCCGGCTCATCTGAAACTGGCAAATGCACCTCCAAAGCTAATGGCACAAAAAGTGGATTTAAAGGCGCATGCCACAGTTTCAGGACACAAAAATGCATCCACAGTCGACTAGCGATCCCA
```

```
"TATA" E1a                      ┌ cap E1a mRNA                                                       start E1a 28K, 25K, 6.8K
                                                                                                            M  R  H  L  R  F  L  P  Q
ATTTAAACCTGACGAGTTCCGTCAAGAGGCCACTCTTGAGTGCCAGCGAGAAGAGTTTTCTCCTCCGCGCCGCAAGTCAGTTCTGCGCTTTGAAAATGAGACACCTGCGCTTCCTGCCAC
        490       500       510       520       530       540       550       560       570       580       590       600
TAAATTTGGACTGCTCAAGGCAGTTCTCCGGTGAGAACTCACGGTCGCTCTTCTCAAAAGAGGAGGCGCGGCGGTTCAGTCAAGACGCGAAACTTTTACTCTGTGGACGCGAAGGACGGTG
```

```
                                        splice─┬E1a mRNA (6.3K)
       E  I  I  S  S  E  T  G  I  E  I  L  E  F  V │V  N  T  L  M  G  D  D  P  E  P  P  V  Q  P  F  D  P  P  T  L  H  D  L  Y
AGGAGATTATCTCCAGTGAGACCGGGATCGAAATACTGGAGTTTGTGGTAAATACCCTAATGGGAGACGACCCGGAACCGCCAGTGCAGCCTTTTGATCCACCTACGCTGCACGATCTGT
        610       620       630       640       650       660       670       680       690       700       710       720
TCCTCTAATAGAGGTCACTCTGGCCCTAGCTTTATGACCTCAAACACCATTTATGGGATTACCCTCTGCTGGGCCTTGGCGGTCACGTCGGAAAACTAGGTGGATGCGACGTGCTAGACA
```

```
       D  L  E  V  D  G  P  E  D  P  N  E  G  A  V  N  G  F  F  T  D  S  M  L  L  A  A  D  E  G  L  D  I  N  P  P  P  E  T  L
ATGATTTAGAGGTAGACGGGCCGGAGGATCCCAATGAGGGAGCTGTGAATGGGTTTTTTTACTGATTCTATGCTGCTAGCTGCCGATGAAGGATTGGACATAAACCCTCCTCCTGAGACCC
        730       740       750       760       770       780       790       800       810       820       830       840
TACTAAATCTCCATCTGCCCGGCCTCCTAGGGTTACTCCCTCGACACTTACCCAAAAAATGACTAAGATACGACGATCGACGGCTACTTCCTAACCTGTATTTGGGAGGAGGACTCTGGG
```

```
       V  T  P  G  V  V  V  E  S  G  R  G  G  K  K  L  P  D  L  G  A  A  E  M  D  L  R  C  Y  E  E  G  F  P  P  S  D  D  E  D
TTGTCACCCCAGGGGTGGTTGTGGAAAGCGGCAGAGGTGGGAAAAAATTGCCTGATCTGGGAGCAGCTGAAATGGACTTGCGTTGTTATGAAGAGGGTTTTCCTCCGAGTGATGATGAAG
        850       860       870       880       890       900       910       920       930       940       950       960
AACAGTGGGGTCCCCACCAACACCTTTCGCCGTCTCCACCCTTTTTAACGGACTAGACCCTCGTCGACTTTACCTGAACGCAACAATACTTCTCCCAAAAGGAGGCTCACTACTACTTC
```

One-letter code for amino acids: A, ala; C, cys; D, asp; E, glu; F, phe; G, gly; H, his; I, ile; K, lys; L, leu; M, met; N, asn; P, pro; Q, gln; R, arg; S, ser; T, thr; V, val; W, trp; Y, tyr

Table 7.1 (Continued)

```
                                                                              splice ─┬─ Ela mRNA(25K)
        G  E  T  E  Q  S  I  H  T  A  V  N  E  G  V  K  A  A  S  D  V  F  K  L  D  C  P  E  L  P  G  H  G │ C  K  S  C  E  F  H
ATGGGGAAACTGAGCAGTCCATCCATACCGCAGTGAATGAGGGAGTAAAAGCTGCCAGCGATGTTTTTAAGTTGGACTGTCCGGAGCTGCCTGGACATGGCTGTAAGTCTTGTGAATTTC
       970       980       990      1000      1010      1020      1030      1040      1050      1060      1070      1080
TACCCCTTTGACTCGTCAGGTAGGTATGGCGTCACTTACTCCCTCATTTTCGACGGTCGCTACAAAAATTCAACCTGACAGGCCTCGACGGACCTGTACCGACATTCAGAACACTTAAAG

                                                                     splice ─┬─ Ela mRNA(28K)
        R  N  N  T  G  M  K  E  L  L  C  S  L  C  Y  M  R  M  H  C  H  F  I  Y │ S
ACAGGAATAACACTGGGATGAAAGAACTATTGTGCTCGCTTTGCTATATGAGAATGCACTGCCACTTTATTTACAGTAAGTGTATTTAAGTGAAATTTAAAGGAATAGTGTAGCTGTTTA
      1090      1100      1110      1120      1130      1140      1150      1160      1170      1180      1190      1200
TGTCCTTATTGTGACCCTACTTTCTTGATAACACGAGCGAAACGATATACTCTTACGTGACGGTGAAATAAATGTCATTCACATAAATTCACTTTAAATTTCCTTATCACATCGACAAAT

                                         splice ─┬─ Ela mRNA
                                         6.8K──→│ V  L  C  L  M  M  S  H  L  L  L  I  Q  L  P  H  L  L  K  F  R  R  P  H
                                       28K,25K─┼─→ P  V  S  D  D  E  S  P  S  P  D  S  T  T  S  P  P  E  I  Q  A  P  A  P
ATAACTGTTGAATGGTAGATTTATGTTTTTTACTTGCGATTTTTTGTAGGTCCTGTGTCTGATGATGAGTCAACCTTCTCCTGATTCAACTACCTCACCTCCTGAAATTCAGGCGCCCGCAC
      1210      1220      1230      1240      1250      1260      1270      1280      1290      1300      1310      1320
TATTGACAACTTACCATCTAAATACAAAAATGAACGCTAAAAAACATCCAGGACACAGACTACTACTCAGTGGAAGAGGACTAAGTTGATGGAGTGGAGGACTTTAAGTCCGCGGGCGTG

                               stop Ela 6.8K *
        L  Q  T  Y  A  S  P  F  L  *
        A  N  V  C  K  P  I  P  V  K  P  K  P  G  K  R  P  A  V  D  K  L  E  D  L  L  E  G  G  D  G  P  L  D  L  S  T  R  K  L
CTGCAAACGTATGCAAGCCCATTCCTGTAAAGCCTAAGCCTGGGAAACGCCCTGCTGTGGATAAGCTTGAGGACTTGTTGGAGGGTGGGGATGGACCTTTGGACCTTAGTACCCGGAAAC
      1330      1340      1350      1360      1370      1380      1390      1400      1410      1420      1430      1440
GACGTTTGCATACGTTCGGGTAAGGACATTTCGGATTCGGACCCTTTGCGGGACGACACCTATTCGAACTCCTGAACAACCTCCCACCCCTACCTGGAAACCTGGAATCATGGGCCTTTG

              stop Ela 28K,25K                                          ┌─ 3'-poly(A) Ela                      "TATA" Elb
        P  R  Q  *
TGCCAAGGCAATGAGTGCCCTGCAGCTGTGTTTATTTAATGTGACGTCATGTAATAAAAATTATGTCAGCTGCTGAGTGTTTTATTACTTCTTGGGTGGGGTCTTGGATATATAAGTAGGA
      1450      1460      1470      1480      1490      1500      1510      1520      1530      1540      1550      1560
ACGGTTCCGTTACTCACGGGACGTCGACACAAATAAATTACACTGCAGTACATTATTTTAATACAGTCGACGACTCACAAAATAATGAAGAACCCACCCCAGAACCTATATATTCATCCT

              ┌─cap Elb                            start Elb 21K
                                                 M  E  V  W  A  I  L  E  D  L  R  Q  T  R  L  L  L  E  N  A  S  D  G  V  S  G  L
GCAGATCTGTGTGGTTAGCTCACAGCAACTTGCTGCCATCCATGGAGGTTTGGGCTATCTTGGAAGACCTCAGACAGACTAGGCTACTACTAGAAAACGCCTCGGACGGAGTCTCTGGCC
      1570      1580      1590      1600      1610      1620      1630      1640      1650      1660      1670      1680
CGTCTAGACACCAATCGAGTGTCGTTGAACGACGGTAGGTACCTCCAAACCCGATAGAACCTTCTGGAGTCTGTCGATCCGATGATGATCTTTTGCGGAGCCTGCCTCAGAGACCGG

        W  R  F  W  F  G  G  D  L  A  R  L  V  F  R  I  K  Q  D  Y  R  E  E  F  E  K  L  L  D  D  I  P  G  L  F  E  A  L  N  L
TTTGGAGATTCTGGTTCGGTGGTGATCTAGCTAGGCTAGTGTTTAGGATAAAACAGGACTACAGGGAAGAATTTGAAAAGTTATTGGACGACATTCCAGGACTTTTTGAAGCTCTTAACT
      1690      1700      1710      1720      1730      1740      1750      1760      1770      1780      1790      1800
AAACCTCTAAGACCAAGCCACCACTAGATCGATCCGATCACAAATCCTATTTTGTCCTGATGTCCCTTCTTAAACTTTTCAATAACCTGCTGTAAGGTCCTGAAAAACTTCGAGAATTGA

                                                                                                  start Elb 55K,9K
                                                                                                        M  D  P  P  N
        G  H  Q  A  H  F  K  E  K  V  L  S  V  L  D  F  S  T  P  G  R  T  A  A  A  V  A  F  L  T  F  I  L  D  K  W  I  R  Q  T
TGGGCCATCAGGCTCATTTTAAGGAGAAGGTTTTATCAGTTTTAGATTTTTCTACTCCTGGTAGAACTGCTGCTGCTGTAGCTTTTCTTACTTTTATATTGGATAAATGGATCCGCCAAA
      1810      1820      1830      1840      1850      1860      1870      1880      1890      1900      1910      1920
ACCCGGTAGTCCGAGTAAAATTCCTCTTCCAAAATAGTCAAAATCTAAAAAGATGAGGACCATCTTGACGACGACGACATCGAAAAGAATGAAAATATAACCTATTTACCTAGGCGGTTT

        S  L  Q  Q  G  I  R  F  G  F  H  S  S  S  F  V  E  M  E  G  S  Q  D  E  D  N  L  R  L  L  A  S  A  A  S  G  S  S  R
        H  F  S  K  G  Y  V  L  D  F  I  A  A  A  L  W  R  T  W  K  A  R  R  M  R  T  I  L  D  Y  W  P  V  Q  P  L  G  V  A  G
CTCACTTCAGCAAGGGATACGTTTTGGATTTCATAGCAGCAGCTTTGTGGAGAACATGGAAGGCTCGCAGGATGAGGACAATCTTAGATTACTGGCCAGTGCAGCCTCTGGGAGTAGCAG
      1930      1940      1950      1960      1970      1980      1990      2000      2010      2020      2030      2040
GAGTGAAGTCGTTCCCTATGCAAAACCTAAAGTATCGTCGTCGAAACACCTCTTGTACCTTCCGAGCGTCCTACTCCTGTTAGAATCTAATGACCGGTCACGTCGGAGACCCTCATCGTC

        D  T  E  T  P  T  D  H  A  S  G  S  A  G  G  A  A  G  G  Q  S  E  S  R  P  G  P  S  G  G  G  V  A  D  L  F  P  E  L  R
        I  L  R  H  P  P  T  M  P  A  V  L  Q  E  E  Q  Q  E  D  N  P  R  A  G  L  D  P  P  V  E  E  *
GGATACTGAGCACCCACCGACCATGCCAGCGGTTCTGCAGGAGGAGCAGCAGGAGGACAATCCGAGAGCCGGCCTGGACCCTCCGGTGGAGGAGTAGCTGACCTGTTTCCTGAACTGCG
      2050      2060      2070      2080      2090      2100      2110      2120      2130      2140      2150      2160
CCTATGACTCGTGGGTGGCTGGTACGGTCGCCAAGACGTCCTCCTCGTCGTCCTCCTGTTAGGCTCTCGGCCGGACCTGGGAGGCCACCTCCTCATCGACTGGACAAAGGACTTGACGC

        ┌─splice Elb mRNA(9K, 21K)
        R│ V  L  T  R  S  T  T  S  G  Q  N  R  G  I  K  R  E  R  N  P  S  G  N  N  S  R  T  E  L  A  L  S  L  M  S  R  R  R  P
ACGGGTGCTTACTAGGTCTACGACCAGTGGACAGAACAGGGGAATTAAGAGGGGAGGGAAATTCCTAGTGGGAATAATTCAAGAACCGAGTTGGCTTTAAGTTTAATGAGCCGCAGGCGTCC
      2170      2180      2190      2200      2210      2220      2230      2240      2250      2260      2270      2280
TGCCCACGAATGATCCAGATGCTGGTCACCTGTCTTGTCCCCTTAATTCTCCCTCTCCTTAGGATCACCCTTATTAAGTTCTTGGCTCAACGAAATTCAAATTACTCGGCGTCCGCAGG

        E  T  V  W  W  H  E  V  Q  S  E  G  R  D  E  V  S  I  L  Q  E  K  Y  S  L  E  Q  L  K  T  C  W  L  E  P  E  D  D  W  E
TGAAACTGTTTGGTGGCATGAGGTTCAGAGCGAAGGCAGGGATGAAGTTTCAATATTGCAGGAGAAATATTCACTAGAACAACTTAAGACCTGTTGGTTGGAACCTGAGGATGATTGGGA
      2290      2300      2310      2320      2330      2340      2350      2360      2370      2380      2390      2400
ACTTTGACAAACCACCGTACTCCAAGTCTCGCTTCCGTCCCTACTTCAAAGTTATAACGTCCTCTTTATAAGTGATCTTGTTGAATTCTGGACAACCAACCTTGGACTCCTACTAACCCT

        V  A  I  R  N  Y  A  K  I  S  L  R  P  D  K  Q  Y  R  I  T  K  K  K  I  N  I  R  N  A  C  Y  I  S  G  N  G  A  E  V  I  I
GGTGGCCATTAGGAATTATGCTAAGATATCTCTGAGGCCTGATAAACAATATAGAATTACTAAGAAGATTAATATTAGAAATGCATGCTACATATCAGGGAATGGGGCAGAGGTTATAAT
      2410      2420      2430      2440      2450      2460      2470      2480      2490      2500      2510      2520
CCACCGGTAATCCTTAATACGATTCTATAGAGACTCCGGACTATTTGTTATATCTTAATGATTCTTCTAATTATAATCTTTACGTACGATGTATAGTCCCTTACCCCGTCTCCAATATTA

        D  T  Q  D  K  A  A  F  R  C  C  M  M  G  M  W  P  G  V  V  G  M  E  A  I  T  L  M  N  I  R  F  R  G  D  G  Y  N  G  I
AGATACAAGATAAAGCAGCTTTTAGATGTTGTATGATGGGTATGTGGCCAGGGGTTGTCGGCATGGAAGCAATAACACTTATGAATATTAGGTTTAGAGGGGATGGGTATAATGGCAT
      2530      2540      2550      2560      2570      2580      2590      2600      2610      2620      2630      2640
TCTATGTGTTCTATTTCGTCGAAAATCTACAACATACTACCCATACACCGGTCCCCAACAGCCGTACCTTCGTTATTGTGAATACTTATAATCCAAATCTCCCCTACCCATATTACCGTA

        V  F  M  A  N  T  K  L  I  L  H  G  C  S  F  F  G  F  N  N  T  C  V  E  A  W  G  Q  V  S  V  R  G  C  S  F  Y  A  C  W
TGTATTTATGGCTAACACTAAGCTGATTCTACATGGTTGTAGCTTTTTTGGGTTTAATAATACGTGTGTAGAAGCTTGGGGGCAAGTTAGTGTGAGGGGTTGTAGTTTTTATGCATGCTG
      2650      2660      2670      2680      2690      2700      2710      2720      2730      2740      2750      2760
ACATAAATACCGATTGTGATTCGACTAAGATGTACCAACATCGAAAAAACCCAAATTATTATGCACACATCTTCGAACCCCCGTTCAATCACACTCCCCAACATCAAAAATACGTACGAC
```

Table 7.1 (Continued)

```
     I  A  T  S  G  R  V  K  S  Q  L  S  V  K  K  C  M  F  E  R  C  N  L  G  I  L  N  E  G  E  A  R  V  R  H  C  A  A  T  E
GATTGCAACATCAGGTAGGGTGAAGAGTCAGTTGTCTGTGTGAAGAAATGCATGTTTGAGAGATGTAATCTTGGCATACTGAATGAAGGTGAAGCAAGGGTCCGCCACTGCGCAGCTACAGA
         2770      2780      2790      2800      2810      2820      2830      2840      2850      2860      2870      2880
CTAACGTTGTAGTCCATCCCACTTCTCAGTCAACAGACACTTCTTTACGTACAAACTCTCTACATTAGAACCGTATGACTTACTTCCACTTCGTTCCCAGGCGGTGACGCGTCGATGTCT
```

```
     T  A  C  F  I  L  I  K  G  N  A  S  V  K  H  N  M  I  C  G  H  S  D  E  R  P  Y  Q  M  L  T  C  A  G  G  H  C  N  I  L
AACTGCCTGCTTCATTCTAATAAAGGGAAATGCCAGTGTGAAGCATAATATGATCTGTGGACATTCGGATGAGAGGCCTTATCAGATGCTAACCTGCGCTGGTGGACATTGCAATATTCT
         2890      2900      2910      2920      2930      2940      2950      2960      2970      2980      2990      3000
TTGACGGACGAAGTAAGATTATTTCCCTTTACGGTCACACTTCGTATTATACTAGACACCTGTAAGCCTACTCTCCGGAATAGTCTACGATTGGACGCGACCACCTGTAACGTTATAAGA
```

```
     A  T  V  H  I  V  S  H  A  R  K  K  W  P  V  F  E  H  N  V  I  T  K  C  T  M  H  I  G  G  R  R  G  M  F  M  P  Y  Q  C
TGCTACCGTGCATATCGTTTCACATGCACGCAAGAAATGGCCTGTATTTGAACATAATGTGATTACCAAGTGCACCATGCATATAGGTGGTCGCAGGGGAATGTTTATGCCTTACCAGTG
         3010      3020      3030      3040      3050      3060      3070      3080      3090      3100      3110      3120
ACGATGGCACGTATAGCAAAGTGTACGTGCGTTCTTTACCGGACATAAACTTGTATTACACTAATGGTTCACGTGGTACGTATATCCACCAGCGTCCCCTTACAAATACGGAATGGTCAC
```

```
     N  M  N  H  V  K  V  M  L  E  P  D  A  F  S  R  V  S  V  T  G  I  F  D  M  N  I  Q  L  W  K  I  L  R  Y  D  D  T  K  P
TAACATGAATCATGTGAAGGTAATGTTGGAACCAGATGCCTTTTCCAGAGTGAGCGTAACAGGAATCTTTGATATGAATATTCAACTATGGAAGATCCTGAGATATGATGACACTAAACC
         3130      3140      3150      3160      3170      3180      3190      3200      3210      3220      3230      3240
ATTGTACTTAGTACACTTCCATTACAACCTTGGTCTACGGAAAAGGTCTCACTCGCATTGTCCTTAGAAACTATACTTATAAGTTGATACCTTCTAGGACTCTATACTACTGTGATTGG
```

```
     R  V  R  A  C  E  C  G  G  K  H  A  R  F  Q  P  V  C  V  D  V  T  E  D  L  R  P  D  H  L  V  L  A  C  T  G  A  E  F  G
AAGGGTGCGCGCATGCGAATGCGGAGGCAAGCATGCTAGATTCCAGCCGGTGTGCGTGGATGTGACTGAAGACCTGAGGCCCGATCATTTGGTGCTTGCCTGCACTGGAGCGGAGTTCGG
         3250      3260      3270      3280      3290      3300      3310      3320      3330      3340      3350      3360
TTCCCACGCGCGTACGCCTCCGTTCGTACGATCTAAGGTCGGCCACACGCACCTACACTGACTTCTGGACTCCGGGCTAGTAAACCACGAACGGACGTGACCTCGCCTCAAGCC
```

                              stop Elb 55K   splice ┌── Elb
                                                                                                                     │   L P
     S S G E E T D *   protein IX mRNA ┬── cap   │
```
                          ┌── splice Elb mRNA                                                             │           │         M
TTCTAGTGGTGAAGAAACTGACTAAAGTAAGTAGTGGGGGCAAAATGTGGATGGGGACTTTCAGGTTGGTAAGGTGGACAAATTGGGTAAATTTTGTTAATTTCTGTCTTGCAGCTGCCA
         3370      3380      3390      3400      3410      3420      3430      3440      3450      3460      3470      3480
AAGATCACCACTTCTTTGACTGATTTCATTCATCACCCCCGTTTTACACCTACCCCTGAAAGTCCAACCATTCCACCTGTTTAACCCATTTAAAACAATTAAAGACAGAACGTCGACGGT
```

stop Elb 9K
start protein IX
   *
     S G S A S F E G G V F S P Y L T G R L P P W A G V R Q N V M G S T V D G R P V Q
```
TGAGTGGAAGCGCTTCTTTTGAGGGGGGAGTATTTAGCCCTTATCTGACGGGCAGGCTCCCACCATGGGCAGGAGTTCGTCAGAATGTCATGGGATCCACTGTGGATGGGAGACCCGTCC
         3490      3500      3510      3520      3530      3540      3550      3560      3570      3580      3590      3600
ACTCACCTTCGCGAAGAAAACTCCCCCCTCATAAATCGGGAATAGACTGCCCGTCCGAGGGTGGTACCCGTCCTCAAGCAGTCTTACAGTACCCTAGGTGACACCTACCCTCTGGGCAGG
```

```
     P  A  N  S  S  T  L  T  Y  A  T  L  S  S  S  P  L  D  A  A  A  A  A  A  T  A  A  A  N  T  I  L  G  M  G  Y  Y  G  S
AGCCCGCCAATTCCTCAACGCTGACCTATGCCACTTTGAGTTCGTCACCATTGGATGCAGCTGCAGCCGCCGCCGCTACTGCTGCCGCCAACACCATCCTTGGAATGGGCTATTACGGAA
         3610      3620      3630      3640      3650      3660      3670      3680      3690      3700      3710      3720
TCGGGCGGTTAAGGAGTTGCGACTGGATACGGTGAAACTCAAGCAGTGGTAACCTACGTCGACGTCGGCGGCGGCGATGACGACGGCGGTTGTGGTAGGAACCTTACCCGATAATGCCTT
```

```
     I  V  A  N  S  S  S  S  N  N  P  S  T  L  A  E  D  K  L  L  V  L  L  A  Q  L  E  A  L  T  Q  R  L  G  E  L  S  K  Q  V
GCATTGTTGCCAATTCCAGTTCCTCTAATAATCCTTCAAACCCTGGCTGAGGACAAAGCTACTTGTTCTCTTGGCTCAGCTCGAGGCCTTAACCCAACGCTTAGGCGAACTGTCTAAGCAGG
         3730      3740      3750      3760      3770      3780      3790      3800      3810      3820      3830      3840
CGTAACAACGGTTAAGGTCAAGGAGATTATTAGGAAGTTGGGACCGACTCCTGTTCGATGAACAAGAGAACCGAGTCGAGCTCCGGAATTGGGTTGCGAATCCGCTTGACAGATTCGTCC
```

                              stop protein IX   ┌─ 3'-poly(A) Elb,pIX mRNAs
     A Q L R E Q T E S A V A T A K S K *   │
```
TGGCCCAGTTGCGTGAGCAAACTGAGTCTGCTGTTGCCACAGCAAAGTCTAAATAAAGATCTCAAATCAATAAATAAAGAAATACTTGTTATAAAAACAAATGAATGTTTATTTGATTTT
         3850      3860      3870      3880      3890      3900      3910      3920      3930      3940      3950      3960
ACCGGGTCAACGCACTCGTTTGACTCAGACGACAACGGTGTCGTTTCAGATTTATTTCTAGAGTTTAGTTATTTATTTCTTTATGAACAATATTTTGTTTACTTACAAATAAACTAAAA
                                                                             *  K  I  K
                                                                   protein IVa2 stop
```

```
TCGCGCGCGGTATGCCCTGGACCATCGGTTTCGATCATTGAGAACTCGGTGGATCTTTTCCAGTACCCTGTAAAGGTGGGATTGAATGTTTAGATACATGGGCATTAGTCCGTCTCGGGG
         3970      3980      3990      4000      4010      4020      4030      4040      4050      4060      4070      4080
AGCGCGCGCCATACGGGACCTGGTAGCCAAAGCTAGTAACTCTTGAGCCACCTAGAAAAGGTCATGGGACATTCTACCCTAACTTACAAATCTATGTACCCGTAATCAGGCAGAGCCCC
     R  A  R  Y  A  R  W  S  R  R  N  D  N  L  V  R  H  I  K  E  L  V  R  Y  L  H  S  Q  I  N  L  Y  P  M  L  G  D  R  P
```

```
GTGGAGATGACTCCATTGAAGAGCCTCTTGCTCCGGGGTAGTGTTATAAATCACCCAGTCATAGCAAGGTCGGAGTGCATGGTGTTGCACAATATCTTTTAGGAGCAGACTAATTGCAAC
         4090      4100      4110      4120      4130      4140      4150      4160      4170      4180      4190      4200
CACCTCTACTGAGGTAACTTCTCGGAGAACGAGGCCCCATCACAATATTTAGTGGGTCAGTATCGTTCCAGCCTCACGTACCACAACGTGTTATAGAAAATCCTCGTCTGATTAACGTTG
     H  L  H  S  W  Q  L  A  E  Q  E  P  T  T  N  Y  I  V  W  D  Y  C  P  R  L  A  H  H  Q  V  I  D  K  L  L  L  S  I  A  V
```

```
GGGGAGGCCCTTAGTGTAGGTGTTTACAAATCTGTTGAGCTGGGACGGGTGCATCCGGGGTGAAATTATATGCATTTTGGACTGGATCTTGAGGTTGGCAATGTTGCCGCCTAGATCCCG
         4210      4220      4230      4240      4250      4260      4270      4280      4290      4300      4310      4320
CCCCTCCGGGAATCACATCCACAAATGTTTAGACAACTCGACCCTGCCCACGTAGGCCCCACTTTAATATACGTAAAACCTGACCTAGAACTCCAACCGTTACAACGGCGGATCTAGGGC
     P  L  G  K  T  Y  T  N  V  F  R  N  L  Q  S  P  H  M  R  P  S  I  I  H  M  K  S  Q  I  K  L  N  A  I  N  G  G  L  D  R
```

```
TCTCGGGTTCATATTGTGCAGGACCACCAAGACAGTGTATCCGGTGCAGTTGGGAAATCTATCATGCAGCTTAGAGGGAAAAGCATGAAAAAATTTGGAGACGCCTTTGTGACCCCCCAG
         4330      4340      4350      4360      4370      4380      4390      4400      4410      4420      4430      4440
AGAGCCCAAGTATAACACGTCCTGGTGGTTCTGTCACATAGGCCACGTGAACCCTTTAGATAGTACGTCGAATCTCCCTTTTCGTACTTTTTTAAACCTCTGCCGGAAACACTGGGGGGTC
     R  P  N  M  N  H  L  V  V  L  V  T  Y  G  T  C  K  P  F  R  D  H  L  K  S  P  F  A  H  F  F  K  S  V  G  K  H  G  G  L
```

```
ATTCTCCATGCACTCATCCCATAATGATAGCGATGGGGCCGTGGGCAGCGGCACGGGCGAACACGTTCCGGGGGTCTGAAACATCATAGTTATGCTCCTGAGTCAGGTCATCATAAGCCAT
         4450      4460      4470      4480      4490      4500      4510      4520      4530      4540      4550      4560
TAAGAGGTACGTGAGTAGGTATTACTATCGCTACCCCGGCACCCGTCGCCGTGCCCGCTTGTGCAAGGCCCCAGACTTTGTAGTATCAATACGAGGACTCAGTCCAGTAGTATTCGGTA
     N  E  M  C  E  D  M  I  I  A  I  P  G  H  A  A  A  A  R  A  F  V  N  R  P  D  S  V  D  Y  N  H  E  Q  T  L  D  D  Y  A  M
```

```
TTTAATAAACTTTGGGCGGAGGGTGCCAGATTGGGGGATGAAAGTTCCCTGTGGCCCGGGAGCATAGTTTCCCTCACATATTTGCATTTCCCAGGCTTTCAGTTCAGAGGGGGGGATCAT
         4570      4580      4590      4600      4610      4620      4630      4640      4650      4660      4670      4680
AAATTATTTGAAACCCGCCTCCCACGGTCTAACCCCCTACTTTCAAGGGACACCGGGCCCTCGTATCAAAGGGAGTGTATAAACGTAAAGGGTCCGAAAGTCAAGTCTCCCCCCCTAGTA
     K  I  F  K  P  R  L  T  G  S  Q  P  I  F  T  G  Q  P  G  P  A  Y  N  G  E  C  I  Q  M  E  W  A  K  L  E  S  P  P  I  M
```

Table 7.1 (Continued)

```
GTCCACCTGCGGGGCTATAAAAAATACCGTTTCTGGAGCCGGGGTGATTAACTGGGATGAGAGCAAATTCCTAAGCAGCTGAGACTTGCCGCACCCGGTGGGACCGTAAATGACCCCAAT
     4690      4700      4710      4720      4730      4740      4750      4760      4770      4780      4790      4800
CAGGTGGACGCCCCGATATTTTTTATGGCAAAGACCTCGGCCCCACTAATTGACCCTACTCTCGTTTAAGGATTCGTCGACTCTGAACGGCGTGGGCCACCCTGGCATTTACTGGGGTTA
 D  V  Q  P  A  I  F  F  V  T  E  P  A  P  T  I  L  Q  S  S  L  L  N  R  L  L  Q  S  K  G  C  G  T  P  G  Y  I  V  G  I


TACGGGTTGCAGATGGTAGTTTAGGGAGCGACAGCTGCCGTCCTCCCGGAGCAGGGGGGCCACTTCGTTCATCATTTCCCTTACATGGATATTTTCCCGCACCAAGTCCGTTAGGAGGCG
     4810      4820      4830      4840      4850      4860      4870      4880      4890      4900      4910      4920
ATGCCCAACGTCTACCATCAAATCCCTCGCTGTCGACGGCAGGAGGGCCTCGTCCCCCCGGTGAAGCAAGTAGTAAAGGGAATGTACCTATAAAAGGGCGTGGTTCAGGCAATCCTCCGC
 V  P  Q  L  H  Y  N  L  S  R  C  S  G  D  E  R  L  L  P  A  V  E  N  M  M  E  R  V  H  I  N  E  R  V  L  D  T  L  L  R


CTCTCCCCCAAGTGATAGAAGCTCCTGGAGCGAGGAGAAGTTTTTCAGCGGCTTCAGCCCGTCAGCCATGGGCATTTTGGAAAGAGTCTGTTGCAAGAGCTCGAGCCGGTCCCAGAGCTC
     4930      4940      4950      4960      4970      4980      4990      5000      5010      5020      5030      5040
GAGAGGGGGTTCACTATCTTCGAGGACCTCGCTCCTCTTCAAAAAGTCGCCGAAGTCGGGCAGTCGGTACCCGTAAAACCTTTCTCAGACAACGTTCTCGAGCTCGGCCAGGGTCTCGAG
 E  G  C  L  S  L  L  E  Q  L  S  S  F  N  K  L  P  K  L  G  D  A  M  P  M  K  S  L  T  Q  Q  L  L  E  L  R  D  W  L  E


                                                                                        start ORF 21K
                                                                                        M  G  V  Q  R  C  Q  G  P  I  L  P  W
GGTGATGTGCTCTATGGCATCTCGATCCAGCAGACCTCCTCGTTTCGCGGGTTGGGACGGCTCCTGGAGTAGGGAATCAGACGATGGGCGTCCAGCGCTGCCAGGGTCCGATCCTTCCAT
     5050      5060      5070      5080      5090      5100      5110      5120      5130      5140      5150      5160
CCACTACACGAGATACCGTAGAGCTAGGTCGTCTGGAGGACGCAAAGCGCCCAACCCTGCCGAGGACCTCATCCCTTAGTCTGCTACCCGCAGGTCGCGACGGTCCCAGGCTAGGAAGGTA
 T  I  H  E  I  A  D  R  D  L  L  G  G  R  K  A  P  Q  S  P  E  Q  L  L  S  D  S  S  P  R  G  A  S  G  P  D  S  G  E  M
   *  P  M  E  I  W  C  V  E  E  N  R  P  N  P  R  S  R  S  Y  P  I  L  R  H  A  D  L  A  A  L  T  R  D  K  W  P
stop E2B 129K


     S  Q  R  P  S  Q  G  C  F  R  H  G  E  G  V  R  A  W  L  G  A  C  E  G  A  L  Q  T  H  P  A  G  R  E  P  L  P  I  G  A
GGTCGCAGCGTCCGAGTCAGGGGTTGTTTCCGTCACGGTGAAGGGGTGCGCGCCTGGTTGGGCGCTTGCGAGGGTGCGCTTCAGACTCATCCTGCTGGTCGAGAACCGCTGCCGATCGGCG
     5170      5180      5190      5200      5210      5220      5230      5240      5250      5260      5270      5280
CCAGCGTCGCAGGCTCAGTCCCAACAAAGGCAGTGCCACTTCCCCACGCGCGGACCAACCCGCGAACGCTCCCACGCGAAGTCTGAGTAGGACGACGACGAGTCTTGGCGACGGCTAGCCGC
 T  A  A  D  S  D  P  N  N  G  D  R  H  L  P  A  R  R  T  P  R  K  R  P  H  A  E  S  E  D  Q  Q  D  L  V  A  A  S  R  R
   R  L  T  R  T  L  T  T  E  T  V  T  F  P  H  A  G  P  Q  A  S  A  L  T  R  K  L  S  M  R  S  T  S  F  R  Q  R  D  A  G


     L  H  V  G  Q  V  A  V  Y  H  K  F  V  V  E  R  L  G  R  V  A  F  G  T  E  L  T  F  G  S  F  M  A  G  R  A  V  D  T  F
CCCTGCATGTCGGCCAGGTAGCAGTTTACCATAAGTTCGTAGTTGAGCGCCTCGGCCGCGTGGCCTTTGGCACGGAGCTTACCTTTGGAAGTTTTATGGCAGGCAGGGCAGTAGATACAT
     5290      5300      5310      5320      5330      5340      5350      5360      5370      5380      5390      5400
GGGACGTACAGCCGGTCCATCGTCAAATGGTATTCAAGCATCAACTCGCGGAGCCGGCGCACCGGAAACCGTGCCTGAATGGAAACCTTCAAAATACCGTCCGTCCCGTCATCTATGTA
 Q  M  D  A  L  Y  C  N  V  M  L  E  Y  N  L  A  E  A  A  H  G  K  A  R  L  K  G  K  S  T  K  H  C  A  P  C  Y  I  C  K
└─splice IVa2 mRNA


     E  G  I  Q  L  G  R  E  E  N  G  F  G  G  V  C  I  R  T  A  G  D  A  D  G  F  A  L  H  K  P  G  Q  I  R  L  I  R  V  K
TTGAGGGCATACAGCTTGGGCGCGAGGAAAATGGATTCGGGGGAGTATGCATCCGCACCGCAGGAGACGCAGACGGTTTCGCACTCCACAAGCCAGGTCAGATCCGGCTCATCAGGGTCA
     5410      5420      5430      5440      5450      5460      5470      5480      5490      5500      5510      5520
AACTCCCGTATGTCGAACCCGCGCTCCTTTTACCTAAGCCCCCTCATACGTAGGCGTGGCGTCCTCTGCGTCTGCCAAAGCGTGAGGTGTTCGGTCCAGTCTAGGCCGAGTAGTCCCAGT
 L  A  Y  L  K  P  A  L  F  I  S  E  P  S  Y  A  D  A  G  C  S  V  C  V  T  E  C  E  V  L  W  T  L  D  P  E  D  P  D  F


     N  K  F  S  A  M  F  F  D  A  F  L  T  F  G  F  H  E  F  V  S  T  L  G  D  K  E  A  V  R  V  P  V  D  R  L  Y  G  P  V
AAAACAAGTTTTCCGCCATGTTTTTTGATGCGTTTCTTACCTTTGGTTTCCATGAGTTCGTGTCCACGCTGGGTGACAAAGAGGCTGTCCGTGTCCCGTAGACCGACTTTATGGGCCTG
     5530      5540      5550      5560      5570      5580      5590      5600      5610      5620      5630      5640
TTTTTGTTCAAAAGGCCGGTACAAAAAACTACGCAAAGAATGGAAACCAAAGGTACTCAAGCACAGGTGCGACCCACTGTTTCTCCGACAGGCACAGGGGCATCTGGCTGAAATACCCGGAC
 V  L  K  G  G  H  K  K  I  R  K  K  G  K  T  E  M  L  E  H  G  R  Q  T  V  F  L  S  D  T  D  G  Y  V  S  K  I  P  R  D
                     splice IVa2 mRNA─┘              start protein IVa2


                                             stop ORF 21K
     L  E  R  S  A  S  V  L  F  V  E  E  S  S  P  L  *
TCCTCGAGCGGAGTGCCTCGGTCCTCTTCGTAGAGGAATCCAGCCCACTCTGATACAAAAGCCGTGTCCAGGCCAGCACAAAGGAGGCCACGTGGGAGGGGTAGCGGTCGTTGTCAACC
     5650      5660      5670      5680      5690      5700      5710      5720      5730      5740      5750      5760
AGGAGCTCGCCTCACGGAGCCAGGAGAAGCATCTCCTTAGGTCGGGTGAGACTATGTTTTCGGCGCACAGGTCCGGTCGTGTTTCCTCCGGTGCACCCTCCCCATCGCCAGCAACAGTTGG
 E  L  P  T  G  R  D  E  E  Y  L  F  G  A  W  E  S  V  F  A  R  T  W  A  L  V  F  S  A  V  H  S  P  Y  R  D  N  D  V  L
                                             cap─┘IVa2 mRNA


                                                                                                  major late "TATA"
AGGGGGATCCACCTTCTCTACGTGTATGTAAACACATGTCCCCCTCCTCCACATCCAAGAATGTGATTGGCTTGTAAGTGTAGGCCACGTGACCAGGGGTCCCCGCCGGGGGGGGTATAAAAG
     5770      5780      5790      5800      5810      5820      5830      5840      5850      5860      5870      5880
TCCCCTAGGTGGAAGAGATGCCATACATTTGTGTACAGGGGGAGGAGGTGTAGGTTCTTACACTAACCGAACATTCACATCCGGTGCACTGGTCCCCAGGGGCGGCCCCCCCATATTTTC
 P  D  V  K  E  V  T  H  L  C  M  D  G  E  E  V  D  L  F  T  I  P  K  Y  T  Y  A  V  H  G  P  T  G  A  P  P  T  Y  F  P


                 ↓ cap major late mRNAs   1st leader 3'─────┬─splice
GGGGCGGACCTCTGTTCGTCCTCACTGTCTTCCGGATCGCTGTCCAGGAGCGCCAGCTGTTGGGGTAGGTATTCCCTCTCGAATGCGGGCATGACCTCTGCACTCAGGTTGTCAGTTTCT
     5890      5900      5910      5920      5930      5940      5950      5960      5970      5980      5990      6000
CCCCGCCTGGAGACAAGCAGGAGTGACAGAAGGCCTAGCGACAGGTCCTCGCGGTCGACAACCCATCCATAAGGGAGAGCTTACGCCCGTACTGGAGACGTGAGTCCAACAGTCAAAGA
 A  S  R  Q  E  D  E  S  D  E  P  D  S  D  L  L  A  L  Q  Q  P  L  Y  E  R  E  F  A  P  M  V  E  A  S  L  N  D  T  E  L


AGGAACGAGGAGGATTTGATATTGACAGTACCAGCAGAGATGCCTTTTATAAGACTCTCGTCCATCTGGTCAGAAAACACAATCTTCTTGTTGTCCAGCTTGGTGGCAAATGATCCATAG
     6010      6020      6030      6040      6050      6060      6070      6080      6090      6100      6110      6120
TCCTTGCTCCTCCTAAACTATAACTGTCATGGTCGTCTCTACGGAAAATATTCTGAGACGCAGGTAGACCAGTCTTTTGTGTTAGAAGAACAACAGGTCGAACCACCGTTTACTAGGATC
 F  S  S  S  K  I  N  V  T  G  A  S  I  G  K  I  L  S  E  D  M  Q  D  S  F  V  I  K  K  N  D  L  K  T  A  F  S  G  Y  L


            start ORF 11.5K
            M  E  R  M  V  W  F  F  S  L  S  A  R  S  L  A  A  M  L  S  W  T  Y  S  R  A  T  H  F  H  S  G
AGGGCGTTGGATAGAAGCTTGGCGATGGAGCGCATGGTTTGGTTCTTTTCCTTGTCCGCGCGCTCCTTGGCGGCGATGTTAAGCTGGACGTACTCGCGCGCCACACATTTCCATTCAGGA
     6130      6140      6150      6160      6170      6180      6190      6200      6210      6220      6230      6240
TCCCGCAACCTATCTTCGAACCGCTACCTCGCGTACCAAACAAGAAAAGGAACAGGCGCGCGAGGAACCGCCGCTACAATTCGACCTGCATGAGCGCGCGGTGTGTAAAGGTAAGTCCT
 A  N  S  L  L  K  A  I  S  R  M  T  Q  N  K  E  K  D  A  R  E  K  A  A  I  N  L  Q  V  Y  E  R  A  V  C  K  W  E  P  F


     K  M  V  V  S  S  S  G  T  I  L  T  R  H  P  L  L  C  R  V  I  R  S  T  V  V  A  T  S  P  R  R  G  S  L  V  Q  Q  S  R
AAGATGGTTGTCAGTTCATCCGGAACTATTCTGACTCGCCATCCCCTATTGTGCAGGGTTATCGATCCACAGTGGTGGCCACCTCGCCTCGGAGGGGCTCATTGGTCCAGCAGAGTCGA
     6250      6260      6270      6280      6290      6300      6310      6320      6330      6340      6350      6360
TTCTACCAACAGTCAAGTAGGCCTTGATAAGACTGAGCGGTAGGGATAACACGTCCCAATAGTCTAGGTGTCACCACCGGTGGAGCGGAGCCTCCCCGAGTAACCAGGTCGTCTCAGCT
     I  T  T  L  E  D  P  V  I  R  V  R  W  G  R  N  H  L  T  I  L  D  V  T  T  A  V  E  G  R  L  P  E  N  T  W  C  L  R  G
```

Table 7.1 (Continued)

```
                                                                                    stop ORF 11.5K
 P  P  F  R  E  Q  K  G  G  R  G  S  S  M  N  S  S  G  G  S  A  S  M  V  N  I  P  G  S  K  S  L  S  K  *
CCTCCTTTTCGTGAACAGAAAGGGGGGAGGGGGTCTAGCATGAACTCATCAGGGGGGTCCGCATCTATGGTAAATATTCCCGGTAGCAAATCTTTGTCAAAATAGCTGATGGTGGCAGGA
     6370      6380      6390      6400      6410      6420      6430      6440      6450      6460      6470      6480
GGAGGAAAAGCACTTGTCTTTCCCCCCTCCCCCAGATCGTACTTGAGTAGTCCCCCCAGGCGTAGATACCATTTATAAGGGCCATCGTTTAGAAACAGTTTTATCGACTACCACCGTCCT
 G  K  R  S  C  F  P  P  P  L  P  D  L  M  F  E  D  P  P  P  D  A  D  I  T  F  I  G  P  L  L  D  K  D  F  Y  S  I  T  A  P  D


TCATCCAAGGTCATCTGCCATTCTCGAACTGCCAGCGCGCGCTCATAGGGGTTAAGAGGGGTGCCCCAGGGCATGGGGTGGGTGAGCGCGGAGGCATACATGCCACAGATATCGTAGACA
     6490      6500      6510      6520      6530      6540      6550      6560      6570      6580      6590      6600
AGTAGGTTCCAGTAGACGGTAAGAGCTTGACGGTCGCGCGCGAGTATCCCCAATTCTCCCCACGGGGTCCCGTACCCCACCCACTCGCGCCTCCGTATGTACGGTGTCTATAGCATCTGT
 D  L  T  M  Q  W  E  R  V  A  L  A  R  E  Y  P  N  L  P  T  G  W  P  M  P  H  T  L  A  S  A  Y  M  G  C  I  D  Y  V  V  Y


TAGAGGGGCTCTTCGAGGATGCCGATGTAAGTGGGATAACAGCGCCCCCCTCTGATGCTTGCTCGCACATAGTCATAGAGTTCATGTGAGGGGGCGAGGAGACCCGGGCCCAGATTGGTG
     6610      6620      6630      6640      6650      6660      6670      6680      6690      6700      6710      6720
ATCTCCCCGAGAAGCTCCTACGGCTACATTCACCCTATTGTCGCGGGGGGAGACTACGAACGAGCGTGTATCAGTATCTCAAGTACACTCCCCCGCTCCTCTGGGCCCGGGTCTAACCAC
 L  P  E  E  L  I  G  I  Y  T  P  Y  C  R  G  G  R  I  S  A  R  V  V  Y  D  Y  L  E  H  S  P  A  L  L  G  P  G  L  N  T  R


CGGTTGGGTTTTTCCGCCCTGTAAACGATTTGGCGAAAGATGGCATGGGAATTGGAAGAAATAGTAGGTCTCTGGAATATGTTAAAATGAACATGAGGTAGGCCTACAGAGTCTCTTATG
     6730      6740      6750      6760      6770      6780      6790      6800      6810      6820      6830      6840
GCCAACCCAAAAAGGCGGGACATTTGCTAAACCGCTTTCTACCGTACCCTTAACCTTCTTTATCATCCAGAGACCTTATACAATTTTACTTGTACTCCATCCGGATGTCTCAGAGAATAC
 N  P  K  E  A  R  Y  V  I  Q  R  F  I  A  H  S  N  S  S  I  T  P  R  Q  F  I  N  F  H  V  H  P  L  G  V  S  D  R  I  F


AAGTGGGCATATGACTCTTGCAGCTTGGCTACCAGCTCTGCGGTGACGAGTACATCCAGGGCACAGTAGTTGAGAGTTTCCTGGATGATGTCATAACGCGGTTGGCTTTTCTTTTCCCAC
     6850      6860      6870      6880      6890      6900      6910      6920      6930      6940      6950      6960
TTCACCCGTATACTGAGAACGTCGAACCGATGGTCGAGACGCCACTGCTCATGTAGGTCCCGTGTCATCAACTCTCAAAGGACCTACTACAGTAGTTGCGCCAACCGAAAAGAAAAGGGTG
                      *  W  S  Q  P  S  S  Y  M  W  P  V  T  T  S  L  K  R  S  S  T  M  V  R  N  A  K  R  K  G  C
 H  A  Y  S  E  Q  L  K  A  V  L  E  A  T  V  L  V  D  L  A  C  Y  N  L  T  E  Q  I  I  D  Y  R  P  Q  S  K  K  E  W  L
                       stop ORF 19K


 ┌splice
 │5' 2nd late leader                                                2nd late leader 3'  ┌── splice
AGCTCGCGGTTGAGAAGGTATTCTTCGTGATCCTTCCAGTACTCTTCGAGGGGAAACCCGTCTTTTTCTGCACGGTAAGAGCCCAACATGTAGAACTGATTGACTGCCTTGTAGGGACAG
     6970      6980      6990      7000      7010      7020      7030      7040      7050      7060      7070      7080
TCGAGCGCCAACTCTTCCATAAGAAGCACTAGGAAGGTCATGAGAAGCTCCCCTTTGGGCAGAAAAAGACGTGCCATTCTCGGGTTGTACATCTTGACTAACTGACGGAACATCCCTGTC
 S  A  T  S  F  T  N  K  T  I  R  G  T  S  K  S  P  F  G  T  K  K  Q  V  T  L  A  W  C  T  S  S  I  S  Q  R  T  P  V  A
 E  R  N  L  L  Y  E  E  H  D  K  W  Y  E  E  L  P  F  G  D  K  E  A  R  Y  S  G  L  M  Y  F  Q  N  V  A  K  Y  P  C  C


                                          start ORF 10K
                                           M  S  E  G  K  S  V  P  D  H  D  F  E  E  L  I  L  E  V  D  V  I  T
CATCCCTTCTCCACTGGGGAGAGAGTATGCTTGGGCTGCATTGCGCAGCGAGGTATGAGTGAGGGCAAAAGTGTCCCTGACCATGACTTTGAGGAATTGATACTTGAAGTCGATGTCATCA
     7090      7100      7110      7120      7130      7140      7150      7160      7170      7180      7190      7200
GTAGGGAAGAGGTGACCCTCTCTCATACGAACCCGACGTAACGCGTCGCTCCATACTCACTCCCGTTTTCACAGGGACTGGTACTGAAACTCCTTAACTATGAACTTCAGCTACAGTAGT
 D  R  R  W  Q  S  L  T  H  K  P  Q  M  A  C  R  P  I  L  S  P  L  L  T  G  V  M  V  K  L  F  Q  Y  K  F  D  I  D  D  C
 G  K  E  V  P  L  S  Y  A  Q  A  A  N  R  L  S  T  H  T  L  A  F  T  D  R  V  M  V  K  L  F  Q  Y  K  F  D  I  D  D  C


 G  P  L  F  P  E  L  E  V  R  P  L  L  V  G  G  I  G  Q  S  E  S  N  I  I  E  E  D  L  T  G  P  G  H  E  I  S  G  D  F
CAGGCCCCCTGTTCCCAGAGTTGGAAGTCCGCCCGCTTCTTGTAGGCGGGATTGGGCAAAGCGAAAGTAACATCATTGAAGAGGATCTCACCGGCCCTGGGCATGAAATTTCGGGTGATT
     7210      7220      7230      7240      7250      7260      7270      7280      7290      7300      7310      7320
GTCCGGGGGACAAGGGTCTCAACCTTCAGGCGGGCGAAGAACATCCGCCCTAACCCGTTTCGCTTTCATTGTAGTAACTTCTCCTAGAGTGGCCGGGACCCGTACTTTAAAGCCCACTAA
 P  G  R  N  G  S  N  S  T  R  G  S  R  T  P  P  I  P  C  L  S  L  L  M  M  S  S  R  V  P  G  P  C  S  I  E  P  S  K
 A  G  Q  E  W  L  Q  F  D  A  R  K  K  Y  A  P  N  P  L  A  F  T  V  D  N  F  L  I  E  G  A  R  P  M  F  N  R  T  I  K


                                                                    stop ORF 10K
 K  R  L  R  D  L  C  S  V  I  D  N  L  S  G  Q  D  D  L  I  K  A  I  D  V  V  P  H  Y  V  Q  F  *
TTAAAAGGCTGAGGGACCTCTGCTCGGTTATTGATAACCTGAGCGGCCAAGACGATCTCATCAAAGCCATTGATGTTGTGCCCCACTATGTACAGTTCTAAGAATCGAGGGGTGCCCCTG
     7330      7340      7350      7360      7370      7380      7390      7400      7410      7420      7430      7440
AATTTTCCGACTCCCTGGAGACGAGCCAATAACTATTGGACTCGCCGGTTCTGCTAGGATAGTTTCGGTAACTACAACACGGGGTGATACATGTCAAGATTCTTAGCTCCCCACGGGGAC
 F  P  Q  P  V  E  A  R  N  N  I  V  Q  A  A  L  V  I  E  D  F  G  N  I  N  H  G  V  I  Y  L  E  L  F  R  P  T  G  R  V
                                                                    start ORF 19K


ACATGAGGCAGCTTCTTGAGTTCTTCAAAAGTGAGATCTGTAGGGTCAGTGAGAGCATAGTGTTCGAGGGCCCATTCGTGCATGTGAGGGTTCGCTTTGAGGAAGGAGGACCAGAGGTCC
     7450      7460      7470      7480      7490      7500      7510      7520      7530      7540      7550      7560
TGTACTCCGTCGAAGAACTCAAGAAGTTTTCACTCTAGACATCCCAGTCACTCTCGTATCACAAGCTCCCGGGTAAGCACGTACACTCCCAAGCGAAACTCCTTCCTCCTGGTCTCCAGG
 H  P  L  K  K  L  E  E  F  T  L  D  T  P  D  T  L  A  Y  H  E  L  A  W  E  H  M  H  P  N  A  K  L  F  S  S  W  L  D  V


ACTGCCAGTGCTGTTTGTAACTGGTCCCGGTACTGACGAAAATGCTGTCCGACTGCCATCTTTTCTGGGGTGATGCAATAGAAGGTTTGGGGGTCCTGCCGCCAGCGATCCCACTTGAGT
     7570      7580      7590      7600      7610      7620      7630      7640      7650      7660      7670      7680
TGACGGTCACGACAAACATTGACCAGGGCCATGACTGCTTTTACGACAGGCTGACGGTAGAAAAGACCCCACTACGTTATCTTCCAAACCCCCAGGACGGCGGTCGCTAGGGTGAACTCA
 A  L  A  T  Q  L  Q  D  R  Y  Q  R  F  H  Q  G  V  A  M  K  E  P  T  I  C  Y  F  T  Q  P  D  Q  R  W  R  D  W  K  L  K


TTCATGGCGATGTCATAGGCGATGTTAACGAGCCGCTGGTCTCCAGAGAGTTTCATGACCAGCATGAAGGGGATTAGCTGCTTGCCAAAGGACCCCATCCAGGTGTAGGTTTCCACATCG
     7690      7700      7710      7720      7730      7740      7750      7760      7770      7780      7790      7800
AAGTACCGCTACAGTATCCGCTACAATTGCTCGGCGACCAGAGGTCTCTCAAAGTACTGGTCGTACTTCCCCTAATCGACGAACGGTTTCCTGGGGTAGGTCCACATCCAAAGGTGTAGC
 M  A  I  D  Y  A  I  N  V  L  R  Q  D  G  S  L  K  M  V  L  M  F  P  I  L  Q  K  G  F  S  G  M  W  T  Y  T  E  V  D  Y


    5' late i leader
 ┌splice                        start 15.3K agnoprotein
 │                               M  R  A  D  R  E  E  L  D  F  L  P  P  V  G  G  M  A  V  D  V  M  E  V  E  L  P  A  T  R  R
TAGGTGAGGAAGAGCCTTTCTGTCGCGAGGATGAGAGCCGATCGGGAAGAACTGGATTTCCTGCCACCAGTTGGAGGAATGGCTGTTGATGTGATGGAAGTAGAACTCCCTGCGACGCGCC
     7810      7820      7830      7840      7850      7860      7870      7880      7890      7900      7910      7920
ATCCACTCCTTCTCGGAAAGACACGCTCCTACTCTCGGCTAGCCCTTCTTGACCTAAAGGACGGTGGTCAACCTCCTTACCGACAACTACACTACCTTCATCTTGAGGGACGCTGCGCGG
 T  L  F  L  R  E  T  R  P  H  S  G  I  P  F  F  Q  I  E  Q  W  W  N  S  S  H  S  N  I  H  H  H  F  Y  F  E  R  R  R  A  S
```

Table 7.1 (Continued)

```
 A  F  M  L  V  L  V  Q  T  A  A  V  L  A  A  I  H  G  M  H  L  M  N  E  L  Y  L  T  S  F  D  E  K  F  Q  W  K  I  E  A
GAGCATTCATGCTTGTGCTTGTACAGACGGCCGCAGTACTCGCAGCGATTCACGGGATGCACCTCATGAATGAGTTGTACCTGACTTCCTTTGACGAGAAATTTCAGTGGAAAATTGAGG
      7930      7940      7950      7960      7970      7980      7990      8000      8010      8020      8030      8040
CTCGTAAGTACGAACACGAACATGTCTGCCGGCGTCATGAGCGTCGCTAAGTGCCCTACGTGGAGTACTTACTCAACATGGACTGAAGGAAACTGCTCTTTAAAGTCACCTTTTAACTCC
 C  E  H  K  H  H  K  Y  L  R  G  C  Y  E  C  R  N  V  P  H  V  E  H  I  L  Q  V  Q  S  G  K  V  L  F  K  L  P  F  N  L  S

 W  R  L  Y  L  A  L  Y  Y  V  V  C  I  G  M  T  I  F  C  L  D  G  G  H  A  D  E  P  S  R  E  A  S  P  D  L  G  A  A  G
CTTGGCGCTTGTACCTCGCGCTCTACTATGTTGTCTGGCATCGGCATGACCATCTTCTGTCTCGATGGTGGTCATGCTGACGAGCCCTCGCGGGAGGCAAGTCCAGACCTCGGCGGCCAG
      8050      8060      8070      8080      8090      8100      8110      8120      8130      8140      8150      8160
GAACCGCGAACATGGAGCGCGAGATGATACAACAGACGTAGCCGTACTGGTAGAAGACAGAGCTACCACCAGTACGACTGCTCGGGAGCGCCCTCCGTTCAGGTCTGGAGCCGCGCCGTC
 P  A  Q  V  E  R  E  V  I  N  D  A  D  A  H  G  D  E  T  E  I  T  T  M  S  V  L  G  R  P  L  C  T  W  V  E  A  R  C  P

                                              late i leader 3'─┬─splice
 A  E  L  E  D  E  S  A  Q  A  G  A  V  Q  G  P  E  T  L  R  S  Q│
GGGCGGAGCTCGAGGACGAGAGCGCGCAGGCCGGAGCTGTCCAGGGTCCTGAGCACGCTGCGGAGTCAGGTTAGTAGGCAGTGTCAGGAGATTGACTTGCATGATCTTTTCGAGGGCGTGA
      8170      8180      8190      8200      8210      8220      8230      8240      8250      8260      8270      8280
CCCGCCTCGAGCTCCTGCTCTCGCGCGTCCGGCCTCGACAGGTCCCAGGACTCTGCGACGCCTCAGTCCAATCATCCGTCACAGTCCTCTAACTGAACGTACTAGAAAAGCTCCCGCACT
                                                                   *  Y  A  T  D  P  S  Q  S  A  H  D  K  R  P  R  S
 R  L  E  L  V  L  A  R  L  G  S  S  D  L  T  R  L  R  Q  P  T  L  N  T  P  L  T  L  L  N  V  Q  M  I  K  E  L  A  H  P
                                                                stop ORF 12.6K

GGGAGGTTCAGATGGTACTTGATCTCCACGGGTCCGTTGGTGGAGATGTCGATGGCTTGCAGGGTTCCGTGCCCCTTGGGCGCTACCACCGTGCCCTTGTTTTTCCTTTTGGGCGGCGGT
      8290      8300      8310      8320      8330      8340      8350      8360      8370      8380      8390      8400
CCCTCCAAGTCTACCATGAACTAGAGGTGCCCAGGCAACCACCTCTAACGGCACCTACCGAACGTCCCAAGGCACGGCGCATGGTGGCACGGGACAAAAAGGAAAACCCGCCGCCA
 P  P  E  S  P  V  Q  D  G  R  T  R  Q  H  L  H  R  H  S  A  P  N  R  A  G  Q  A  S  G  H  G  Q  K  E  K  Q  A  A  T
 L  N  L  H  Y  K  I  E  V  P  G  N  T  S  I  D  I  A  Q  L  T  G  H  G  K  P  A  V  V  T  G  K  N  K  R  K  P  P  P  P

GGCTCTGTTGCTTCTTGCATGTTTAGAAGCGGTGTCGAGGGCGCGCACCGGGCGGCAGGGGCGGCTCGGGACCCGGCGGCATGGCTGGCAGTGGTACGTCGGCACCGCGCGCGGGTAGGT
      8410      8420      8430      8440      8450      8460      8470      8480      8490      8500      8510      8520
CCGAGACAACGAAGAACGTACAAATCTTCGCCACAGCTCCCGCGCTGGCCCGCCGTCCCCGCCGAGCCCTGGGCGCCGTACCGACCGTCACCATGCAGCCGTGGCGCGCGCCCATCCA
 A  R  N  S  R  A  H  K  S  A  T  D  L  A  R  V  P  R  C  P  R  S  P  V  R  R  C  P  Q  C  H  Y  T  P  V  A  R  P  Y  T
                 *  F  R  H  R  P  R  A  G  P  P  L  P  P  E  P  G  P  P  M  A  P  L  P  V  D  A  G  R  A  P  L  N
 E  T  A  E  Q  M
 E2b 129K start
           stop E2b pTP 74K


                   start ORF 14K
                   M  R  D  D  A  A  V  D  I  L  D  L  T  P  L  G  E  S  Y  R  P  R  E  L  E  P  E  R  E  F  N
TCTGGTACTGCGCCCTGAGAAGACTCGCATGCGCGACGACGCGGCGGTTGACATCCTGGATCTGACGCCTCTGGGTGAAAGCTACCGGCCCCGTGAGCTTGAACCTGAAAGAGAGTTCAA
      8530      8540      8550      8560      8570      8580      8590      8600      8610      8620      8630      8640
AGACCATGACGCGGGACTCTTCTGAGCGTACGCGCTGCTGCGCCAACTGTAGGACCTAGACTGCGGAGACCCACTTTCGATGGCCGGGGCACTCGAACTTGGACTTTCTCTCAAGTT
 R  T  S  R  G  G  S  F  V  R  M  R  S  S  A  A  T  S  M
 Q  Y  Q  A  R  L  L  S  A  H  A  V  V  R  R  N  V  D  Q  I  Q  R  R  Q  T  F  A  V  P  G  T  L  K  F  R  F  S  L  E  V
                                          start ORF 12.6K

 R  I  N  L  G  I  V  D  G  G  L  P  K  D  F  L  H  V  A  R  V  V  L  V  G  D  L  G  H  E  L  L  D  L  F  L  L  E  I  S
CAGAATCAATCTCGGTATCGTTGACGGCGGCTTGCCTAAGGATTTCTTGCACGTCGCCAGAGTTGTCCTGGTAGGCGATCTCGGCCATGAACTGCTCGATCTCTTCCTCTTGGAGATCTC
      8650      8660      8670      8680      8690      8700      8710      8720      8730      8740      8750      8760
GTCTTAGTTAGAGCCATAGCAACTGCCGCCGAACGGATTCCTAAAGAACGTGCAGCGGTCTCAACAGGACCATCCGCTAGAGCCGGTACTTGACGAGCTAGAGAAGGAGAACCTCTAGAG
 S  D  I  E  T  D  N  V  A  A  Q  R  L  I  E  Q  V  D  G  S  N  D  Q  Y  A  I  E  A  M  F  Q  E  I  E  E  E  Q  L  D  G

 A  A  R  S  L  D  G  G  R  E  V  V  G  D  A  P  N  E  L  R  E  S  I  H  A  R  L  V  P  D  A  A  V  D  H  S  P  H  G  I
CGCGGCCCGCTCTCTCGACGGTGGCCGCGAGGTCGTTGGAGATGCGCCCAATGAGTTGAGAGAAAGCATTCATGCCCGCCTCGTTCCAGACGCGGCTGTAGACCACAGCCCCCACGGGAT
      8770      8780      8790      8800      8810      8820      8830      8840      8850      8860      8870      8880
GCGCCGGGCGAGAGAGCTGCCACCGGCGCTCCAGCAACCTCTACGCGGGTTACTCAACTCTCTTTCGTAAGTACGGGCGGAGCAAGGTCTGCGCCGACATCTGGTGTCGGGGGTGCCCTA
 R  G  A  R  E  V  T  A  A  L  D  N  S  I  R  G  I  L  Q  S  F  A  N  M  G  A  E  N  W  V  R  S  Y  V  V  A  G  V  P  D

                                     stop ORF 14K
 S  R  A  H  D  H  L  G  E  V  E  L  H  V  A  G  E  D  R  I  V  A  *
CTCTCGCGCGCCATGACCACCTGGGCGAGGTTGAGCTCCACGTGGCGGGTGAAGACCGCATAGTTGCATAGGCGCTGGAAAAGGTAGTTGAGTGTGGTGGCGATGTGCTCGGTGACGAAGA
      8890      8900      8910      8920      8930      8940      8950      8960      8970      8980      8990      9000
GAGAGCGCGCGGTACTGGTGGACCCGCTCCAACTCGAGGTGCACCGCCCACTTCTGGCGTATCAACGTATCCGCGACCTTTCCATCAACTCACACCACCGCTACACGAGCCACTGCTTCT
 R  A  R  M  V  V  Q  A  L  N  L  E  V  H  R  T  F  V  A  Y  N  C  L  R  Q  F  L  Y  N  L  T  T  A  I  H  E  T  V  F  F

AATACATGATCCATCGTCTCAGCGGCATCTCGCTGACATCGCCCAGCGCTTCCAAGCGCTCCATGGCCTCGTAGAAGTTCACGGCAAAGTTGAAAAACTGGGAGTTACGCGCGGACACGG
      9010      9020      9030      9040      9050      9060      9070      9080      9090      9100      9110      9120
TTATGTACTAGGTAGCAGAGTCGCCGTAGAGCGACTGTAGCGGGTCGCGAAGGTTCGCGAGGTACCGGAGCATCTTCAAGTGCCGTTTCAACTTTTTGACCCTCAATGCGCGCCTGTGCC
 Y  M  I  W  R  R  L  P  M  E  S  V  D  G  L  A  E  L  R  E  M  A  E  Y  F  N  V  A  F  N  F  F  Q  S  N  R  A  S  V  T

TCAACTCCTCTTCCAGAAGACGGATAAGTTCGGCGATGGTGGTGCGCACCTCGCGCTCGAAAGCTCCTAGGATTTCTTCCTCAATCTCTTCTTCCTCCTAACATCTCTTCCTCTTCAG
      9130      9140      9150      9160      9170      9180      9190      9200      9210      9220      9230      9240
AGTTGAGGAGAAGGTCTTCTGCCTATTCAAGCCGCTACCACCACGCGTGGAGCGCGAGCTTTCGAGGATCCTAAAGAAGGAGTTAGAGAAGAAGAAGGTGATTGTAGAGAAGGAGAAGTC
 L  E  E  E  L  L  R  I  L  E  A  I  T  T  R  V  E  R  E  F  A  G  L  I  E  E  E  I  E  E  E  E  V  L  M  E  E  E  E  P

GTGGGGCTGCAGGAGGAGGGGGAACGCGGCGACGCCGGCGGCGCACGGGCAGACGGTCGATGAATCTTTCAATGACCTCTCCGCGGCGGCGGCGCATAGTCTCGGTGACGGCACGACCGT
      9250      9260      9270      9280      9290      9300      9310      9320      9330      9340      9350      9360
CACCCCGACGTCCTCCTCCCCCTTGCGCCGGCTGCGGCCGCGCGTGCCCGTCTGCCAGCTACTTGAAAGTTACTGGAGAGGCGCCGCCGCCGCGCGTATCAGAGCCACTGCCGTGCCGGCA
 P  A  A  P  P  P  P  V  R  R  R  R  R  R  R  V  P  L  R  D  I  F  R  E  I  V  E  G  R  R  R  R  R  M  T  E  T  V  A  R  G  N

                                                                                              splice ─┬─
                                                                                                      │V
TCTCCCTGGGTCTCAGAGTGAAGACGCCTCCGCGCATCTCCCTGAAGTGGTGACTGGGAGGCTCTCCGTTGGGCAGGGACACCGCGCTGATTATGCATTTTATCAATTGCCCCGTAGGTA
      9370      9380      9390      9400      9410      9420      9430      9440      9450      9460      9470      9480
AGAGGGACCCAGAGTCTCACTTCTGCGGAGGCGCGTAGAGGGACTTCACCACTGACCCTCCGAGAGGCAACCCGTCCCTGTGGCGCGACTAATACGTAAAATAGTTAACGGGGCATCCAT
 E  R  P  R  L  T  F  V  G  G  R  M  E  R  F  H  H  S  P  P  E  G  N  P  L  S  V  A  S  I  I  C  K  I  L  Q  G  T  P  V
```

Table 7.1 (Continued)

```
-5' 3rd late leader
           stop agnoprotein 15.3K                              3rd late leader 3'┌─splice
  L R A R T   *                                    5' 3rd late leader 3'┐
CTCCGCGCAAGGACCTGATTGTCTCAAGATCCACGGGATCTGAAAACCTTTCGACGAAAGCGTCTAACCAGTCGCAATCGCAAGGTAGGCTGAGCACTGTTTCTTGCGGGCGGGGGCGGC
      9490      9500      9510      9520      9530      9540      9550      9560      9570      9580      9590      9600
GAGGCGCGTTCCTGGACTAACAGAGTTCTAGGTGCCCTAGACTTTTGGAAAGCTGCTTTCGCAGATTGGTCAGCGTTAGCGTTCCATCCGACTCGTGACAAAGAACGCCCGCCCCGCCG
                                                                        *  G T A I A L Y A S C Q K K R A P A A
  G R L S R I T E L D V P D S F R E V F A D L W D C D C P L S L V T E Q P R P R S
                                  ORF 11K stop
```

```
TAGACGCTCGGTCGGGGTTCTCTCTTTCTTCTTCCTTCCCCCTCTTGCGAGGGTGAGACGATGCTGCTGGTGATGAAATTAAAATAGGCAGTTTTAAGACGGCGGATGGTGGCGAGGAGCA
      9610      9620      9630      9640      9650      9660      9670      9680      9690      9700      9710      9720
ATCTGCGAGCCAGCCCCAAGAGAGAAAGAAGAGGAAGGGGGGAGAACGCTCCCACTCTGCTACGACGAACCACTACTTTAATTTTATCCGTCAAAATTCTGCCGCCTACCACCGCTCCTCGT
  L R E T P T R E K K K E K G R K R P H S S A A P S S I L I P L K L V A S P P S S C
  S A R D P N E R E E G E G E Q S P S V I S S T I F N F Y A T K L R R I T A L L V
```

```
                start ORF 10K
                M S H P P S I I L T S G Q I F I V V L H E S F H G H F F
CCAAGTCTTTGGGTCCGGCTTGTTGGATGCGCAGGCGATGAGCCATCCCCCAAGCATCATCCTGACATCTGGCCAGATCTTTATAGTAGTCTTGCATGAGTCGTTCCACGGGCACTTCTT
      9730      9740      9750      9760      9770      9780      9790      9800      9810      9820      9830      9840
GGTTCAGAAACCCAGGCCGAACAACCTACGCGTCCGCTACTCGGTAGGGGGTTCGTAGTAGGACGTGTAGACCGGTCTAGAAATATCATCAGAACGTACTCAGCAAGGTGCCCGTGAAGAA
  W T K P D P K N S A C A I L W G G L M M R V D P W I K I T T K C S D N W P C K K
  L D K P G A Q Q I R L R H A M G W A D D Q C R A L D K Y Y D Q M L R E V P V E E
```

```
  F A R P A M H A S D P E P A H G L D K C Q L R Y N P F G E D G L L H L G E G G L
CTTCGCCCGCCCTGCCATGCATGCGAGTGATCCCGAACCCGCGCATGGGCTGGACAAGTGCCAGCTCCGCTACAACCCTTTCGGCGAGGATGGCTTGCTGCACCTGGGTGAGGGTGGCTT
      9850      9860      9870      9880      9890      9900      9910      9920      9930      9940      9950      9960
GAAGCGGGCGGGACGGTACGTACGCTCACTAGGGCTTGGGCGCGTACCCGACCTGTTCACGGTCGAGGCGATGTTGGGAAAGCCGCTCCTACCGAACGACGTGGACCCACTCCACCGAA
  K A R G A M
  E G A R G H M R T I G F G R M P Q V L A L E A V V R E A L I A Q Q V Q T L T A Q
       start ORF 11K
```

```
                                              stop ORF 10K
  K V V V K V H E A V V G P G V D C V G A V G H D   *
GAAAGTCGTCAAAGTCCACGAAGCGGTGGTAGGCCCCGGTGTTGATTGTGTAGGAGCAGTTGGCCATGACTGACCAGTTGACTGTCTGGTGCCCAGGGCGCACGAGCTCGGTGTACTTCA
      9970      9980      9990      10000     10010     10020     10030     10040     10050     10060     10070     10080
CTTTCAGCAGTTTCAGGTGCTTCGCCACCATCCGGGGCCACAACTAACACATCCTCGTCAACCGGTACTGACTGGTCAACTGACAGACCACGGGTCCCGCGTGCTCGAGCCACATGAAGT
  F D D F D V F R H Y A G T N I T Y S C N A M V S W N V T Q H G P R V L E T Y K L
```

```
GGCGCGAGTATGCGCGCGTGTCAAAGATGTAATCGTTGCAGGTGCGCACCAGGTACTGGTAGCCGATGAGAAAGTGTGGCGATGGCTGGCGGTACAGGGGCCATCGCTCGTAGCCGGGG
      10090     10100     10110     10120     10130     10140     10150     10160     10170     10180     10190     10200
CCGCGCTCATACGCGCGCACAGTTTCTACATTAGCAACGTCCACGCGTGGTCCATGACCATCGGCTACTCTTTCACACCGCTACCGACCGCCATGTCCCCGGTAGCGAGACATCGGCCCC
  R S Y A R T D F I Y D N C T R V L Y Q Y G I L F H P S P Q R Y L P W R E T A P A
```

```
CTCCGGGGGCGAGGTCTTCCAGCATGAGGCGGTGGTAGCCGTAGATGTACCTGGACATCCAGGTGATACCGGAGGCGGTGGTGGATGCACGTGGGAACTCGCGCACGCGGTTCCAGATGT
      10210     10220     10230     10240     10250     10260     10270     10280     10290     10300     10310     10320
GAGGCCCCCGCTCCAGAAGGTCGTACTCCGCCACCATCGGCATCTACATGGACCTGTAGGTCCACTATGGCCTCCGCCACCACCTACGTGCACCCTTGAGCGCGTGCGCCAAGGTCTACA
  G P A L D E L M L R H Y G Y I Y R S M W T I G S A T T S A R P F E R V R N W I N
```

```
                                                                                    ┌─5' VA1 RNA
TGCGCAGCGGCATGAAGTAGTTCATGGTAGGCACGGTCTGGCCAGTGAGGCGCGCGCAGTCATTGACGCTCTGTAGACACGGAGAAAACGAAAGCGATGAGCGGCTCGACTCCGTGGCCT
      10330     10340     10350     10360     10370     10380     10390     10400     10410     10420     10430     10440
ACGCGTCGCCGTACTTCATCAGTACCATCCGTGCCAGACCGGTCACTCCGCGCGCGTCAGTAACTGCGAGACATCTGTGCCTCTTTTGCTTTCGCTACTCGCCGAGCTGAGGCACCGGA
  R L P M F Y N M T P V T Q G T L R A C D N V S Q L C P S F S L S S R S S E T A Q
     start E2b pTP 74K? (as in Ad5)
```

```
GGGGGAACGTGGACGGGTTGGGTCGCGGTGTACCCCGGTTCGAGTCCAAAGCTAAGCAATCACACTCGGATCGGCCGGAGCCGCGGCTAACGTGGTATTGGCTATCCCGTCTCGACCCAG
      10450     10460     10470     10480     10490     10500     10510     10520     10530     10540     10550     10560
CCCCCTTGCACCTGCCCAACCCAGCGCCACATGGGGCCAAGCTCAGGTTTCGATTCGTTAGTGTGAGCCTAGCCGGCCTCGGCGCCGATTGCACCATAACCGATAGGGCAGAGCTGGGTC
  P F T S P N P R P T G R N S D L A L C D C E S R G S G R S V H Y Q S D R R S G A
```

```
                3' VA1 RNA ┬┬┬┬                                                  ┌─5' VA2 RNA
CCGACGAATATCCAGGGTACGGAGTAGAGTCGTTTTTGCTGCTTTTTTTCCTGGACGTGTGCCATTGCCACGTCAAGCTTTACAACGCTCAGTTCTCGGGCCGTGAGTGGCTCGCGCCCGT
      10570     10580     10590     10600     10610     10620     10630     10640     10650     10660     10670     10680
GGCTGCTTATAGGTCCCATGCCTCATCTCAGCAAAAACGACGAAAAAAGGACCTGCACACGGTACGGTGCAGTTCGAAATGTTGCGAGTCAAGAGCCCGGCACTCACCGAGCGCGGGCA
  S S Y G P Y P T S D N K S S K E Q V H A M
                                      start E2b pTP ??
```

```
AGTCTGGAGAATCAGTCGCCAGGGTTGCGTTGCGGTATGCCCCCGGTTCGAGCCTAAGCGCGGCTCGTATCGGCCGGTTTCCGCGACAAGCGAGGGTTTGGCAGCCCAGTCATTTCCAAG
      10690     10700     10710     10720     10730     10740     10750     10760     10770     10780     10790     10800
TCAGACCTCTTAGTCAGCGGTCCCAACGCAACGCCATACGGGGGCCAAGCTCGGATTCGCGCCGGCATAGCCGGCCAAAGGCGCTGTTCGCTCCCAAACCGTCGGGTCAGTAAAGGTTC
```

```
                VA2 RNA 3' ┬┬┬┬              splice├
                                                   start L1 55,52K?
                                         M H P V L R Q M R P Q Q Q A P S Q Q
ACCCCCGCCAGCCGACTTCTCCAGTTTACGGGAGCGAGCCCTTTTTTTTTTTTTGTTTTTGTCGCCCAGATGCATCCAGTGCTGCGACAGATGCGCCCCAGCAACAGGCCCCTTCTCAGCA
      10810     10820     10830     10840     10850     10860     10870     10880     10890     10900     10910     10920
TGGGGCGGTCGGCTGAAGAGGTCAAATGCCCTCGCTCGGGAAAAAAAAAAAAACAAAAACAGCGGGTCTACGTAGGTCACGACGCTGTCTACGCGGGGGTCGTTGTCGGGGAAGAGTCGT
```

```
   Q P Q K A L L A P
ACAGCCACAAAAGGCTCTTCTTGCTCCT
      10930     10940
TGTCGGTGTTTTCCGAGAAGAACGAGGA
```

Table 7.2. Landmarks in the Ad7 DNA sequence 0–30.2%

Strand, nucleotide		Sequence	Identity
r	l		
	T136		end ITR
	T480	TATTTAAA	"TATA" box E1A
	A512		cap site E1A mRNAs
	A576	ATG	start E1A proteins
	G647		splice donor E1A mRNA
	G746		*Bam*HI 2.1%
	T1062		splice donor E1A mRNA
	A1155		splice donor E1A mRNA
	G1249		splice acceptor E1A mRNAs
	T1348	TAA	stop E1A 6.8K protein
	A1383	AAGCTT	*Hin*dIII 3.8%
	T1452	TGA	stop E1A 28K, 25K proteins
	A1493	AATAAA	3'-poly(A) signal E1A
	T1510		3'-poly(A) attachment site E1A mRNAs
	T1548	TATATAA	"TATA" box
	A1563	AGATCT	*Bgl*II 4.3%
	G1578		cap site E1B mRNAs
	A1602	ATG	start E1B 21K protein
	A1907	ATG	start E1B 55K, 9.0K proteins
	G1909	GGATCC	*Bam*HI 5.3%
	T2136	TAG	stop E1B protein
	G2164		splice donor E1B mRNA
	A2712	AAGCTT	*Hin*dIII 7.5%
	T3383	TAA	stop E1B protein
	A3386		splice donor E1B mRNA
	A3460		cap site protein IX mRNA (no "TATA" box!)
	A3480	ATG	start protein IX
	T3481	TGA	stop E1B 9.0K protein
	G3573	GGATCC	*Bam*HI 9.9%
	C3798	CTCGAG	*Xho*I 10.5%
	T3894	TAA	stop protein IX
	A3897	AGATCT	*Bgl*II 10.8%
	A3892	AATAAA	
	A3908	AATAAA	3'-poly(A) signals E1B, protein IX mRNAs
	A3913	AATAAA	
	C3938		3'-poly(A) attachment site E1B, protein IX mRNAs
T3951		TAA	stop protein IVa2
A3953		AATAAA	3'-poly(A) signal IVa2, E2B mRNAs
	C4615	CCCGGG	*Sma*I 12.7%
	C5020	CTCGAG	*Xho*I 13.9%
T5054		TAG	stop E2B 129K DNA polymerase
	A5124	ATG	start ORF 21K
G5282			splice acceptor IVa2 mRNA
G5561			splice donor IVa2 mRNA
A5573		ATG	start protein IVa2
	C5643	CTCGAG	*Xho*I 15.6%
	T5691	TGA	stop ORF 21K
A5691			cap sites IVa2 mRNA
T5693			

Table 7.2 (Continued)

Strans, nucleotide		Sequence	Identity
r	l		
	G5764	GGATCC	*Bam*HI 15.9%
	T5873	TATAAAA	"TATA" box major late mRNAs
	A5904		cap site major late mRNAs (1st leader)
	G5944		splice donor 1st late leader
	A6135	AAGCTT	*Hind*III 16.9%
	A6145	ATG	start ORF 11.5K
	G6356	GTCGAC	*Sal*I 17.6%
	T6463	TAG	stop ORF 11.5K
	C6703	CCCGGG	*Sma*I 18.5%
T6871		TAG	stop ORF 19K
	C6963		splice acceptor 2nd late leader
	G7034		splice donor 2nd late leader
	A7134	ATG	start ORF 10K
A7390		ATG	start ORF 19K
	T7419	TAA	stop ORF 10K
	A7474	AGATCT	*Bgl*II 20.6%
	G7704	GTTAAC	*Hpa*I 21.3%
	G7804		splice acceptor late i leader
	A7830	ATG	start agnoprotein 15.3K
	C8169	CTCGAG	*Xho*I 22.6%
	G8228		splice donor late i leader
T8232		TAA	stop ORF 12.6K
A8420		ATG	start E2B 129K DNA polymerase
T8425		TAA	stop E2B pTP 74K
	A8549	ATG	start ORF 14K
A8574		ATG	start ORF 12.6K
	A8754	AGATCT	*Bgl*II 24.2%
	T8948	TAG	stop ORF 14K
	G9478		splice acceptor 3rd late leader
	T9496	TGA	stop agnoprotein 15.3K
T9546		TAG	stop ORF 11K
	G9564		splice acceptor 3rd late leader
	A9758	ATG	start ORF 10K
	A9795	AGATCT	*Bgl*II 27.1%
A9858		ATG	start ORF 11K
	T10031	TGA	stop ORF 10K
A10345		ATG	start E2B pTP (in analogy with Ad5)
	G10423		5'-end VA1 RNA
	T1059		heterogeneous 3'-end VA1
	to		
	T10597		
A10624		ATG	potential start E2B pTB (84K)
	A10634	AAGCTT	*Hind*III 29.4%
	G10668		5'-end VA2 RNA
	T10841–		heterogeneous 3'-end VA2 RNA
	T10846		
	A10868		splice acceptor L1 mRNAs
	A10868	ATG	start L1 55,52K?

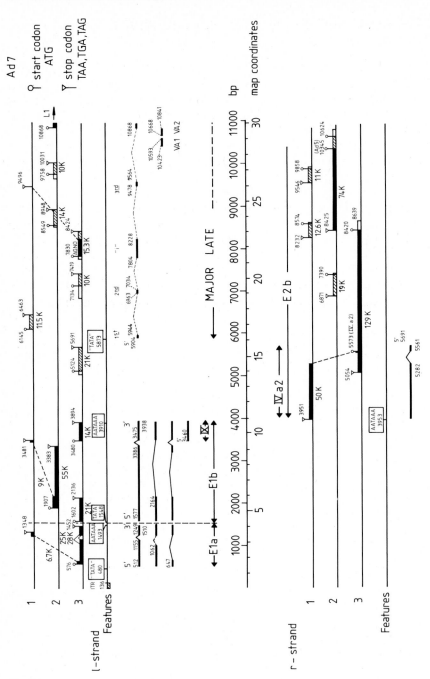

Fig. 7.1

8 DNA Sequence of Human Ad12 (Subgroup A) Between Coordinates 0.0 and 11

The sequence (Table 8.2) was determined by Shinagawa and Padmanabhan (1980; ITR), Sugisaki et al. (1980; nucleotides 1–2323), Bos et al. (1981; nucleo-tides 1400–3814), Kimura et al. (1981; nucleotides 1487–3860), and R. Bernards (personal communication; nucleotides 3861–3957). It is given in double-stranded format with 120 nucleotides per line, with the numbering (starting at the left terminus of Ad12 DNA) between the two strand sequences. Each number refers to the position above and below its last zero. The following features are marked: the end of the ITR, RNA 5′ termini (cap sites), "TATA" boxes and 3′-poly(A) attachment sites (AATAAA; underlined), and predicted initiation and termina-tion codons (Table 8.2) (Sugisaki et al. 1980; Bos et al. 1981; Kimura et al. 1981; Perricaudet et al. 1980b; Virtanen et al. 1982b). The splice donor resi-due G588 was determined by J.L. Bos (personal communication). Above the l-strand sequence is given the predicted primary structure (in one-letter code; see footnote to Table 8.1) for the E1A and E1B proteins and for viral protein IX (Sugisaki et al. 1980; Bos et al. 1981; Kimura et al. 1981). The Ad12 DNA between coordinates contains no unidentified ORFs of appreciable length.

Table 8.1. Ad12 DNA sequence 0–11%

```
CTATATATATAATATACCTTATACTGGACTAGTGCCAATATTAAAATGAAGTGGGCGTAGTGTGTAATTTGATTGGGTGGAGGTGTGGCTTTGGCGTGCTTGTAAGTTTGGGCGGATGAG
        10        20        30        40        50        60        70        80        90       100       110       120
GATATATATATTTATATGGAATATGACCTGATCACGGTTATAATTTTACTTCACCCGCATCACACATTAAACTAACCCACCTCCACACCGAAACCGCACGAACATTCAAACCCGCCTACTC

                                                    ┌ end ITR
GAAGTGGGGCGCGGCGTGGGAGCCGGGCGCGCCGGATGTGACGT TTTAGACGCCATTTTACACGGAAATGATGTTTTTTGGGCGTTGTTTGTGCAAATTTTGTGTTTTAGGCGCGAAAAC
       130       140       150       160       170       180       190       200       210       220       230       240
CTTCACCCCGCGCCGCCACCCTCGGCCCGCGCGGCCTACACTGCAAAATCTGCGGTAAAATGTGCCTTTACTACAAAAAACCCGCAACAAACACGTTTAAAACACAAAATCCGCGCTTTTG

              alternative "TATA" E1a
TGAAATGCGGAAGTGAAAATTGATGACGGCAATTTTATTATAGGCGCGGAATATTTACCGAGGGCAGAGTGAACTCTGAGCCTCTACGTGTGGGTTTCGATACGTGAGCGACGGGAAAC
       250       260       270       280       290       300       310       320       330       340       350       360
ACTTTACGCCTTCACTTTTAACTACTGCCGTTAAAATAATATCCGCGCCTTATAAATGGCTCCCGTCTCACTTGAGACTCGGAGATGCACACCCAAAGCTATGCACTCGCTGCCCCTTTG
```

One-letter code for amino acids: A, ala; C, cys; D, asp; E, glu; F, phe; G, gly; H, his; I, ile; K, lys; L, leu; M, met; N, asn; P, pro; Q, gln; R, arg; S, ser; T, thr; V, val; W, trp; Y, tyr

◀

Fig. 7.1. Schematic representation of RNA coordinates and of identified and unidentified reading frames in Ad7 DNA between coordinates 0.0 and 30.2. The map scale in the *center* of the figure reflects a conversion factor of 362 bp, which corresponds to 1% of the viral genome. Immediately *above* and *below* the scale, the locations of the various transcription units are indicated. The *continuous lines* above the transcription unit designations represent the segments of rightward transcripts present in mature RNAs; *interrupted carets* connecting the lines denote RNA splices. The coordinates of the RNA 5′ caps and 3′-poly(A) attachment sites and of splice donor and acceptor sites are also given in this part of the figure. On the *next line above* a number of RNA expression signals have been drawn: "TATA" boxes and 3′-poly(A) signals (AATAAA). Lines 1, 2, and 3 in the *upper part* of the figure represent the three possible frames in which the DNA l-strand can be read. Tracts open for translation are indicated as *solid bars* for known genes and as *hatched bars* for unidentified translatable regions. The open frames are flanked by the symbols ⌐ and ⌐, denoting initiation (ATG) or termination (TAA, TAG or TGA) codons respectively. The *numbers* next to these codons are their coordinates, and the *numbers in larger type* refer to the predicted MW of the translation products. *Interrupted lines* connecting solid bars show how open frames are linked due to RNA splicing.

In the *bottom* half of the figure are the open frames in the DNA r-strand for known genes (*solid bars*) and potential (unidentified) polypeptides (*hatched bars*), *below* them a schematic represen-tation of the mRNAs transcribed from the l-strand (as far as they are known at the nucleotide level)

Table 8.1 (Continued)

```
                                           "TATA" Ela              ┌ cap Ela mRNA
TCCACGTTGCGCTCAAAGGGCGCGTTTATTGTTCTGTCAGCTGATCGTTTGGGTATTTAATGCCGCCGTGTTCGTCAAGAGGCCACTCTTGAGTGCCAGCGAGAAGAGTTTTCTCTGCCA
   370       380       390       400       410       420       430       440       450       460       470       480
AGGTGCAACGCGAGTTTCCCGCGCAAATAACAAGACAGTCGACTAGCAAACCCATAAATTACGGCGGCACAAGCAGTTCTCCGGTGAGAACTCACGGTCGCTCTTCTCAAAAGAGACGGT


            start Ela proteins 29K, 26K 6.2K                                                    splice Ela mRNA (6.2K)
              M  R  T  E  M  T  P  L  V  L  S  Y  Q  E  A  D  D  I  L  E  H  L  V  D  N  F  F  N  E│V  P  S  D
GCTCATTTTCACGGCGCCATTATGAGAACTGAAATGACTCCCTTGGTCCTGTCGTATCAGGAAGCTGACGACATATTGGAGCATTTGGTGGACAACTTTTTTAACGAGGTACCCAGTGAT
   490       500       510       520       530       540       550       560       570       580       590       600
CGAGTAAAAGTGCCGCGGTAATACTCTTGACTTTACTGAGGGAACCAGGACAGCATAGTCCTTCGACTGCTGTATAACCTCGTAAACCACCTGTTGAAAAAATTGCTCCATGGGTCACTA


        D  D  L  Y  V  P  S  L  Y  E  L  Y  D  L  D  V  E  S  A  G  E  D  N  N  E  Q  A  V  N  E  F  F  P  E  S  L  I  L  A  A
GATGATCTTTATGTTCCGTCTCTTTACGAACTGTATGATCTTGATGTGGAGTCTGCCGGTGAAGATAATAATGAACAGGCGGTGAATGAGTTTTTTCCCGAATCGCTTATTTTAGCTGCC
   610       620       630       640       650       660       670       680       690       700       710       720
CTACTAGAAATACAAGGCAGAGAAATGCTTGACATACTAGAACTACACCTCAGACGGCCACTTCTATTATTACTTGTCCGCCACTTACTCAAAAAAGGGCTTAGCGAATAAAATCGACGG


        S  E  G  L  F  L  P  E  P  P  V  L  S  P  V  C  E  P  I  G  G  E  C  M  P  Q  L  H  P  E  D  M  D  L  L  C  Y  E  M  G
AGTGAGGGGTTGTTTTTACCGGAGCCTCCTGTACTTTCTCCTGTCGTGAGCCATTGGGGGCGAATGTATGCCACAACTGCACCCTGAAGATATGGATTTATTGTGCTACGAGATGGGC
   730       740       750       760       770       780       790       800       810       820       830       840
TCACTCCCCAACAAAAATGGCCTCGGAGGACATGAAAGAGGACAGACACTCGGATAACCCCCGCTTACATACGGTGTTGACGTGGGACTTCTATACCTAAATAACACGATGCTCTACCCG


        F  P  C  S  D  S  E  D  E  Q  D  E  N  G  M  A  H  V  S  A  S  A  A  A  A  A  A  D  R  E  R  E  E  F  Q  L  D  H  P  E
TTTCCCTGTAGCGATTCGGAAGACGAGCAAGACGAACGGAATGGCCGCATGTTTCTGCATCCGCAGCTGCTGCTGCCGCTGATAGGGAACGTGAGGAGTTTCAGTTAGACCATCCAGAG
   850       860       870       880       890       900       910       920       930       940       950       960
AAAGGGACATCGCTAAGCCTTCTGCTCGTTCTGCTCTTGCCTTACCGGCGTACAAAGACGTAGGCGTCGACGACGACGGCGACTATCCCTTGCACTCCTCAAAGTCAATCTGGTAGGTCTC


                                                                                                              (29K)
       splice─┬─Ela mRNA (26K)                                                                        splice─┬─Ela mRNA
       L  P  G  H  N│C  K  S  C  E  H  H  R  N  S  T  G  N  T  D  L  M  C  S  L  C  Y  L  R  A  Y  N  M  F  I  Y│S
TTGCCCGGACACAATTGTAAGTCCTGTGAGCACCACCGGAATAGTACTGGAAATACTGACTTAATGTGCTCTTTGTGCTATCTGCGAGCCTACAACATGTTCATTTACAGTAAGTGTGCT
   970       980       990      1000      1010      1020      1030      1040      1050      1060      1070      1080
AACGGGCCTGTGTTAACATTCAGGACACTCGTGGTGGCCTTATCATGACCTTTATGACTGAATTACACGAGAAACACGATAGACGCTCGGATGTTGTACAAGTAAATGTCATTCACACGA


                               splice─┬─Ela mRNA
                               6.2K───>│V  L  F  P  I  M  S  L  N  L  I  A  L  W  M  A  M  S  D
                               29K, 26K──┤>  P  V  S  D  N  E  P  E  P  N  S  T  L  D  G  D  E  R  P
ATGGGAGGTGGGAGGTGATTTTTTTTTCTTAAGCAGTGAAAAATAATATTTTGTTGTTTTTAGGTCCTGTTTCCGATAATGAGCCTGAACCTAATAGCACTTTGGATGGCGATGAGCGAC
  1090      1100      1110      1120      1130      1140      1150      1160      1170      1180      1190      1200
TACCCTCCACCCTCCACTAAAAAAAAAGAATTCGTCACTTTTTATTATAAAACAACAAAAATCCAGGACAAAGGCTATTACTCGGACTTGGATTATCGTGAAACCTACCGCTACTCGCTG


         stop Ela 6.2K
     P  H  P  R  N  *
     S  P  P  K  L  G  S  A  V  P  E  G  V  I  K  P  V  P  Q  R  V  T  G  R  R  R  C  A  V  E  S  I  L  D  L  I  Q  E  E  E
CCTCACCCCCGAAACTAGGAAGTGCGGTTCCAGAAGGAGTAATAAAACCTGTGCCTCAGCGGGTGACTGGGAGGCGTAGATGTGCTGTGGAAAGCATTTTGGATTTGATTCAAGAGGAAG
  1210      1220      1230      1240      1250      1260      1270      1280      1290      1300      1310      1320
GGAGTGGGGGCTTTGATCCTTCACGCCAAGGTCTTCCTCCATTATTTTGGACACGGAGTCGCCCACTGACCCTCCGCATCTACACGACACCTTTCGTAAAACCTAAACTAAGTTCTCCTTC


                                                  stop Ela 29K, 26K
     R  E  Q  T  V  P  V  D  L  S  V  K  R  P  R  C  N  *
AAAGAGAACAAACAGTGCCTGTTGATCTGTCAGTGAAACGCCCTAGATGTAATTAATGGACTTTGAGCACCTGGGCAATAAAATAGGGGTAATGTGGTTTTTGTGAGTCATGTATAATAA
  1330      1340      1350      1360      1370      1380      1390      1400      1410      1420      1430      1440
TTTCTCTTGTTTGTCACGGACAACTAGACAGTCACTTTGCGGGATCTACATTAATTACCTGAAACTCGTGGACCCGTTATTTTATCCCATTACACCAAAAACACTCAGTACATATTATT


      ┌ 3'-poly(A) Ela                              "TATA" Elb           cap─┬─Elb         start Elb 19K
                                                                                     M  E  L  E  T  V  L
AACTGGTTTCGGTTGAAGTGTCTTGTTAATGTTTGTTTGGGCGTGGTTAAACAGGGATATAAAGCTGGGTTGGTGTTGCTTTGAATAGTTCATCTTAGTAATGGAGTTGGAAACTGTGCT
  1450      1460      1470      1480      1490      1500      1510      1520      1530      1540      1550      1560
TTGACCAAAGCCAACTTCACAGAACAATTACAAACAAACCCGCACCAATTTGTCCCTATATTTCGACCCAACCACAACGAAACTTATCAAGTAGAATCATTACCTCAACCTTTGACACGA


     Q  S  F  Q  S  V  R  Q  L  L  Q  Y  T  S  K  N  T  S  G  F  W  R  Y  L  F  G  S  T  L  S  K  V  V  N  R  V  K  E  D  Y
GCAAAGTTTTCAGAGCGTTCGCCAGCTCTTGCAGTATACCTCTAAAAACACTTCAGGTTTTTGGAGGTATCTGTTTGGCTCTACCTTAAGCAAGGTGGTAAATAGGGTGAAAGAAGACTA
  1570      1580      1590      1600      1610      1620      1630      1640      1650      1660      1670      1680
CGTTTCAAAAGTCTCGCAAGCGGTCGAGAACGTCATATGGAGATTTTTGTGAAGTCCAAAAACCTCCATAGACAAACCGAGATGGAATTCGTTCCACCATTTATCCCACTTTCTTCTGAT


     R  E  E  F  E  N  I  L  A  D  C  P  G  L  L  A  S  L  D  L  C  Y  H  L  V  F  Q  E  K  V  V  R  S  L  D  F  S  S  V  G
TAGAGAGGAATTTGAAAACATATTGGCCGACTGTCCAGGGCTTTTGGCTTCACTAGACCTTTGTTACCACTTGGTGTTTCAGGAAAAAGTGGTCAGATCCTTAGATTTTTCATCTGTGGG
  1690      1700      1710      1720      1730      1740      1750      1760      1770      1780      1790      1800
ATCTCTCCTTAAACTTTTGTATAACCGGCTGACAGGTCCCGAAAACCGAAGTGATCTGGAAACAATGGTGAACCACAAAGTCCTTTTTCACCAGTCTAGGAATCTAAAAAGTAGACACCC


                         start Elb 54K, 8.4K, 11.6K
                           M  E  R  E  I  P  P  E  L  G  L  H  A  G  L  H  V  N  A  A  V  E  G  M  A
     R  T  V  A  S  I  A  F  L  A  T  I  L  D  K  W  S  E  K  S  H  L  S  W  D  Y  M  L  D  Y  M  S  M  Q  L  W  R  A  W  L
ACGAACGGTTGCTTCTATTGCTTTTTTGGCAACCATATTGGATAAATGGAGCGAGAAATCCCACCTGAGTTGGGATTACATGCTGGATTACATGTCAATGCAGCTGTGGAGGGCATGGCT
  1810      1820      1830      1840      1850      1860      1870      1880      1890      1900      1910      1920
TGCTTGCCAACGAAGATAACGAAAAAACCGTTGGTATAACCTATTTACCTCGCTCTTTAGGGTGGACTCAACCCTAATGTACGACCTAATGTACAGTTACGTCGACACCTCCCGTACCGA


                                                                                                   Elb 19K stop
     E  E  E  G  L  H  L  L  A  G  A  A  F  D  H  A  A  A  A  D  V  A  R  G  E  G  G  G  A  E  P  C  G  G  G  E  V  N  M  E
     K  R  R  V  C  I  Y  S  L  A  R  P  L  T  M  P  P  L  P  T  L  Q  E  E  K  E  E  E  R  N  P  A  V  V  E  K  *
GAAGAGGAGGGGTTTGCATTTACTCGCTGGCGCGGCCTTTGACCATGCCGCCGCTGCCGACGTTGCAAGAGGACGAAGGAGGAGGAGCGGAACCCTGCGGTGGTGGAGAAGTAAACATGGAA
  1930      1940      1950      1960      1970      1980      1990      2000      2010      2020      2030      2040
CTTCTCCTCCCAAACGTAAATGAGCGACCGCGCCGGAAACTGGTACGGCGGCGACGGCTGCAACGTTCTCCTCTTCCTCCTCCTCGCCTTGGGACGCCACCACCTCTTCATTTGTACCTT


      ┌ splice Elb mRNA (19K, 8.4K, 11.6K)
     Q  Q│V  Q  E  G  H  V  L  D  S  G  E  G  P  S  C  A  D  D  R  D  K  Q  E  K  K  E  S  L  K  E  A  A  V  L  S  R  L  T
CAACAGGTGCAAGAAGGCCATGTACTTGACTCTGGCGAAGGGCCTAGTTGCGCAGATGATAGAGATAAGCAGGAAAAAAAAGAAAGTTTAAAGGAAGCTGCTGTTCTTAGTAGGCTAACT
  2050      2060      2070      2080      2090      2100      2110      2120      2130      2140      2150      2160
GTTGTCCACGTTCTTCCGGTACATGAACTGAGACCGCTTCCCGGATCAACGCGTCTACTATCTCTATTCGTCCTTTTTTTTTCTTTCAAATTTCCTTCGACGACAAGAATCATCCGATTGA
```

Table 8.1 (Continued)

```
 V  N  L  M  S  R  P  R  L  E  T  V  Y  W  Q  E  L  Q  D  E  F  Q  R  G  D  M  H  L  Q  Y  K  Y  S  F  E  Q  L  K  T  H
GTTAATCTGATGTCCCGCCCGCGTTTGGGAAACTGTATATTGGCAGGAGTTGCAGGATGAATTTCAGCGGGGTGATATGCATTTACAGTACAAATACAGTTTTGAACAATTAAAAACCCAC
    2170      2180      2190      2200      2210      2220      2230      2240      2250      2260      2270      2280
CAATTAGACTACAGGGCGGGCGCAAACCTTTGACATATAACCGTCCTCAACGTCCTACTTAAAGTCGCCCCACTATACGTAAATGTCATGTTTATGTCAAAACTTGTTAATTTTTGGGTG


 W  L  E  P  W  E  D  M  E  C  A  I  K  A  F  A  K  L  A  L  R  P  D  C  S  Y  R  I  T  K  T  V  T  I  T  S  C  A  Y  I
TGGTTAGAGCCATGGGAGGATATGGAGTGTGCTATTAAAGCTTTTGCTAAATTGGCCTTACGTCCTGATTGTAGCTACAGAATTACTAAAACAGTAACCATTACTTCATGCGCCTATATT
    2290      2300      2310      2320      2330      2340      2350      2360      2370      2380      2390      2400
ACCAATCTCGGTACCCTCCTATACCTCACACGATAATTTCGAAAACGATTTAACCGGAATGCAGGACTAACATCGATGTCTTAATGATTTTGTCATTGGTAATGAAGTACGCGGATATAA


 I  G  N  G  A  I  V  E  V  D  T  S  D  R  V  A  F  R  C  R  M  Q  G  M  G  P  G  V  V  G  L  D  G  I  T  F  I  N  V  R
ATAGGTAACGGGGCAATAGTTGAGGTAGATACAAGCGACAGAGTTGCTTTTAGATGTCGAATGCAGGGTATGGGCCCAGGGGTGGTGGGTTTGGATGGAATTACATTTATAAATGTTAGG
    2410      2420      2430      2440      2450      2460      2470      2480      2490      2500      2510      2520
TATCCATTGCCCCGTTATCAACTCCATCTATGTTCGCTGTCTCAACGAAAATCTACAGCTTACGTCCCATACCCGGGTCCCCACCACCCAAACCTACCTTAATGTAAATATTTACAATCC


 F  A  G  D  K  F  K  G  I  M  F  E  A  N  T  C  L  V  L  H  G  V  Y  F  L  N  F  S  N  I  C  V  E  S  W  N  K  V  S  A
TTTGCTGGAGATAAGTTTAAAGGCATTATGTTCGAAGCTAATACCTGTCTTGTCTTGCATGGTGTTTACTTTCTTAACTTTAGTAACATTTGTGTAGAGTCTTGGAATAAGGTTTCTGCT
    2530      2540      2550      2560      2570      2580      2590      2600      2610      2620      2630      2640
AAACGACCTCTATTCAAATTTCCGTAATACAAGCTTCGATTATGGACAGAACAGAACGTACCACAAATGAAAGAATTGAAATCATTGTAAACACATCTCAGAACCTTATTCCAAAGACGA


 R  G  C  T  F  Y  G  C  W  K  G  L  V  G  R  P  K  S  K  L  S  V  K  K  C  L  F  E  K  C  V  L  A  L  I  V  E  G  D  A
AGGGGCTGTACTTTTTATGGATGTTGGAAGGGTTTGGTGGGTAGACCAAAAAGTAAACTGTCTGTAAAAAAGTGTTTGTTTGAAAAATGTGTACTTGCTTTAATTGTAGAGGGGGATGCA
    2650      2660      2670      2680      2690      2700      2710      2720      2730      2740      2750      2760
TCCCCGACATGAAAAATACCTACAACCTTCCCAAACCACCCATCTGGTTTTTCATTTGACAGACATTTTTTCACAAACAAACTTTTTACACATGAACGAAATTAACATCTCCCCCTACGT


 H  I  R  H  N  A  A  S  E  N  A  C  F  V  L  L  K  G  M  A  I  L  K  H  N  M  V  C  G  V  S  D  Q  T  M  R  R  F  V  T
CATATTAGGCATAATGCAGCTTCAGAAAATGCCTGTTTTGTATTATTGAAGGGAATGGCTATTTTAAAGCATAATATGGTTTGTGGGGTGTCTGATCAAACTATGCGACGTTTTGTTACC
    2770      2780      2790      2800      2810      2820      2830      2840      2850      2860      2870      2880
GTATAATCCGTATTACGTCGAAGTCTTTTACGGACAAAACATAATAACTTCCCTTACCGATAAAATTTCGTATTATACCAAACACCCCACAGACTAGTTTGATACGTGCAAAACAATGG


 C  A  D  G  N  C  H  T  L  K  T  V  H  I  V  S  H  S  R  H  C  W  P  V  C  D  H  N  M  F  M  R  C  T  I  H  L  G  L  R
TGTGCTGATGGAAATTGTCATACCTTAAAAACTGTTCATATTGTGAGCCACAGTAGACATTGTTGGCCTGTATGTGATCATAACATGTTTATGCGCTGTACCATACATTTAGGCTTAAGG
    2890      2900      2910      2920      2930      2940      2950      2960      2970      2980      2990      3000
ACACGACTACCTTTAACAGTATGGAATTTTTGACAAGTATAACACTCGGTGTCATCTGTAACAACCGGACATACACTAGTATTGTACAAATACGCGACATGGTATGTAAATCCGAATTCC


 R  G  M  F  R  P  S  Q  C  N  F  S  H  S  N  I  M  L  E  P  E  V  F  S  R  V  C  L  N  G  V  F  D  L  S  V  E  L  C  K
CGGGGTATGTTTAGACCTTCCCAATGTAACTTCAGCCACTCAAACATTATGCTGGAACCTGAAGTGTTTTCTAGAGTGTGTTTAAATGGGGTATTTGATTTATCTGTGGAATTATGTAAG
    3010      3020      3030      3040      3050      3060      3070      3080      3090      3100      3110      3120
GCCCCATACAAATCTGGAAGGGTTACATTGAAGTCGGTGAGTTTGTAATACGACCTTGGACTTCACAAAAGATCTCACACAAATTTACCCCATAAACTAAATAGACACCTTAATACATTC
```

                                                                  splice ─┬─ E1b mRNA (11.6K)

```
 V  I  R  Y  N  D  D  T  R  H  R  C  R  Q  C  E  C  G  S  S  H  L  E  L  R  P  I  V  L  N  V  T  E  E  L  R  S  D  H  L
GTTATAAGATATAATGATGATACTCGACATCGTTGCCGACAGTGTGAGTGTGGTAGCAGTCATCTAGAACTTCGTCCCATTGTGCTAAATGTAACTGAGGAGCTGAGAAGTGACCACCTT
    3130      3140      3150      3160      3170      3180      3190      3200      3210      3220      3230      3240
CAATATTCTATATTACTACTATGAGCTGTAGCAACGGCTGTCACACTCACACCATCGTCAGTAGATCTTGAAGCAGGGTAACACGATTTACATTGACTCCTCGACTCTTCACTGGTGGAA
```

                               11.6K
                          E1b 54K stop ─┬─ splice E1b mRNA   "TATA" mRNA IX   cap ─┬─mRNA IX

```
 T  L  S  C  L  R  T  D  Y  E  S  S  D  E  D  D  N  *
ACCCTGTCTTGCCTGCGGACTGACTATGAGTCAAGTGATGAAGACGACAACTCGAGGTAAGTGGGTGGGAGCTAGGTGGGATTATAAAAGGCTGGAAGTCAACTAAAAATTGTTTTTGTTCT
    3250      3260      3270      3280      3290      3300      3310      3320      3330      3340      3350      3360
TGGGACAGAACGGACGCCTGACTGATACTCAGTTCACTACTTCTGCTGTTGACTCCATTCACCCACCTCGATCCACCCTAATATTTTCCGACCTTCAGTTGATTTTTAACAAAACAAGA
```

splice ─┬─ E1b mRNA
    │ start protein IX   stop E1b 8.4K   Alternative splice ─┬─E1b mRNA
    │   M N G T T Q N N A A L F D G G V F S P Y L T S R L P Y W A G V R Q N V V
    H D E R N Y S E Q R C A F *

```
TTTAACAGCACGATGAACGGAACTACTCAGAACAACGCTGCGCCTTTTGATGTGGAGGGGTTTTTAGCCCTTATTTGACTTCCAGGTTACCATATTGGGCCGGAGTACGTCAGAATGTGGTA
    3370      3380      3390      3400      3410      3420      3430      3440      3450      3460      3470      3480
AAATTGTCGTGCTACTTGCCTTGATGAGTCTTGTTGCGACGCGAAAAACTACCTCCCCAAAAATCGGGAATAAACTGAAGGTCCAATGGTATAACCCGGCCTCATGCAGTCTTACACCAT


 G  S  T  V  D  G  R  P  V  A  P  A  N  S  S  T  L  T  Y  A  T  I  G  P  S  P  L  D  T  A  A  A  A  A  A  S  A  A  A  S
GGATCTACAGTGGACGGTCGACCTGTGGCACCTGCAAATTCATCAACATTAACCTATGCAACTATTGGACCCTCGCCTTTGGATACCGCCGCCGCCGCTGCAGCTTCCGCGGCCGCTTCT
    3490      3500      3510      3520      3530      3540      3550      3560      3570      3580      3590      3600
CCTAGATGTCACCTGCCAGCTGGACACCGTGGACGTTTAAGTAGTTGTAATTGGATACGTTGATAACCTGGGAGCGGAAACCTATGGCGGCGGCGGCGACGTCGAAGGCGCCGGCGAAGA


 T  A  R  S  M  A  A  D  F  S  F  Y  N  H  L  A  S  N  A  V  T  R  T  A  V  R  E  D  I  L  T  V  M  L  A  K  L  E  T  L
ACGGCTCGCAGTATGGCAGCTGATTTCAGCTTCTACAATCACTTGGCTTCGAATGCTGTGACACGCACCGCAGTTCGAGAGGACATTCTGACTGTTATGCTTGCCAAGCTTGAAACTCTA
    3610      3620      3630      3640      3650      3660      3670      3680      3690      3700      3710      3720
TGCCGAGCGTCATACCGTCGACTAAAGTCGAAGATGTTAGTGAACGAAGCTTACGACACTGTGCGTGGCGTCAAGCTCTCCTGTAAGACTGACAATACGAACGGTTCGAACTTTGAGAT
```

                                                              IX stop   3'-poly(A) ─┬─ E1b, IX

```
 T  A  Q  L  E  E  L  S  Q  K  V  E  E  L  A  D  A  T  T  H  T  P  A  Q  P  V  T  Q  *
ACTGCTCAGCTGGAAGAGCTATCGCAAAAGGTTGAGGAATTAGCTGATGCTACTACCCATACCCCAGCCCAACCTGTAACCCAATAAAGAAAAAACTTAAATTGAGATGGTGTTATGAAT
    3730      3740      3750      3760      3770      3780      3790      3800      3810      3820      3830      3840
TGACGAGTCGACCTTCTCGATAGCGTTTTCCAACTCCTTAATCGACTACGATGATGGGTATGGGGTCGGGTTGGACATTGGGTTATTCTTTTTTGAATTTAACTCTACCACAATACTTA


CTTTATTGATACTTGTTTTTTCTGACATGGTAAGCTTCTTGACCACCGTTCCCTATCATTAAGAACACGGTGAATGTGTTCCAGTATTTTGTAAAGATGAGCCTGTATATTAAGGTAC
    3850      3860      3870      3880      3890      3900      3910      3920      3930      3940      3950
GAAATAACTATGAACAAAAAAGACTGTACCATTCGAGAACTGGTGGCAAGGGAGTAGTAATTCTTGTGCCACTTACACAAGGTCATAAAACATTTCTACTCGGACATATAATTCCATG
 *  Q  Y  K  N  K  R  V  H  Y  A  R  S  W  R  E  R  D  N  L  V  R  H  I  H  E  L  I  K  Y  L  H  A  Q  I  N  L  Y  R
stop protein IVa2
```

Table 8.2. Landmarks in the Ad12 DNA sequence 0–11%

Strand, nucleotide		Sequence	Identity
r	l		
	T164		end ITR
	T276		alternative "TATA" box E1A
	T414		"TATA" box E1A
	A445		cap site E1A mRNAs
	A502	ATG	start E1A proteins
	G588	GGTACC	*Kpn*I 1.7%
	G588		splice donor E1A mRNA
	T976		splice donor E1A mRNA
	A1069		splice donor E1A mRNA
	G1144		splice acceptor E1A mRNAs
	T1216	TAG	stop E1A 6.2K protein
	T1374	TAA	stop E1A 30K, 26K proteins
	A1397	AATAAA	3′-poly(A) signals E1A
	A1436	AATAAA	
	G1455		3′-poly(A) attachment site E1A mRNAs
	T1498	TATATAAT	"TATA" box E1B
	A1525		cap sites E1B mRNAs
	G1528		
	A1541	ATG	start E1B 19K protein
	G1594	GTATAC	end transforming *Acc*IH fragment 4.6%
	A1846	ATG	start E1B 54K, 11.6K, 8.4K proteins
	T2030	TGA	stop E1B 19K protein
	G2046		splice donor E1B mRNA
	A2318	AAGCTT	*Hind*III 6.6%
	T3163		alternative splice acceptor E1B mRNA
	T3292	TGA	stop E1B 54K, 11.6K proteins
	G3295		splice donor E1B mRNA
	T3321	TATAAAA	"TATA" box protein IX mRNA
	G3350		cap site protein IX mRNA
	C3369		splice acceptor E1B mRNA
	A3373	ATG	start protein IX
	T3408	TGA	stop E1B 8.4K protein
	G3444		alternative splice acceptor E1B mRNA
	G3497	GTCGAC	*Sal*I 10.0%
	A3706	AAGCTT	*Hind*III 10.6%
	A3803	AATAAA	3′-poly(A) signal E1B, protein IX mRNAs
	T3805	TAA	stop protein IX
	G3824		3′-poly(A) attachment site E1B, IX
T3845		TAA	stop protein IVa2
A3847		AATAAA	3′-poly(A) signal E2B, IVa2 mRNAs

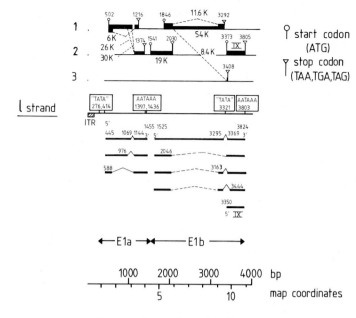

No open frames in r strand

Fig. 8.1. Schematic representation of identified and unidentified reading frames and RNA coordinates in Ad12 DNA between coordinates 0.0 and 11. The map scale reflects a conversion factor of 350 bp, which corresponds to 1% of the viral genome. Immediately *above* the scale, the locations of the various transcription units are indicated. The *continuous lines* above the transcription unit designations represent the segments of rightward transcripts present in mature RNAs; *interrupted carets* connecting the lines denote RNA splices. The coordinates of the RNA 5′ caps and 3′-poly(A) attachment sites, and of splice donor and acceptor sites are also given in this part of the figure. On the *next line above* a number of RNA expression signals have been drawn: "TATA" boxes and 3′-poly(A) signals (AATAAA). Lines 1, 2, and 3 in the *upper part* of the figure represent the three possible frames in which the DNA l-strand can be read. Tracts open for translation are indicated as *solid bars* for known genes. The open frames are flanked by the symbols ⋔ and ⋎, denoting initiation (ATG) and termination (TAA, TAG or TGA) codons respectively. The *numbers* next to the codons are their coordinates, and the *numbers in larger type* refer to the predicted MW of the translation products. *Interrupted lines* connecting solid bars show how open frames are linked due to RNA splicing. Neither strand of the Ad12 DNA between coordinates 0 and 11 contains unidentified ORFs of appreciable length

9 DNA Sequence of Human Ad12 (Subgroup A) Between Coordinates 61 and 67

The sequence (Table 9.1) was determined by KRUIJER et al. (1983). It is given in double-stranded format with 120 nucleotides per line, the numbering starting at a Sau96I site within the *Bam*HI C fragment. Each number refers to the positions above and below its last zero. The following features are marked: predicted initiation and termination codons (underlined), 3′-poly(A) signals (AATAAA; underlined), and splice points (Table 9.2) (KRUIJER et al. 1983;

KRUIJER 1983). Above or below the DNA sequence (sense strand), the predicted amino acid sequence (in one-letter code; see footnote to Table 9.1) is given for the C-terminal residues of the L3 23K protein, the E2A DBP and the N-terminus of the L4 100K protein. Apart from the genes for these proteins, a hitherto unidentified ORF has been found in the sequence; the amino acid sequence of its hypothetical translation product is also given.

Table 9.1. Ad12 DNA sequence 61–67%

```
 D  L  L  T  G  V  P  N  C  M  L  Q  S  P  Q  V  V  G  T  L  Q  R  N  Q  N  E  L  Y  K  F  L  N  N  L  S  P  Y  F  R  H
GACCTACTTACTGGGGTGCCTAATTGTATGCTACAAAGTCCTCAGGTAGTGGGCACATTGCAACGCAATCAGAATGAATTGTATAAATTCTTAAACAATCTGTCCCCTTACTTTCGTCAC
        10        20        30        40        50        60        70        80        90       100       110       120
CTGGATGAATGACCCCACGGATTAACATACGATGTTTCAGGAGTCCATCACCCGTGTAACGTTGCGTTAGTCTTACTTAACATATTTAAGAATTTGTTAGACAGGGGAATGAAAGCAGTG

                                                                        stop L3 23K?
 N  R  E  R  I  E  K  A  T  S  F  T  K  M  Q  N  G  L  K  *
AACCGCGAGCGCATAGAAAAAGCTACATCTTTTACTAAAATGCAAAATGGACTCAAATAAACGTGTACACAATGCATTAATAATAAAACCATTTTATTAGCTCATTGGAGTACAAGCTTG
        130       140       150       160       170       180       190       200       210       220       230       240
TTGGCGCTCGCGTATCTTTTTCGATGTAGAAAATGATTTTACGTTTTACCTGAGTTTATTTGCACATGTGTTACGTAATTATTATTTTGGTAAAATAATCGAGTAACCTCATGTTCGAAC

ACTGTTTTATTAAAAATCAAATGGCTCTTCGCGACAGTCGCCGTGGTTGGTGGGCAGGGATATGTTTCTGTACTGCAAACGCTGATGCCACTTGAATTCTGGAATAACAAGCCTAGGGGG
        250       260       270       280       290       300       310       320       330       340       350       360
TGACAAAATAATTTTTAGTTTACCGAGAAGCGCTGTCAGCGGCACCAACCACCCGTCCCTATACAAAGACATGACGTTTGCGACTACGGTGAACTTAAGACCTTATTGTTCGGATCCCCC
          *      F  D  F  P  E  E  R  C  D  G  H  N  T  P  L  S  I  N  R  Y  Q  L  R  Q  H  W  K  F  E  P  I  V  L  R  P  P
     stop E2a DBP

GGAGCCGTCAAAATTTTCTCCCCACAGCTGGCGCACAAGTTGCAGGGCGCCCATAACATCAGGAGCAGAAATCTTGAAGTCGCAATTAGGGCCAGCATTGCCGCGCGCATTGCGATAAAC
        370       380       390       400       410       420       430       440       450       460       470       480
CCTCGGCAGTTTTAAAAGAGGGGTGTCGACCGCGTGTTCAACGTCCCGCGGGTATTGTAGTCCTCGTCTTTAGAACTTCAGCGTTAATCCCGGTCGTAACGGCGCGCGTAACGCTATTTG
 S  G  D  F  N  E  G  W  L  Q  R  V  L  Q  L  A  G  M  V  D  P  A  S  I  K  F  D  C  N  P  G  A  N  G  R  A  N  R  Y  V

TGGATTTGCGCACTGAAAAACCAACAAACACGGATACTTAATACTGGCTAACGCTCCAGGGTCGGTTACTTCGTTGATATCAATGTTATCCACATTGCTGAGGTTAAAAGGAGTGATTTT
        490       500       510       520       530       540       550       560       570       580       590       600
ACCTAAACGCGTGACTTTTTGGTTGTTTGTGCCTATGAATTATGACCGATTGCGAGGTCCCAGCCAATGAAGCAACTATAGTTACAATAGGTGTAACGACTCCAATTTTCCTCACTAAAA
 P  N  A  C  Q  F  V  L  L  C  P  Y  K  I  S  A  L  A  G  P  D  T  V  E  N  I  D  I  N  D  V  N  S  L  N  F  P  T  I  K

                                                                  start ORF 21K
                                                                  M  S  H  V  R  V  V  G  Q  H  K  S
ACACAGTTGACGCCCCATCCGTGGCAGGCCATCTTGCTTGTTTAAACATTCGCAGCGCACTGGCATAAGGAGACGTTTTTGCCCATGTCGCATGTGAGGGTAGTCGGCCAGCATAAAAGC
        610       620       630       640       650       660       670       680       690       700       710       720
TGTGTCAACTGCGGGGTAGGCACCGTCCGGTAGAACGAACAAATTTGTAAGCGTCGCGTGACCGTATTCCTCTGCAAAAACGGGTACAGCGTACACTCCCATCAGCCGGTCGTATTTTCG
 C  L  Q  R  G  M  R  P  L  G  D  Q  K  N  L  C  E  C  R  V  P  M  L  L  R  K  Q  G  H  R  M  H  P  Y  D  A  L  M  F  A

 F  N  L  P  K  S  Y  L  S  L  H  S  F  R  I  K  Q  A  A  G  L  S  G  E  R  I  I  P  A  A  N  I  M  K  T  A  A  G  I  V
TTCAATTTGCCTAAAAGCTATTTGAGCCTTCATTCCTTCAGAATAAAACAAGCCGCAGACTTTCCGGAGAAAGAATTATTCCCGCAGCCAACATCATGAAAACAGCAGCGGGCATCGTC
        730       740       750       760       770       780       790       800       810       820       830       840
AAGTTAAACGGATTTTCGATAAACTCGGAAGTAAGGAAGTCTTATTTTGTTCGGCGTCCTGAAAGGCCTCTTTCTTAATAAGGGCGTCGGTTGTAGTACTTTTGTCGTCGCCCGTAGCAG
 E  I  Q  R  F  A  I  Q  A  K  M  G  E  S  Y  F  L  G  C  S  K  G  S  F  S  N  N  G  C  G  V  D  H  F  C  C  R  A  D  D

 V  F  N  L  N  Y  I  T  P  P  A  V  L  R  H  L  G  F  R  G  V  L  F  Q  R  S  L  P  T  F  A  G  Y  I  H  F  H  Q  M  L
GTTTTTAATTTGAACTACATTACCGCCCCCAGCGGTTTTGCGCCACCTTGGCTTTCGAGGGGGTTCTCTTTCAACGCTCGTTGCCCACTTTCGCTGGTTACATCCATTTCCACCAAATGCTC
        850       860       870       880       890       900       910       920       930       940       950       960
CAAAAATTAAACTTGATGTAATGCGGGGGTCGCCAAAACGCGGTGAACCGAAAGCTCCCCAAGAGAAAGTTGCGAGCAACGGGTGAAAGCGACCAATGTAGGTAAAGGTGGTTTACGAG
 N  K  I  Q  V  V  N  R  G  W  R  N  Q  A  V  K  A  K  S  P  N  E  K  L  A  R  Q  G  S  E  S  T  V  D  M  E  V  L  H  E

 F  A  H  H  L  H  S  M  Q  A  S  K  L  P  F  A  L  G  T  L  M  L  P  H  A  A  T  G  G  F  P  G  I  L  L  D  T  G  I  S
TTTGCGCACCATCTCCATTCCATGCAGGCATCTAAGCTCCCCTTCGCGCTCGGTACCTTATGCTCCCACACGCAGCAACCGGTGGGTTCCCAGGAATTCTGTTGGACACCGGCATAAGC
        970       980       990      1000      1010      1020      1030      1040      1050      1060      1070      1080
AAACGCGTGGTAGAGGTAAGGTACGTCCGTAGATTCGAGGGGAAGCGCGAGCCATGTGAATACGAGGGTGTGCGTCGTTGGCCACCCAAGGGTCCTTAAGACAACCTGTGGCCGTATTCG
 K  R  V  M  E  M  G  H  L  C  R  L  E  G  E  R  E  T  C  K  H  E  W  V  C  C  G  T  P  E  W  S  N  Q  Q  V  G  A  Y  A

 L  H  I  S  L  Q  K  A  S  H  E  L  L  K  G  F  L  G  R  K  S  Q  L  Q  T  A  L  F  V  E  P  C  C  A  Y  F  L  V  H
TTGCATATATCCTTGCAAAAAGCGTCCCATGAGCTCCTGAAAGGTTTTTTGGGACGAAAAAGTCAGCTGCAAACCGCGCTTTTCTTCGTTGAGCCATGTTGTGCATATTTTCTTGTACAC
       1090      1100      1110      1120      1130      1140      1150      1160      1170      1180      1190      1200
AACGTATATAGGAACGTTTTTCGCAGGGTACTCGAGGACTTTCCAAAAAACCCTGCTTTTTCAGTCGACGTTTGGCGCGAAAAGAAGCAACTCGGTACAACACGTATAAAAGAACATGTG
 Q  M  Y  G  L  F  R  G  M  L  E  Q  F  T  K  Q  S  S  F  T  L  Q  L  G  R  K  E  E  N  L  W  T  T  C  I  K  K  Y  V

                                                    stop ORF 21K
 A  A  L  I  R  Q  K  T  K  G  G  A  L  V  V  I  H  M  V  L  F  H  *
GCTGCCCTGATCCGGCAAAAAACGAAAGGTGGCGCGCTCGTCGTGATCCACATGGTACTTTTCCATTAGCATAGCCATGGCTTCCATGCCTTTTTCCCAAGCTGAAACTAGGGGCTGGCT
       1210      1220      1230      1240      1250      1260      1270      1280      1290      1300      1310      1320
CGACGGGACTAGGCCGTTTTTGCTTTGCCACCGCGCGAGCAGCACTAGGTGTACCATGAAAAGGTAATCGTATCGGTACCGAAGGTACGGAAAAAGGGTTCGACTTTGATCCCCGACCGA
 S  G  Q  D  P  L  F  R  F  T  A  R  E  D  H  D  V  H  Y  K  E  M  L  M  A  M  A  E  M  G  K  E  W  A  S  V  L  P  Q  S
```

One-letter code for amino acids: A, ala; C, cys; D, asp; E, glu; F, phe; G, gly; H, his; I, ile; K, lys; L, leu; M, met; N, asn; P, pro; Q, gln; R, arg; S, ser; T, thr; V, val; W, trp; Y, tyr

Table 9.1 (Continued)

```
TGCCGGATTGCGAACAACAACAACATTCTTTTCATTTTCGTCGCTGTTTTGAGCGGAAGCCTTCAAAACGTGTACCTGCCTGGTTTCCATTTTTTGAAAAGACTGAGAACCGTCTGCATG
       1330      1340      1350      1360      1370      1380      1390      1400      1410      1420      1430      1440
ACGGCCTAACGCTTGTTGTTGTTGTTAAGAAAAGTAAAAGCAGCGACAAAACTCGCCTTCGGAAGTTTTGCACATGGACGGACCAAAGGTAAAAAACTTTTCTGACTCTTGGCAGACGTAC
 A  P  N  R  V  V  V  V  N  K  E  N  E  D  S  N  Q  A  S  A  K  L  V  H  V  Q  R  T  E  M  K  Q  F  S  Q  S  G  D  A  H

ATGCATAATGCGGACGGGCGGCATGCTGAAACCCATTACTCCTAAAACTGCTCTTGGTGGTTCTGCCTCTTCTTCTTCTGCACTCTCTGGGGAAAGAGGTATCGCAGCCATAGATTTCTT
       1450      1460      1470      1480      1490      1500      1510      1520      1530      1540      1550      1560
TACGTATTACGCCTGCCCGCCGTACGACTTTGGGTAATGAGGATTTTGACGAGAACCACCAAGACGGAGAAGAAGAAGACGTGAGAGACCCCTTTCTCCATAGCGTCGGTATCTAAAGAA
 H  M  I  R  V  P  P  M  S  F  G  M  V  G  L  V  A  R  P  P  E  A  E  E  E  E  A  S  E  P  S  L  P  I  A  A  M  S  K  K

GACTTTTTTCTTTGGAGGTAAAGGCACAGCTTCCAGTTCTTCTTCGCTTTCGGAATCCAGAAAGTATCTGCCCATTTTTGGCGGCGGCGGCTGAGCGCTGCGGTCTGGGGTGCGCTCCCT
       1570      1580      1590      1600      1610      1620      1630      1640      1650      1660      1670      1680
CTGAAAAAGAAACCTCCATTTCCGTGTCGAAGGTCAAGAAGAAGCGAAAGCCTTAGGTCTTTCATAGACGGGTAAAAACCGCCGCCGCCGACTCGCGACGCCAGACCCCACGCGAGGGA
 V  K  K  K  P  P  L  P  V  A  E  L  E  E  E  S  E  S  D  L  F  Y  R  G  M  K  P  P  P  P  Q  A  S  R  D  P  T  R  E  R
```

```
                 L4 mRNA splice ─┐                start L4 100K?
                                 │      M  M  D  L  E  P  Q  E  S  L  T  A  P  T  A  P  A  I  G  A  T  A  V  M
CTGTGAGTGCTGATTGCTGGCCATTATTTAATCCTAGGCAAAGAAACACATGATGGATCTGGAGCCACAGGAAAGCTTAACCGCCCCCACCGCTCCCGCCATTGGCGCTACGGCTGTCAT
       1690      1700      1710      1720      1730      1740      1750      1760      1770      1780      1790      1800
GACACTCACGACTAACGACCGGTAATAAATTAGGATCCGTTTCTTTGTGTACTACCTAGACCTCGGTGTCCTTTCGAATTGGCGGGGGTGGCGAGGGCGGTAACCGCGATGCCGACAGTA
 Q  S  H  Q  N  S  A  M                 │
          E2a DBP start                 └─splice E2a mRNA
```

```
  E  K  D  K  S  L  L  I  P  Q  D  A  P  V  E  Q  N  L  G  Y  E  T  P  P  E  E  F  E  G  F  L  Q  I  Q  K  Q  P  N  E  Q
GGAGAAGGACAAAAGTCTACTCATACCCCAAGACGCACCGGTTGAGCAGAACTTGGGCTACGAGACTCCCCCCGAGGAATTTGAAGGCTTTCTTCAAATCCAAAAGCAACCAAATGAGCA
       1810      1820      1830      1840      1850      1860      1870      1880      1890      1900      1910      1920
CCTCTTCCTGTTTTCAGATGAGTATGGGGTTCTGCGTGGCCAACTCGTCTTGAACCCGATGCTCTGAGGGGGGCTCCTTAAACTTCCGAAAGAAGTTTAGGTTTTCGTTGGTTTACTCGT
```

```
  N  A  G  L  E
AAACGCTGGGCTCGAG
       1930
TTTGCGACCCGAGCTC
```

Table 9.2. Landmarks in the Ad12 DNA sequence 61–67%

Strans, nucleotide		Sequence	Identity
r	l		
	A176	AATAAA	3′-poly(A) signal L3 mRNA?
	T178	TAA	stop L3 23K protein
	A202	AATAAA	3′-poly(A) signal L3 mRNA?
A218		AATAAA	3′-poly(A) signal E2A mRNA
A252		TAA	stop E2A DBP
	A685	ATG	start ORF 21K
	T1267	TAG	stop ORF 21K
A1704		ATG	start E2A DBP
G1713			acceptor E2A mRNA splice
	G1718		acceptor L4 mRNA splice
	A1730	ATG	start L4 100K protein

10 Comparison of the Left-terminal DNA Sequences of Human of Ad2, Ad5, Ad7, and Ad12

The left-terminal sequences of Ad5 (Sect. 2; top row), Ad7 (Sect. 7; middle row) and Ad12 (Sect. 8; bottom row) have been shifted to obtain maximum homology; resulting gaps have been filled in with dashes (Table 10.1). Dashes above and below the sequences indicate positions of three-strain homology. Additional (two-strain) homologies are indicated by asterisks (between top and

Table 10.1. Comparison of the left-terminal DNA sequences of Ad5, Ad7, and Ad12 (from the l-strands)

```
         -    *-  ┌─see Section 1
         -   --  ---------- ----   -  ------ -- * ------  _ *** * - ** * -- * **  -- - - *   --*-
     1   CATCATCAAT AATATACCTT ATTT-TGGAT TGAAGCCAAT ATGATAATGA GG-GGGTGGA GTTT-GTG-A CGTGGCGCGG GGCGTGGGAA C--GGGGCGG 5
                            *                         *        *  *       *  **   ** ** *       * *   *
     1   CTCTCTATAT AATATACCTT ATAGATGGAA TGGTGCCAAC ATGTAAATGA GG-TAATTTA AAAAAGTGCG CGCTGTGTGG TGATTGGCTG T--GGGGTGA 7
           *  * **                     *             **        *         *          *        *   *   *
     1   CTATATATAT AATATACCTT ATAC-TGGAC TAGTGCCAAT ATTAAATGA AGTGGGCGTA GTGT-GTA-A TTTGATTGGG TGGAGGTGTG GCTTTGGCGT 12
         -  :   -  --  ---------- -- : ----:  - ----- -- ----- - - : -- :-- -:: -  :  -- -:


            *      _**    *  ---- -* * -  *  --  **  *     *  *
    95   GTGACGTAGT A-GTGTGGCG GAAGTGTGA- TGTTGCAAGT GTGGCG---- -------GAA CACATGTAAG CGACGGATGT GGCAAAAGTG ACGTTTTGG
         ****                              *                        * * ****         ** ** *** *** **** **
    98   ATGACTAACA -T----GGGCG GGGCGGCCG- TGGGAAAATG ACGTGACTTA TGTGGGAGGA GTTATGTTGC AAGTTATTGC GGTAAATGTG ACGTAAAAGG
           **       *                       *                             *
    98   GCTTGTAAGT TTG---GGCG GATGAGGAAG TGGGGCGCGG CGTGGGA--- ---------- ---------- ---------- ---------- ----------
          -             ----  - : :-:: --          ::


             t   g     - - - --   --- --- --- -*-  --***  ** -*  --  -  - ------ --*       a     tg
   182   TGTGCGCCGG TGTACACAGG AAGT-GACAA TTTTCGCGCG GTTTTAGGCG GATGTTGTAG TAAATTTGGG CGTAACCGAG TAAGATTTGG CCATTTTCGC
          *         * * *      *    *     **  *     *       *             * ** *                 *** ***
   193   AGGTGTGGTT TGAACAC-GG AAGTAGACAG TTTTCCCACG CTTACTGATA GGATATGAGG TAGTTTTGGG CGGATGCAAG TGAAAATTCT CCATTTTCGC
                             *                       *    * * *   *                            *
   142   ------GCCG GGCGCGCCGG ATGT-GACGT TTTAGACGCC ATTTTACACG GAA-ATGATG TT-TTTTGGG CGTTGTTTGT GCAAATTTTG TGTTTTAGGC
          :       -: : -- -- --- : --- : --- --       - --     -- - : :    :  - - -: --- --


         - --------- -- - --- ------*   ---  -*         * *-* -     -*-*- - *-----   - ------ - - -*** --- - ------
   281   GGGAAAACTG AATAAGAGGA AGTGAAA-TC TGAATAATTT TGTGTTACTC ATAGCGCGTA ATATTTGTCT AGGGCGCGG GGACTTTGAC CGTTTACGTG
                          *  *         **  * ****  *  * *              *        *       *    *    *  * *
   292   GCGAAAACTG AAT--GAGGA AGTGAATTTC TGAGTCATTT CGCGGTTATG ACAGGGTGGA GTATTTGCCG AGGGCCGAGT AGACTTTGAC CGTTTACGTG
          *                              *                                 *        * *        * *
   233   GCGAAAACTG AAAT-GCGGA AGTGAAA-AT TGATGACGGC AATTTTATTA TAGGCGCGGA ATATTTACCG AGGGCAGAGT GAACTCTGAG CCTCTACGTG
         - --------- -- - --- ------   ---:         :  - :-:  - - ------ - - ------


                                                                                                        "TATA" Ela
                                                                                                         c c
         - -             ---           - **    --- -- -* *-  ---  ---    -*- --- *** -*  -------- -- - - ------
   380   GAGACTCGCC CAG--GTGTT TTTCTCAGGT GTTTTCCGCG TTCCGGGTCA AAGTTG-GCG TTTTATTATT ATAGTCAGCT GACGTGTAGT GTATTTATAC
          **         ** **** *                      *     *   *      *   *           *             *          **
   390   GAGGTTTCGA TTACCGTGTT TTTCACCTAA A-TTTCCGCG TACGGTGTCA AAGTCCTGTG TTTTTACGTA GGTGTCAGCT GATCGCTAGG GTATTTAAAC
          ** **** *  *                      *                     *                   *         *       ***  *    *
   331   TGGGTTTCGA T--ACGTGAG CG--ACGGGG AAACTCCACG TTGCGC-TCA AAGGGC-GCG TTT-ATTGTT C-TGTCAGCT GATCGTTTGG GTATTTAATG
         - -         ---        --:  :     --- - --  -:- ---  --- -  -  -  -  - - -- - :-  - -- -------


                                    ┌─cap  Ela                                             Ela protein start
         -*-  ---- -  ------ ----┐         - **   -------- -- ------  ---- -- * -- *    ** * - *  -- * - * *
   477   CCGGTGAGTT CC-TCAAGAG GCCACTCTTG AGTGCCAGCG AGTAGAGTTT TCTCCTCCGA GCCGCTCCGA CACCGGGAC- -TGAAAATG AGACATATTA
          *          *           ↓          *                      ** *   **         ** **    ***  *    *
   489   CTGACGAGTT CCGTCAAGAG GCCACTCTTG AGTGCCAGCG AGAAGAGTTT TCTCCTCCGC GCCGCAAGTC AGTTCTGCGC TTTGAAAATG AGACACCTGC
          *                    ↓          *                           **          *           *
   423   CCGCCGTGTT C-GTCAAGAG GCCACTCTTG AGTGCCAGCG AGAAGAGTTT TCTCTGCC-A GCTCATTTTC -ACGGCGCC- ----ATTATG AGAACTGAAA
         - -:  -  :            - -:  : -  - ::-: :-  - --- --   :::   : :-  ---  --- :  :


          *     - --- -    ------  --        - --* *  -    - *-  --- **  --  - *- *   -  -   -  *   * * *
   573   T----CTGCC ACGGAGGTGT TATTACCGAA GAAATGGCCG CCAGTCTTTT GGACCAGCTG ATCGAAGAGG TACTGGCTGA TAATCTT--- CCACCTCCT-
          ****** ** *  **     *     **         * *                       *  * ** *   *              *  ** **
   589   GCTTCCTGCC ACAGGAGA-T TATCTCCAGT GAGACCGGGA TCGAACTACT GGAGTTTGTG GTAAATACCC TAATGGGAGA CGACCCGGAA CCGCCAGTGC
                                     *                           * *** *   *    * *                 **
   515   TGACTCCCTT G-------GT CCTGTCGTAT CAGGAAGCTG ACGACATATT GGAGCATTTG GTGGACAACT TTTTT---AA CGAGGTACCC AGTGATGAT-
         - -:  -    - -:  : : - : -- :  - ::-: :- - -- ---  :-- -: - : - :-:   :   : -:: :  :


          - -- --  - - - --* ----*  ----------  - --- --*  *  -**    --*----  - --  **-- *-- *-  -----*-*-
   665   AGCCATTTTG AACCCACCTAC CCTTCACGAA CTGTATGATT TAGACGTGAC G---GCCCCG GAAGATCCCA ACGAGGAGGC GGTTTCGCAG ATTTTTCCCG
          ***    *   *  *** **          *           *     * *          **          ***       **
   688   AGCC-TTTTG ATCCACCTAC GCTGCACGAT CTGTATGATT TAGAGGTAGA C---GGGCCG GAGGATCCCA ATGAGGGAGC TGTGAATGGG TTTTTTACTG
            *                              *                          **              *          *****  *
   604   GATCTTTATG TT---CCGTC TCTTTACGAA CTGTATGATC TTGATGTGGA GTCTGCCGGT GAAGATAATA ATGAACAGGC GGTGAATGAG TTTTTTCCCG
         - --  --  - --  :-- --  - -           :-:      -- - -    - --  - : - ------: :-- -- -:


             g                                    t
         - --   - *-  *- -- -   -- --*  -  *--*  ----      **-*--- _        *   *   **   --- -  *
   762   ACTCTGTAAT GTTGGCGGTG CAGGAAGGGA TTGACTTACT CACTTTTCCG CCGGCGCCCG GTTCTCCGGA GCCGCTCAC CTTTCCCGGC AGCCCGAGCA
          *           *          *       *   **       ** **      * * * *              * * *      * *          ** *
   784   ATTTCTATGCT GCTAGCTGCC GATGAAGGAT TGGACATAAA CCCTCCTCCT GAGACCCTTG TCACCCCAGG GGTGGTTGTG GAAAGC-GGC AGAGGTGGGA
              * ** *            *         *            ** * *                         *                  * **
   701   AATCGCTTAT TTTTAGCTGCC AGTGAGGGGT TGTTTTTACC GGAGCCTCCT GTACT----- -TTCTCCTGT CTGTGAGCCT ATTGGG-GGC GAATGTA---
         -:-:  :-:  - - - -:   - - -  ::  :     :      :  :            : :    - --:-:  :: :  : ::  :   - :


                                                          g
          *   -  --    *- -     *---      *--- --  -- * -     --*   -*--*   - -*-----   -- --
   862   GCCGGAGCAG AGAGCCTTGG GTCCGGTTTC TATGCCAAAC CTTGTACCGG AGGTGATCGA TCTTACCTGC CACGAGGCTG GCTTTCCACC CAGTGACGAC
          *   -  --   *  *       *          *   *                   --  - * -  --* _ - *-----  -- --
   883   AAAAATTGCC TGATC--TGG GAGCAGCTGA AATG------ ---------- --------GA CTTGCGTTGT TATGAAGAGG GTTTTCCTCC GAGTGATGAT
          ****                  **
   791   ------TGCC ACAAC--TGC ACCCTGAAGA TATG------ ---------- --------GA TTTATTGTGC TACGAGATGG GCTTTCCCTG TAGCGATTCG
         -:-:  -- -  : -:-: ---                              -- -:::::--   - --  : - - -----:  :-- --  :
```

Table 10.1 (Continued)

```
                                                                  ┌splice Ela Ad5
      -- -- -*                                                  - * ┌-*--*-* *---  ---* -- *-   _
 962  GAGGATGAA- ---------- ---------- ---------- ---------- ---------G AGGGTGAGGA GTTTGTGTTA GATTATGTGG
        *                                                                                         *  *
 957  GAAGATGGGG AAACTGAGCA GTCCA----- -------TCC ATACCGCAGT GAATGAGGGA GTAAAAGCTG CCAGCGATGT TTTTAAGTTG GACTGTCCGG
        *      *  * **  *** *    *                   ******   ** *   *  *                 *      *  *    * **
 859  GAAGACGAGC AAGACGAGAA CGGAATGGCG CATGTTTCTG CATCCGCAGC TGCTGCTGCC GCTGATAGGG AACGTGAGGA GTTTCAGTTA GACCATCCAG
      -- -- -                                                          - ::- -- -   ---: -- -   -   -

                 ┌splice Ela Ad7, Ad12
      -- --*--  --*  *-- ┌ --- --- * ---*-- -- - *-- -- * * - - *---- -- - --- --- -- * *** -**
1002  AGCACCCCGG GCACGGTTGC AGGTCTTGTC ATTATCACCG GAGGAATACG GGGGACCCAG ATATTATGTG TTCGCTTTGC TATATGAGGA CCTGTGGCAT
        *           **       *       *    * *        *         *      *   *       *      ** *  *  *  *      *
1045  AGCTGCCTGG ACATGGCTGT AAGTCTTGTG AATTTCACAG GAATAACACT GGGATGAAAG AACTATTGTG CTCGCTTTGC TATATGAGAA TGCACTGCCA
        **      *  *          *         *     **  * *   *     *    *      *        *   *      *  *
 959  AGTTGCCCGG ACACAATTGT AAGTCCTGTG AGCACCACCG GAATAGTACT GGAAATACTG ACTTAATGTG CTCTTTGTGC TATCTGCGAG CCTACAACAT
      -- -- --     -- -- - --- ---  -: --- --- - -- - :    - -::- ---- --- -   :  -

                 ┌splice Ela                c
      *-- - --- ┌------- --                                      *-* * * * *  *- *-***-* *-*   -*   ***-      *
1102  GTTTGTCTAC AGTAAGTGAA AATTATGGGC AGTGGGTGAT AGAGTGGTGG GTTTGGTGTG GTAATTTTTT TTTTAATTTT TACAGTTTTG TGGTTTAAAG
        *                       *   *  * *   *   * ****      **           *  * *          * * *
1145  CTTTATTTAC AGTAAGTGTA TTTAAGTGAA ATTTAAAGGA ATAGTGTAGC TGTTTAATAA CTGTTGAATG GTAGATTTAT GTTTTTAC-- ----------
        *  *                *      *                 *   *                      *   *
1059  GTTCATTTAC AGTAAGTGTG CTA------- ---------- -------TGG GAGGTGGGAG GTGATTTTTT TTT---CTTA AGCAGTGAAA AATAAT----
      -- -- ------- :                              - :    :     - - -  - -    :   :: --: :

                        ^  ┌splice Ela
      ******         --    ┌ -- ---- -- -- ******- -- *-                                    g           t
1202  AATTTTGTAT TGTGATTTTT TTAAAAGGTC CTGTGTCTGA ACCTGAGCCT GAGCCCGAGC CAGAACCGGA GCCTGCAAGA CCTACCCGCC GTCCTAAAAT
        * *** *   * ** **      *    *    * *
1233  ---------T TGCGA--TTT TTTGTAGGTC CTGTGTCTGA TGA------T GAGTCACC-- ---------- ---------- ---------- ----------
                                      * *    * *
1128  -ATTTTG--- -------TTG TTTTTAGGTC CTGTTTCCGA TAATGAGCCT GAACCT---- ---------- ---------- ---------- ----------
      -- -- :  ----- ---- -- --  :        - -- -:

        t                                                  * **** * _   *--- ** * **        - - --- --   -
1302  GGCGCCTGCT ATCCTGAGAC GCCCGACATC ACCTGTGTCT AGAGAATGCA ATAGTAGTAC GGATAGCGT GACTCCGGTC CTTCTAACAC ACCTCCTGAG
                                                                   *       * ***    * **        * **
1274  ---------- ---------- ---------- ---------- ---------- ----TTCTCC TGAT------ ---------T CAACTACCTC ACCTCCTGAA
                                                                        *                     * * *      *
1173  ---------- ---------- ---------- ---------- ---------A ATAGCACTTT GGATGGCGAT GAGCGA---- -----CCCTC -- --- -- -
                                                                        -:   ---
```

```
       -*     *  *-* --     *   **  --*--- *-  _ * * ** -** --*** -  -------- * * *-  - -- --- -*
1402  ACGAGCCTGG GCAA------ ------CCTT TGGACTTGAG CTGTAAACGC CCCAGGCCA- -*- * ---- --- - --- - --- ---
```


```
       _ * * ** _   * _* --                                 * **** * _  *--- ** *  **        - - --- -- _
1402  ATACACCCGG TGGTCCCGCT GTGCCCCATT AAACCAGTTG CCGTGAGAGT ---TGG---T GGGCGTCGCC AGGCTGTGGA ATGTATCGAG GACTTGCTTA
        * ** **                              * *      *     *    * **    * *         *   *  *         ** *
1305  ATTCAGGCGC CCGCACCTGC AAACGTATGC AAGCCCATTC CTGTAAAGCC ---TAAGCCT GGGAAACGCC CTGCTGTGGA TAAGCTTGAG GACTTGTTGG
        *   *      *   ***      *   *    *    *    *                    *  *              *       *
1215  CTAGGAAGTG CGGTTCCAGA AGGAGTAATA AAACCTGTGC CTCACGGGGT GACTGG---G AGGCGTAGAT GTGCTGTGGA AAGCATTTTG GATTTGATTC
      -  ::      - :--:: :  :               : -- --:  -        -         --   - :  -------- : - - --- ---:- :

                                                               Ela proteins stop
       _ - -** *                  ---  _ -- _* ***** _* **         -*- *        ** *     * *       - *
1496  ACGAGCCTGG GCAA------ ------CCTT TGGACTTGAG CTGTAAACGC CCCAGGCCA- -*- * AAACCTGTGA TTGCGTGTGT GGTTAACGCC
        *    *                       * * *  **        *              AATGAGTGCC C--------- -TGCAGCTGT GTTTA-----
1402  AGGGTGGGGA TGGA------ ------CCTT TGGACCTTAG TACCCGGAAA CTGCCAAGGC AATGAGTGCC C--------- -TGCAGCTGT GTTTA-----
        *        *                     *                * *   * *     *   *   * *
1312  AAGAGGAAGA AAGAGAACAA ACAGTGCCTG TTGATCTGTC AGTGAAACGC CCTAGATGTA ATTAATGGAC T---TTGAGC ACCTGGGCAA TAAAATAGGG
      -:- ---    ::- ::  -                --- - --  *   :::       - :  --    ==  : :
```


```
                  "AAUAAA" Ela                                                                    Elb "TATA"
       * * ** -        -- -- _ * *- _ ------- *         ** * ** *    - -** *  - ---* - -- * ** -* ------
1581  TTTGTTTGCT GAATGAGTTG ATGTAAGTT- AATAAAGGGT GAGATAATGT TTAACTTG-- CATGGCGTGT TAAATGGGGC GGGGCTTAAA GGGTATAAA
        **       **       *  *** *                *         **         *     *   ** *           *  * *    * *
1475  --------TT TAATG---TG ACGTCA-TGT AATAAAA--- --TTATGCAG CTGCTGAG-- TGTTTTATTA CTTCTTGGGT GGGG--TCTT GGATATAAA
        *                               AATAAAA-            * *  * *   ** ** *     * *
1409  GTAATGTGGT TTTTG---TG AGTCATGTAT AATAAAACTG GTTTCG--GT TGAAGTGTCT TGTTA-ATGT TTGTTTGGGC GTGGTTAAAC AGGGATAAA
      -:- -- --  --:   -       ---: ---   ======        -   - :      ::: --- - --   : - ------

                        ┌cap Elb                      start Elb 20K
       **    -* - *   **_    ┌         ***- _ *    -- -----              -- -- **-*      ** *-   *  - -*
1679  TGCGCCGTGG GCTAACTTG GTTA------ ------CATC TGACCT-CAT GGAGGCTTGG GAGTGTTTGG AAGATTTTTC TGCTGTGCGT AACTTGCTGG
        *           *       *  **                             * * * *  * ***** *  *  *   **           *    * *
1555  GTAGGAGCAG A-TCTGTGTG GTTAGCTCAC AGCAACTTGC TGCCATCCAT GGAGGTTTGG GCTACTTGG AAGACCTCAG ACAGACTAGG CTACTACTAG
        *   **             *          *                             *             * *  *         * *    *  *
1503  AGCTGGGTTG GTGTTGCTTT GA-ATAGTT- ------CATC TTAG--TAAT GGAGTTGGAA ACTGTGCTGC AAAGTTTTCA GAGCGTTCGC CAGCTCTTGC
      :   :- :-   :           -     -             -  ==  ---- :  --  -- -  :: ::::  -: : -: -

       _ _ * --- **- * **  -- - *--- ----*- *** -- --*** **       - *- - -- -- - -- *- -- -- -  *-----
1766  AACAGAGCTC TAACAGTACC TCTTGGTTTT GGAGGTTTCT GTGGGGCTCA TCCCAGGCAA AGTTAGTCTG CAGAATTAAG GAGGATTACA AGTGGGAATT
        *          *         *                                 *          * **     *         *  *       * *
1654  AAAACGCCTC GGACGGAGTC TCTGGCCTTT GGAGATTCTG GTTCGGTGGT GATCTAGCTA GGCTAGTGTT TAGGATAAAA CAGGACTACA GGGAAGAATT
        *   *             *             *          *           *  *       *  **     *      *    * *    * * **
1593  AGTATACCTC TAAAAACACT TCAGGTTTTT GGAGGTATCT GTTTGGCTCT ACCTTAAGCA AGGTGGTAAA TAGGGTGAAA GAAGACTATA GAGAGGAATT
      - :-: ---   - :       -- -: --- ---- -      -- :--   :       :-  -:- --: : -- --:-- -- - -    -----
```

Table 10.1 (Continued)

```
      ----  -  ---     -*  *-  _  *--    -- _ **-     -  * _*-      _* -*-_     *  * --  *-   -- -- --     -**   *  -  ----
1866  TGAAGAGCTT TTGAAATCCT GTGGTGAGCT GTTTGATTCT TTGAATCTGG GTCACCAGGC GCTTTTCCAA GAGAAGGTCA TCAAGACTTT GGATTTTTCC
         *          *          *  *  *   *   *   **   *   ***  ***   * *            * *       *
1754  TGAAAAGTTA TTGGACGACA TTCCAGGACT TTTTGAAGCT CTTAACTTGG GCCATCAGGC TCATTTTAAG GAGAAGGTTT TATCAGTTTT AGATTTTTCT
         *    *      * ***     *** *        *                        *             *    *             *
1693  TGAAAACATA TTGGCCGACT GTCCAGGGCT TTTGGCTTCA CTAGACCTTT GTTACCACTT GGTGTTTCAG AAAAAGTGG TCAGATCCTT AGATTTTTCA
      ----  - :- ---       -  ---    -:  - --  -     -:  - -- -- --::   - :  :  --  --------:

                                                                         start Elb 55K
      _  *-- *   _  _  _  _ -- -*---  ---*-*    --- ---  --------*- **  --  _-_  - *-*-_  *  --  --- -*  *------
1966  ACACCGGGGC GCGCTGCGGC TGCTGTTGCT TTTTTGAGTT TTATAAAGGA TAAATGGAGC GAAGAAACCC ATCTGAGCGG GGGGTACCTG CTGGATTTTC
      *  **      *  *   *   *   *           * **  **         *   *                 *          *              *
1854  ACTCCTGGTA GAACTGCTGC TGCTGTAGCT TTTCTTACTT TTATATTGGA TAAATGGATC CGCCAAACTC ACTTCAGCAA GGGATACGTT TTGGATTTCA
         *         *  **     *   *        *         **                  *                                    **
1793  TCTGTGGGAC GAACGGTTGC TTCTATTGCT TTTTTGGCAA CCATATTGGA TAAATGGAGC GAGAAATCCC ACCTGAGTTG GGATTACATG CTGGATTACA
       -  --:-  ---    --- -    ---  --  ---     ---  --- :::- - - - -  -  --  --:---:-   ------
```

Table 10.1 (Continued)

```
           c                                                                               g
     * ----*-- - * -----  * -- ---- **-* ****  * -- - **   --*-- *        -- - -- -- -     -----*- - - --    - -
2857 TTCGGGGCTG TGCCTTTTAC TGCTGCTGGA AGGGGGTGGT GTGTCGCCCC AAAAGCAGGG CTTCAATTAA GAAATGCCTC TTTGAAAGGT GTACCTTGGG
                       *                                                          * * *          * * *  *
2733 TGAGGGGTTG TAGTTTTTAT GCATGCTGGA TTGCAACATC AGGTAGGGTG AAGAGTCAGT TGTCTGTGAA GAAATGCATG TTTGAGAGAT GTAATCTTGG
        *               ** *   * * *                       * *          * *  ** **          *              *   * *
2639 CTAGGGGCTG TACTTTTTAT GGATGTTGGA AGGGTTTGGT GGGTAGACCA AAAAGTAAAC TGTCTGTAAA AAAGTGTTTG TTTGAAAAAT GTGTACTTGC
     ---- - - :: -- ---- -- - ::      -- -: : -- --: --     -- ---:-- -- -- -- :: - -


     * -  -      --*-- - -  -   -- ***-  -- *-- --   -- -- --   - -- -* -- - **- -* * - --  ------ ---
2957 TATCCTGTCT GAGGGTAACT CCAGGGTGCG CCACAAATGG GCCTCCGACT GTGGTTGCTT CATGCTAGTG AAAAGCGTGG CTGTGATTAA GCATAACATG
     * * * *          **** *  * *                 *  * *   ** *         ** **  * *
2833 CATACTGAAT GAAGGTGAAG CAAGGGTCCG CCACTGCGCA GCTACAGAAA CTGCCTGCTT CATTCTAATA AAGGGAAATG CCAGTGTGAA GCATAATATG
        *                               **  * *  ** **                ** ** * *            *
2739 TTTAATTGTA GAGGGGGATG CACATATTAG GCATAATGCA GCTTCAGAAA ATGCCTGTTT TGTATTATTG AAGGGAATGG CTATTTTAAA GCATAATATG
     - - :: -- -- --: -- -: --   -- -- -- :-- -- -- --: --:-- -- -- :-: -- ------ ---


       g -----      - -- - -          - -  - ---- - -*  -- *- --*  t  - * * -- -*--- - - *** --* * -
3057 GTATGTGGCA ACTGCGAGGA CAGGGCCTCT CAGATGCTGA CCTGCTCGGA CGGCAACTGT CACCTGCTGA AGACCATTCA CGTAGCCAGC CACTCTCGCA
             *             * * * * ** * *** **   * *   * *    * *                * *              ** *     * * **
2933 ATCTGTGGAC ATTCGGATGA GAGGCCTTAT CAGATGCTAA CCTGCGCTGG TGGACATTGC AATATTCTTG CTACCGTGCA TATCGTTTCA CATGCACGCA
                                 *  * * *  *   * * *    *                 * *        * *           ** *
2839 GTTTGTGGGG TGTCTGATCA AACTATGCGA CGTTTTGTTA CCTGTGCTGA TGGAAATTGT CATACCTTAA AAACTGTTCA TATTGTGAGC CACAGTAGAC
     -:------:: :- :-- - :- :: : :      -- -:-- --     - : -: :-- -- -- -:-: : -- -: -


     -  -----   -- - ---     c           - - ***-- * -- --- *- -- *  - * -*  ---- - --- *--- - ---*-- - - *- -* -
3157 AGGCCTGGCC AGTGTTTGAG CATAACATAC TGACCCGCTG TTCCTTGCAT TTGGGTAACA GGAGGGGGGT GTTCCTACCT TACCAATGCA ATTTGAGTCA
         *                       **-*             *           *              * **             *     *
3033 AGAAATGGCC TGTATTTGAA CATAATGTGA TTACCAAGTG CACCATGCAT ATAGGTGGTC GCAGGGGAAT GTTTATGCCT TACCAGTGTA ACATGAATCA
          * *             * *         * *   * *        *                * *            *       * *       *
2939 ATTGTTGGCC TGTATGTGAT CATAACATGT TTATGCGCTG TACCATACAT TTAGGCTTAA GGCGGGGTAT GTTTAGACCT TCCCAATGTA ACTTCAGCCA
     - :::----- -- ---: :-   ----- - : :    -- -- --     :- - :- -  --:--- :- :- - :- -  -: :- -- -- --- ---


     * * -- -*-  --*-- - - --      - -- - ---   - -* - --**- -----   - *  -* - - : - -- --*- - -- --    ---
3257 CACTAAGATA TTGCTTGAGC CCGAGAGCAT GTCCAAGGTG AACCTGAACG GGGTGTTTGA CATGACCATG AAGATCTGGA AGGTGCTGAG GTAC---GAT
         * *            *          * *   *                * ** *          * *     *           * *
3133 TGTGAAGGTA ATGTTGGAAC CAGATGCCTT TTCCAGAGTG AGCGTAACAG GAATCTTTGA TATGAATATT CAACTATGGA AGATCCTGAG ATAT---GAT
         *  *           * *   * *   * * *   *    *  *     * *           *        *          * *         *
3039 CTCAAACATT ATGCTGGAAC CTGAAGTGTT TTCTAGAGTG TGTTTAAATG GGGTATTTGA TTTATCTGTG GAATTATGTA AGGTTATAAG ATATAATGAT
     : :-- -- : -- - : - -- :    - -- - -- :- - :- -- : - - -:-----   : -- :- -- -: : -- -- --   ---


     -- -- **  - *** - ** -- --* --*-- - -   --- * ***   - --  - ***-  ---- -- - *--*----- -- --*
3354 GAGACCCGCA CCAGGTGCAG ACCCTGCGAG TGTGGCGGTA AACATATTAG GAACCAGCCT GTGATGCTGG ATGTGACCGA GGAGCTGAGG CCCGATCACT
         * * *             * * *         *               ***  * **     **        *            * *** - *
3230 GACACTAAAC CAAGGGTGCG CGCATGCGAA TGCGGAGGCA AGCATGCTAG ATTCCAGCCG GTGTGCGTGG ATGTGACTGA AGACCTGAGG CCCGATCATT
        * **              *                        *        * *                  *
3139 GATACTGGAC ATCGTTGCCG ACAGTGTGAG TGTGGTAGCA GTCATCTAGA ACTTCGTCCC ATTGTGCTAA ATGTAACTGA GGAGCTGAGA AGTGACCACC
     --:-- -    : -      -  :-- -- -- --:-- -:  -- - -- -- --: -- -- - --    --- ---


                                                       Elb 55K stop ⌐ splice Elb
     -   --* -  ---   *-  -*-- - *-  -- -- --*  ------  - --*-*---               - ****    * -*--- -*   _**
3454 TGGTGCTGGC CTGCACCCGC GCTGAGTTTG GCTCTAGCGA TGAAGATACA GATTGAGGTA CTGAAATGTG TGGGCGTGGC TTAAGGGTGG GAAAGAATAT
     ****  * **         * *  * *  *  *              ** *     ⌡         *  *** ** *    * *       *
3330 TGGTGCTTGC CTGCACTGGA GCGGAGTTCG GTTCTAGTGG TGAAGAAACT GACTAAAGTA AGACAG---GTG GGGGCAAAA- -TGTGGATGG GG-ACTTTCA
                                                       *   *  ⌡          ***
3239 TTACCCTGTC TTGCCTGCGG ACTGACTATG AGTCAAGTGA TGAAGACGAC AACTGAGGTA AGT------- ---GGGTGGA GCTA-GGTGG GA----TTAT
     -  -- -  --- : -:  - -- - - :-- - - -- ------:: - :  - ----  -      : - --- -   -


                                 Elb splice ⌐                      start IX
     *     --- - --- ***        c     * -  * ----  -  - --     -- -*  - ----* -         g
3554 A-----TAAG G-TGGGGGTC TT----ATGT AG-TTTTGTA ----TCTGTT TTGCAGCAGC CGCCGCCGCC ATGAGCACCA AC------- ----------
         *  * *      * *   **     *  *          *        *  ⌡         * *  *    *     *
3424 GGTTGGTAAG G-TGGACAAA TT----GGGT AAATTTTGTT AATTTCGTC TTGCAGCTG- --------CC ATGAGTGGAA GC-------- -------GCT
             *                         * *           *  ⌡               ***
3324 A-----AAAG GCTGGGAAGTC AACTAAAAAT TG-TTTTTGT ----TCT-TT TAACAGCA-- --------CG ATGAACGGAA CTACTCAGAA CAACGCTGCG
     --- - --- :    -    : - ----   --- : - ---       --- - :


     -----*- -* - -*    - --- - --- *----- *     - - --      -----*-- -- -------- ---* - -- -    - -- --*- -
3621 TCGTTTGATG GAAGCATTGT GAGCTCATAT TTGACAACGC GCATGCCCCC ATGGGCCGGG GTGCGTCAGA ATGTGATGGG CTCCAGCATT GATGGTCGCC
       **                              *                               * *                     * *
3495 TCTTTTGAGG GGGGAGTATT TAGCCCTTAT CTGACGGGCA GGCTCCCACC ATGGGCAGGA GTTCGTCAGA ATGTCATGGG ATCCACTGTG GATGGGAGAC
      *           *           *                              *                   *     *       *   * ** *
3403 CTTTTTGATG GAGGGGTTTT TAGCCCTTAT TTGACTTCCA GGTTACCATA TTGGGCCGGA GTACGTCAGA ATGTGGTAGG ATCTACAGTG GACGGTCGAC
     ----- - -:  - -- -   --- --- ----:: - :-:-- ----- -- --:------ ---- - -- --- - : -  - -- --:-  -- --:: --


     - --   -- --*-- --   - -- *- - ---- - --    -     -*-- ---- - *- -- -- * ----- --   ---*- - - -- *  --
3721 CCGTCCTGCC CGGCAAACTCT ACTACCTTGA CCTACGAGAC CGTGTCTGGA ACGCCGTTGG AGACTGCAGC CTCCGCCGCC GCTTCAGCCG CTGCAGCCAC
       * * ***              *            * *                *            *         * *          * *  *
3595 CCGTCCAGCC CGCCAATTCC TCAACGCTGA CCTATGCCAC TTTGAGTTCG TCACCATTGG ATGCAGCTGC AGCCGCCGCC GCTACTGCTG CCGCCAACAC
                *             **   * *    * *                   * *      *  *         * *
3503 CTGTGGCACC TGCAAATTCA TCAACATTAA CCTATGCAAC TATTGGACCC TCGCCTTTGG ATACCGCCGC CGCCGCTGCA GCTTCCGCGG CCGCTTCTAC
     - -- :  - -- -- --:  --:-:-- - :-- - :-: :  --:--:--   -:-:--  -- ---- --- :--:-- : - --::   --
```

Table 10.1 (Continued)

```
         ** _** -  -- *  *** - -*   **    -  *   * *-    *   **_ *   -*  -  - * ** -- --- -*** - - -             a
3821 CGCCCGCGGG ATTGTGACTG ACTTTGCTTT CCTGAGCCCG CTTGCAAGCA GTGCAGCTTC CCGTTCATCC GCCCGCGATG ACAAGTTGAC GGCTCTTTTG
         *  *       *       *        *    *  *   ** **  *                 *      ** *         * *  *
3695 CATCCTTGGA ATG---GGCT ATTACGGAAG CATTGTTGCC AATTCCAGTT CCTCTAATAA TCCTTCAACC CTGGCTGAGG ACAAGCTACT TGTTCTCTTG
         *   *   *    * *     *  *    *           *         *        *  *          *        *  *
3603 GGCTCGCAGT ATGGCAGCTG ATTTCAGCTT CTACAATCAC TTGGCTTCGA ATGCTGTGAC ACGCACCGCA GTTCGAGAGG ACATTCTGAC TGTTATGCTT
         - -: --     - -    -- :    -:: :    :   -: :  : : - :    :- - :: :     : :-- --- -  - -:- --


       -- - - - - -* - --    * *-  *  - - - - *- -- -  **- -                            *    - **
3921 GCACAATTGG ATTCTTTGAC CCGGGAACTT AATGTCGTTT CTCAGCAGCT GTTGGATCTG CGC------C AGCAGGTTTC TGCCCTGAAG ---GCTTCCT
         *         *   **         *      *  **    *  **       * **  *  **  * *  * ** *** *  *  *
3792 GCTCAGCTCG AGGCCTTAAC CCAACGCTTA GGCGAACTGT CTAAGCAGGT GGCCCAGTTG CGTGAG---C AAACTGAGTC TGCTGTTGCC ACAGCAAAGT
         **         *    *         *   * * *      *    *   *   *   *   *** ***     **          ** *
3703 GCCAAGCTTG AAACTCTAAC TGCTCAGCTG GAAGAGCTAT CGCAAAAGGT TGAGGAATTA GCTGATGCTA CTACC----- -------CAT ACCCCAGCCC
         --:  - -:- -:-  --    :- :  -:- - -:- - -    :  -: -              : :        : :


              stop IX           "AAUAAA" E1b                                    "AAUAAA", stop IVa2
       *** *      - *          - -   ----  -                              *   **** --  ---- - -        t
4012 CCCCTCCCAA TGCGGTTTAA A-------AC ATAAATAAAA AACCAGACTC TGTTTGGATT TGGATCAAGC AAGTGTCTTG CTGTCTTTAT TTAGG---GG
     *           * **                ** **       *** * *  *  * ***                                *
3889 CT-------- -AAATAAAGA TCTCAAATCA ATAAATAAAG AAATAC---- ---TTGTTAT AAAAACAA-- -------ATG AATG-TTTAT TT------GA
     ****** *                         *                                                 * ***
3791 AACCTGTAAC CCAATAAAGA A--------A AAACTTAAAT TGAGATG--- ---------- ---------- --GTGTTATG AAT-CTTTAT TGATACTTGT
     :           :         :        -   - ----: :-:                              --    ----- -       -:


       ---- -  -   ---- -- - ----- - -* -- -- -- -    - --- -- - ------ -  * ------ --* *--
4102 TTTTGCGCGC CGGTAGGCCC CGGGACCAGC GGTCTCGGTC GTTGAGGGTC CTGTGTATTT TTTCCAGGAC GTGGTAAAGG TGACTCTGGA TGTTCAGATA  5
        *** **     *       *   *    *  * * *   *       *     *   *    *       *    *          * **** *****
3957 TTTTTGCGC GCGGTATGCC CTGGACCATC GGTTTCGATC ATTGAGAACT CGGTGGATCT TTTCCAGTAC CCTGTAAAGG TGGGATTGAA TGTTTAGATA  7
        *               *            *    * **  *  ***  *             *    *       *
3857 TTTTTCTGAC ATGGTAAGCT CTTGACCACC GTTCCCTATC ATTAAGAACA CGGTGAATGT GTTCCAGTAT TTTGTAAAGA TGAGCCTGT
        ---- -      ----:-- :    - ----:-- - -     : - ---:--:-  ------ -  -- : --:


4202 CATGGGCATA AGCCCGTCTC TGGGGTGGAG GTAGCACCAC TGCAGAGCTT CATGCTGCGG GGTGGTGTTG TAGATGATCC AGTCGTAGCA GGAGCGCTGG
     ********* ** ******* ******** * **** * **** * *** ***** * *** ** *** *****  ** ** *** **** ***** *  ** *
4057 CATGGGCATT AGTCCGTCTC GGGGGTGGAG ATGACTCCAT TGAAGAGCCT CTTGCTCCGG GGTAGTGTTA TAAATCACCC AGTCATAGCA AGGTCGGAGT


4302 GCGTGGTGCC TAAAAATGTC TTTCAGTAGC AAGCTGATTG CCAGGGGCAG GCCCTTGGTG TAAGTGTTTA CAAAGCGGTT AAGCTGGGAT GGGTGCATAC
     ** *****   *  *** ** *** ** ***  *  * **** * *** * *** ** ***** *** *  ***** **** * *** ******** ******** *
4157 GCATGGTGTT GCACAATATC TTTTAGGAGC AGACTAATTG CAACGGGGAG GCCCTTAGTG TAGGTGTTTA CAAATCTGTT GAGCTGGGAC GGGTGCATCC


4402 GTGGGGATAT GAGATGCATC TTGGCTGTA TTTTTAGGTT GGCTATGTTC CCAGCCATAT CCCTCCGGGG ATTCATGTTG TGCAGAACCA CCAGCACAGT
     * ** *** *  * ****** ********* * *** ***** * *** **** **  * *** * ** ***** **** **** **** ****** *** *****
4257 GGGGTGAAAT TATATGCATT TTGGACTGGA TCTTGAGGTT GGCAATGTTC CCGCCTAGAT CCCGTCTCGG GTTCATATTG TGCAGGACCA CCAAGACAGT


                                                                                       g
4502 GTATCCGGTG CACTTGGGAA ATTTGTCATG TAGCTTAGAA GGAAATGCGT GGAAGAACTT GGAGACGCCC TTGTGACCTC CAAGATTTTC CATGCATTCG
     ********* ********** ** ****** *  **  ***** ******** * **  **  **  ********* ********  * ** *** ** * ****** *
4357 GTATCCGGTG CACTTGGGAA ATCTATCATG CAGCTTAGAG GGAAAAGCAT GAAAAAATTT GGAGACGCCT TTGTGACCCC CCAGATTCTC CATGCACTCA


4602 TCCATAATGA TGGCAATGGG CCCACGGGCG GCGGCCTGGG CGAAGATATT TCTGGGATCA CTAACGTCAT AGTTGTGTTC CAGGATGAGA TCGTCATAGG
     ********* ** ** ***** ** **** *****  *** **** ** *    *  ******* ********** ********** ********** **********
4457 TCCATAATGA TAGCGATGGG GCCGTGGGCA GCGGCACGGG CGAACACGTT CCGGGGATCA CTAACGTCAG AGTTGTGTTC CAGGATGAGA TCGTCATAGG


                                                          g
4702 CCATTTTTAC AAAGCGCGGG CGGAGGGTGC CAGACTGCGG TATAATGGTT CCATCCGGCC CAGGGGCGTA GTTACCCTCA CAGATTTGCA TTTCCCACGC
     ********* *** * ***  ********** **** ** ** ** * *** *  *  ** **** * ** ***** *** ****** ** ******* ********* *
4557 CCATTTTTAC AAACTTTGGG CGGAGGGTGC CAGATTGGGG GATGAAAGTT CCCTGTGGCC CGGGAGCATA GTTTCCCTCA CATATTTGCA TTTCCCAGGC


4802 TTTGAGTTCA GATGGGGGGA TCATGTCTAC CTGCGGGGCG ATGAAGAAAA CGGTTTCCGG GGTAGGGGAG ATCAGCTGGG AAGAAAGCAG GTTCCTGAGC
     *** ****** ** ******* ******* ** ********** ** ** ** * * **** **   * **** ** ** **** ** ** **** ***** ****
4657 TTTCAGTTCA GAGGGGGGGA TCATGTCCAC CTGCGGGGCT ATAAAAAAATA CCGTTTCTGG AGCCGGGGTG ATTAACTGGG ATGAGAGCAA ATTCCTAAGC


4902 AGCTGCGACT TACCGCAGCC GGTGGGCCCG TAAATCACAC CTATTACCGG GTGCAACTGG TAGTTAAGAG AGCTGCAGCT GCCGTCATCC CTGAGCAGGG
     ***** **** * ****** * ******* *** * **** *  ** ** ***  *** **** ** ***** * *** *** ***** *** ** * ********
4757 AGCTGAGACT TGCCGCACCC GGTGGGACCG TAAATGACCC CAATTACGGG TTGCAGATGG TAGTTTAGGG AGCGACAGCT GCCGTCCTCC CGGAGCAGGG


                     t                                   g
5002 GGGCCACTTC GTTAAGCATG TCCCTGACTC GCATGTTTTC CCTGACCAAA TCCGCCAGAA GCGCTCGCC GCCCAGCGAT AGCAGTTCTT GCAAGGAAGC
     ********** ** *** *** ***** **  * ** ***** ** ***** *  ***** **** **** ** *** *** ** * *** ** * ** * **** *
4857 GGGCCACTTC GTTCATCATT TCCCTTACAT GGATATTTTC CCGCACCAAG TCCGTTAGGA GGCGCTCTCC CCCAAGTGAT AGAAGCTCCT GGAGCGAGGA


                                                                                            E2b 100K stop
                          g                                                                       g
5102 AAAGTTTTTC AACGGTTTGA GACCGTCCGC CGTAGGCATG CTTTTGAGCG TTTGACCAAG CAGTTCCAGG CGGTCCCACA GCTCGGTCAC CTGCTCTACG
     ********** * *** ** ** * ****** ** * * ***** *      *  ** ** **      ** ** ** ********* * ***** * * ***** *
4957 GAAGTTTTTC AGCGGCTTCA GCCCGTCAGC CATGGGCATT TTGGAAAGAG TCTGTTGCAA GAGCTCGAGC CGGTCCCAGA GCTCGGTGAT GTGCTCTATG


5202 GCATCTCGAT CCAGCATATC TCCTCGTTTC GCGGGTTGGG GCGGCTTTCG CTGTACGGCA GTAGTCGGTG CTCGTCCAGA CGGGCCAGGG TCATGTCTTT
     ********** ****** * * ********** ** ** ** *  ********* *   *** **  ** ** **  ******* *   ****** ** ** ** ***
5057 GCATCTCGAT CCAGCAGACC TCCTCGTTTC GCGGGTTGGG ACGGCTCCTG GAGTAGGGAA TCAGACGATG GGCGTCCAGC GCTGCCAGGG TCCGATCCTT
```

Table 10.1 (Continued)

```
5302 CCACGGGCGC AGGGTCCTCG TCAGCGTAGT CTGGGTCACG GTGAAGGGGT GCGCTCCGGG CTGCGCGCTG GCCAGGGTGC GCTTGAGGCT GGTCCTGCTG
     *** ** *** ** **** *  **** ** **  *  ***** ********** **** ** **  ** ***** ** ******* **** ** **  ********
5157 CCATGGTCGC AGCGTCCGAG TCAGGGTTGT TTCCGTCACG GTGAAGGGGT GCGCGCCTGG TTGGGCGCTT GCGAGGGTGC GCTTCAGACT CATCCTGCTG

                               ┌ splice IVa2
5402 GTGCTGAAGC GCTGCCGGTC TTCGCCCTGC GCGTCGGCCA GGTAGCATTT GACCATGGTG TCATAGTCCA GCCCCTCCGC GGCGTGGCCC TTGGCGCGCA
     **   *** * ******* **  ********   ******** ******* **  *****   ** **** * ** **** ** ********  ***** ** *
5257 GTCGAGAACC GCTGCCGATC GGCGCCCTGC ATGTCGGCCA GGTAGCAGTT TACCATAAGT TCGTAGTTGA GCGCCTCGGC CGCGTGGCCT TTGGCACGGA

                                                      a
5502 GCTTGCCCTT GGAGGAGGCG CCGCACGAGG GGCAGTGCAG ACTTTTGAGG GCGTAGAGCT TGGGCGCGAG AAATACCGAT TCCGGGGAGT AGGCATCCGC
     **** ** ** *** *      *** *  ****** *  ** ******* ** ** **** ********** ** *  *** ** ******* * ********
5357 GCTTACCTTT GGAAGTTTTA TGGCAGGCAG GGCAGTAGAT ACATTTGAGG GCATACAGCT TGGGCGCGAG AAAATGGAT TCGGGGGAGT ATGCATCCGC

5602 GCCGCAGGCC CCGCAGACGG TCTCGCATTC CACGAGCCAG GTGAGCTCTG GCCGTTCGGG GTCAAAAACC AGGTTTCCCC CATGCTTTTT GATGCGTTTC
     *******   ********** *  **** ** *** ****** ** ** ** **  **  ** ** ********  ** ***** *  **** ***** **********
5457 ACCGCAGGAG ACGCAGACGG TTTCGCACTC CACAAGCCAG GTCAGATCCG GCTCATCAGG GTCAAAAAGA AGTTTTCCGC CATGTTTTTT GATGCGTTTC

       ┌ splice, start IVa2
5702 TTACCTCTGG TTTCCATGAG CCGGTGTCCA CGCTCGGTGA CGAAAAGGCT GTCCGTGTCC CCGTATACAG ACTTGAGAGG CCTGTCCTCG AGCGGTGTTC
     ****** *** **********  * ******* **** ***** * ** ***** ********** ***** ** * **** *  ** ********** ***** ** *
5557 TTACCTTTTG TTTCCATGAG TTCGTGTCCA CGCTCGGGTGA CAAAGAGGCT GTCCGTGTCC CCGTAGACCG ACTTTATGGG CCTGTCCTCG AGCGGAGTGC

              IVa2 cap ┌┐
                       │g
5802 CGCGGTCCTC CTCGTATAGA AACTCGGACC ACTCTGAGAC AAAGGCTCGC GTCCAGGCCA GCACGAAGGA GGCTAAGTGG GAGGGGTAGC GGTCGTTGTC
     * ****** * ***** ** ** *  ***** ****** **** ** ** *   ********** ********** *** * **** ********** **********
5657 CTCGGTCCTC TTCGTAGAGG AATCCAGCCC ACTCTGATAC AAAAGCGCGT GTCCAGGCCA GCACAAAGGA GGCCACGTGG GAGGGGTAGC GGTCGTTGTC

                                                                                       a
5902 CACTAGGGGG TCCACTCGCT CCAGGGTGTG AAGACACATG TCGCCCTCTT CGGCATCAAG GAAGGTGATT GGTTTGTAGG TGTAGGCCAC GTGACCGGGT
     ** ***** **** * ** * ** *** ***  ******* ** ***** * *** ** ***** * **** ***** ********** ********** *********
5757 AACCAGGGGA TCCACCTTCT CTACGGTATG TAAACACATG TCCCCCTCCT CCACATCCAA GAATGTGATT GGCTTGTAAG TGTAGGCCAC GTGACCAGGG

           "TATA" major late                           ┌ cap major late            1st leader  3'┐
6002 GTTCCTGAAG GGGGGCTATA AAAGGGGGTG GGGGCGCGTT CGTCCTCACT CTCTTCCGCA TCGCTGTCTG CGAGGGCCAG CTGTTGGGGT GAGTACTCCC
     ** ** * ** *  * ***** **** ******** * *   *** ********** ******* * ********   *** ***** ********** *** ****
5857 GTCCCCGCCG GGGGGGTATA AAGGGGGCG GACCTCTGTT CGTCCTCACT GTCTTCCGGA TCGCTGTCCA GGAGCGCCAG CTGTTGGGGT AGGTATTCCC

         c
6102 TCTGAAAAGC GGGCATGACT TCTGCGCTAA GATTGTCAGT TTCCAAAAAC GAGGAGGATT TGATATTCAC CTGGCCCGCG GTGATGCCTT TGAGGGTGGC
     *** ** ** ********** **** ** * ** ******** *** * *** ********** ****** ** ** ** *  ******** * *
5957 TCTCTAATGC GGGCATGACC TCTGCACTCA GGTTGTCAGT TTCTAGGAAC GAGGAGGATT TGATATTGAC AGTACCAGCA GAGATGCCTT TTATAAGACT

      g                                  g
6202 CGCATCCATC TGGTCAGAAA AGACAATCTT TTTGTTGTCA AGCTTGGTGG CAAACGACCC GTAGAGGGCG TTGGACAGCA ACTTGGCGAT GGAGCGCAGG
     * * ***** ********** * ********  ********* ********** **** ** ** ********** ***** ** *  ********* ******** *
6057 CTCGTCCATC TGGTCAGAAA ACACAATCTT CTTGTTGTCC AGCTTGGTGG CAAATGATCC ATAGAGGGCG TTGGATAGAA GCTTGGCGAT GGAGCGCATG

6302 GTTTGGTTTT TGTCGCGATC GGCGCGCTCC TTGGCCGCGA TGTTTAGCTG CACGTATTCG CGCGCAACGC ACCGCCATTC GGGAAAGACG GTGGTGCGCT
     ******** * ** **   ** ********** ***** **** *  *** *** ** **** ** * *  ****** * ** ****** ********** **** *
6157 GTTTGGTTCT TTTCCTTGTC CGCGCGCTCC TTGGCGGCGA TGTTAAGCTG GACGTACTCG CGCGCCACAC ATTTCCATTC AGGAAAGATG GTTGTCAGTT

                                                                         a
6402 CGTCGGGCAC CAGGTGCACG CGCCAACCGC GGTTGTGCAG GGTGACAAGG TCAACGCTGG TGGCTACCTC TCCGCGTAGG CGCTCGTTGG TCCAGCAGAG
     * ** ** ** *  ** ***** ** * ** ******** ** *** *  ** ** ** *** **** ***** ** ** *** **** **** **********
6257 CATCCGGAAC TATTCTGACT CGCCATCCCC TATTGTGCAG GGTTATCAGA TCCACAGTGG TGGCCACCTC GCCTCGGAGG GGCTCATTGG TCCAGCAGAG

              a             t
6502 GCGGCCGCCC TTGCGCGAGC AGAATGGCGG TAGGGGGTCT AGCTGCGTCT CGTCCGGGGG GTCTGCGTCC ACGGTAAAGA CCCCGGGCAG CAGGCGCGCG
     ** ** ** ** ** ** *  **** ** ** ********** ***  ** ** *** ** ** *  ** ****** * ** ****** * ** ** ** **    *
6357 TCGACCTCCT TTTCGTGAAC AGAAAGGGGG GAGGGGGTCT AGCATGAACT CATCAGGGGG GTCCGCATCT ATGGTAAATA TTCCCGGTAG CAAATCTTTG

6602 TCGAAGTAGT CTATCTTGCA TCCTTGCAAG TCTAGCGCCT GCTGCCATGC GCGGGCGGCA AGCGCGCGCT CGTATGGGTT GAGTGGGGGA CCCCATGGCA
     ** ** **** ** *     ** *  * ***  ** *  ** * ** ** ********** *  *** ***** * **** ***** *****  ****
6457 TCAAAATAGC TGAT---GGT GGCAGGATCA TCCAAGGTCA TCTGCCATTC TCGAACTGCC AGCGCGCGCT CATAGGGGTT AAGAGGGGTG CCCCAGGGCA

6702 TGGGGTGGGT GAGCGCGGAG GCGTACATGC CGCAAATGTC GTAAACGTAG AGGGGCTCTC TGAGTATTCC AAGATATGTA GGGTAGCATC TTCCACCGCG
     ********** ********** ** ******* * ** ** ** ** ** *** ********** *** ** ** * ** ** ** ** ** ** * ** ** *
6554 TGGGGTGGGT GAGCGCGGAG GCATACATGC CACAGATATC GTAGACATAG AGGGGCTCTT CGAGGATGCC GATGTAAGTG GGATAACAGC GCCCCCCTCT

6802 GATGCTGGCG CGCACGTAAT CGTATAGTTC GTGCGAGGGA GCGAGGAGGT CGGGACCGAG GTTGCTACGG GCGGGCTGCT CTGCTCGGAA GACTATCTGC
     ****** *** ***** ** * ** ***** ******** ** **** ** ** * ** ** ** * *  ** * * * ** ** ** ** ** **
6654 GATGCTTGCT CGCACATAGT CATAGAGTTC ATGTGAGGGG GCGAGGAGAC CCGGGCCCAG ATTGGTGCGG TTGGGTTTTT CCGCCCTGTA AACGATTTGG

6902 CTGAAGATGG CATGTGAGTT GGATGATATG GTTGGACGCT GGAAGACGTT GAAGCTGGCG TCTGTGAGAC CTACCGCGTC ACGCACGAAG GAGGCGTAGG
     * ******** **** ** ** *** ** ** ** ** * ** **** * *** **  * * ** ** **** * ** *** *  * **** ** *
6754 CGAAAGATGG CATGGGAATT GGAAGAAATA GTAGGTCTCT GGAATATGTT AAAATGAACA TGAGGTAGGC CTACAGAGTC TCTTATGAAG TGGGCATATG

7002 AGTCGCGCAG CTTGTTGACC AGCTCGGCGG TGACCTGCAC GTCTAGGGCG CAGTAGTCCA GGGTTTCCTT GATGATGTCA TACTTATCCT GTCCCTTTTT
     * ** **** **** *** ** *** *** ** ** * ** ** ** *** ** ** ****** ********* * * ** ***** ** *    * * * ** **
6854 ACTCTTGCAG CTTGGCTACC AGCTCTGCGG TGACGAGTAC ATCCAGGGCA CAGTAGTTGA GAGTTTCCTG GATGATGTCA TAACGCGGTT GGCTTTTCTT
```

Table 10.1 (Continued)

```
                 ┌5' 2nd late leader                                    2nd late leader 3'┐
7102  TTTCCACAGC TCGCGGTTGA GGACAAACTC TTCGCGGTCT TTCCAGTACT CTTGGATCGG AAACCCGTCG GCCTCCGAAC GGTAAGAGCC TAGCATGTAG
      ** ******* ********** **  *   * ** **** * ** ********** *** ** ** ********* ** ** ** ********* *** * *******
6954  TTCCCACAGC TCGCGGTTGA GAAGGTATTC TTCGTGATCC TTCCAGTACT CTTCGAGGGG AAACCCGTCT TTTTCTGCAC GGTAAGAGCC CAACATGTAG

7202  AACTGGTTGA CGGCCTGGTA GGCGCAGCAT CCCTTTTCTA CGGGTAGCGC GTATGCCTGC GCGGCCTTCC GGAGCGAGGT GTGGGTGAGC GCAAAGGTGT
      ********** * **** *** ** ****** ***** ***** *  ***** ** **** * *  ** ** ** * ******** ** ***** ***** **** *
7054  AACTGATTGA CTGCCTTGTA GGGACAGCAT CCCTTCTCCA CTGGGAGAGA GTATGCTTGG GCTGCATTGC GCAGCGAGGT ATGAGTGAGG GCAAAAGTGT

        a                                                                                                      g
7302  CCCTGACCAT GACTTTGAGG TACTGGTATT TGAAGTCAGT GTCGTCGCAT CCGCCCTGCT CCCAGAGCAA AAAGTCCGTG CGCTTTTTGG AACGCGGATT
      ********** ********** * ** ** * ******** * *** ** ** * ***** * ******* ******* ***** *** *  *****
7154  CCCTGACCAT GACTTTGAGG AATTGATACT TGAAGTCGAT GTCATCACAG GCCCCCTGTT CCCAGAGTTG GAAGTCCGCC CGCTTCTTGT AGGCGGGATT

                              a
7402  TGGCAGGGCG AAGGTGACAT CGTTGAAGAG TATCTTTCCC GCGCGAGGCA TAAAGTTGCG TGTGATGCGG AAGGGTCCCG GCACCTCGGA ACGGTTGTTA
      ****  *** ** *** **** * ****** **** **  *  **** ** * ** **** ** **** ****  * ** **  *** **** ***** *
7254  GGGCAAAGCG AAAGTAACAT CATTGAAGAG GATCTCACCG GCCCTGGGCA TGAAATTTCG GGTGATTTTA AAAGGCTGAG GGACCTCTGC TCGGTTATTG

                              g                              g                           g              g
7502  ATTACCTGGG CGGCGAGCAC GATCTCGTCA AAGCCGTTGA TGTTGTGGCC CACAATGTAA AGTTCCAAGA AGCGCGGGAT GCCCTTGATG GAAGGCAATT
      ** ***** ** **** *** ** ****** ** ***** ***  ****** ** *** ***** ***** **** ** ****** *** *  *   ***** *
7354  ATAACCTGAG CGGCCAAGAC GATCTCATCA AAGCCATTGA TGTTGTGCCC CACTATGTAC AGTTCTAAGA ATCGAGGGGT GCCCCTGACA TGAGGCAGCT

                          c.             t        c
7602  TTTTAAGTTC CTCGTAGGTG AGCTCTTCAG GGGAGCTGAG CCCGTGCTCT GAAAGGGCCC AGTCTGCAAG ATGAGGGTTG GAAGCGACGA ATGAGCTCCA
      * ** ***** ** ****  *  *** ** ** *** ***** ** ***  ** ** ****** **** *** ** ** ***** * ** ** * **** * * **
7454  TCTTGAGTTC TTCAAAAGTG AGATCTGTAG GGTCAGTGAG AGCATAGTGT TCGAGGGCCC ATTCGTGCAT GTGAGGGTTC GCTTTGAGGA AGGAGGACCA

7702  CAGGTCACGG GCCATTAGCA TTTGCAGGTG GTCGCGAAAG GTCCTAAACT GGCGACCTAT GGCCATTTTT TCTGGGGTGA TGCAGTAGAA GGTAAGCAGG
      *****      **** *     **** *  ** *** ** *    * **** *  ** *  * *  ***** *** ********** **** ***** *** * ***
7554  GAGGTCCACT GCCAGTGCTG TTTGTAACTG GTCCCGGTAC TGACGAAAAT GCTGTCCGAC TGCCATCTTT TCTGGGGTGA TGCAATAGAA GGTTTGGGGG

                              c  a               g   c           g              a
7802  TCTTGTTCCC AGCGGTCCCA TCCAAGGTTC GCGGCTAGGT CTCGCGCGGC AGTCACTAGA GGCTCATCTC CGCCGAACTT CATGACCAGC ATGAAGGGCA
      ** **  ** **** ***** ** ** ****  *** * * *  ***   * ** * ** ** *** **** * ** *** **** *  * ********* ******** *
7654  TCCTGCCGCC AGCGATCCCA CTTGAGTTTC ATGGCGATGT CATAGGCGAT GTTAACGAGC CGCTGGTCTC CAGAGAGTTT CATGACCAGC ATGAAGGGGA

                                                      ┌5' late i leader         start agnoprotein
7902  CGAGCTGCTT CCCAAAGGCC CCCATCCAAG TATAGGTCTC TACATCGTAG GTGACAAAGA GACGCTCGGT GCGAGGATGC GAGCCGATCG GGAAGAACTG
      ********  ******* *  ********  *  * ***** ** *********  ***  **** ** * ** *** ** **** ********** ********** **********
7754  TTAGCTGCTT GCCAAAGGAC CCCATCCAGG TGTAGGTTTC CACATCGTAG GTGAGGAAGA GCCTTTCTGT GCGAGGATGA GAGCCGATCG GGAAGAACTG

                 g             g
8002  GATCTCCCGC CACCAATTGG AGGAGTGGCT ATTGATGTGG TGAAAGTAGA AGTCCCTGCG ACGGGCCGAA CACTCGTGCT GGCTTTTGTA AAAACGTGCG
      *** *** ** ******** *  ***  **** *** ** * *  ********* *** **** * *** **** *  ** **** * ***** * ** *** ** ***
7854  GATTTCCTGC CACCAGTTGG AGGAATGGCT GTTGATGTGA TGGAAGTAGA ACTCCCTGCG ACGCGCCGAG CATTCATGCT TGTGCTTGTA CAGACGGCCG

8102  CAGTACTGGC AGCGGTGCAC GGGCTGTACA TCCTGCACGA GGTTGACCTG ACGACCGCGC ACAAGGAAGC AGAGTGGGAA TTTGAGCCCC TCGCCTGGCG
      ******* ** **** * *** **  ** *  ** ** ** *  ***** ** *  ** ** **  ***** **  ***** ** ** ***** * *   ** *****
7954  CAGTACTCGC AGCGATTCAC GGGATGCACC TCATGAATGA GTTGTACCTG ACTTCCTTTG ACGAGAAATT TCAGTGGAAA ATTGAG---- --GCTTGGCG

                                                    t
8202  GGTTTGGCTG GTGGTCTTCT ACTTCGGCTG CTTGTCCTTG ACCGTCTGGC TGCTCGAGGG GAGTTACGGT GGATCGGACC ACCACGCCGC GCGAGCCCAA
      * *  ** ** *  * *** *  * ****** *  *  ** **  * ***  * *   *****    *** **  *   ** * ** * **** * *       *
8048  CTTGTACCTC GCGCTCTACT ATGTTGTCTG CATCGGCATG ACCATCTTCT GTCTCGAT-- -------GGT GGTCATGCTG ACGAGCCCTC GCGGGAGGCA

                             Ad5 E2b 120K start          late i leader 3'┐
                                                                   a
8302  AGTCCAGATG TCCGCGCGCG GCGGTCGGAG CTTGATGACA ACATCGCGCA GATGGGAGCT GTCCATGGTC TGGAGCTCCC GCGGCGTCAG GTCAGGCGGG
      ********  ** *****   ** ***** ** ****** *** * * ****** *  ****** *  ***** ***** ****  *** *  **** ***** ** ** **
8139  AGTCCAGACC TCGGCGCGGC AGGGGCGGAG CTCGAGGACG AGAGCGCGCA GGCCGGAGCT GTCCAGGGTC CTGAGACGCT GCGGAGTCAG GTTAGTAGGC

          cg            c                    g           g                                               a
8402  AGCTCCTGCA GGTTTACCTC GCATAGACGG GTCAGGGCGC GGGCTAGATC CAGGTGATAC CTAATTTCCA GGGGCTGGTT GGTGGCGGCG TCGATGGCTT
      ** * *** *** ** * *  *            ****** **  *** *** ** *** ** *** * *  ***** *   *** *** *    **** ** **********
8239  AGTGTCAGGA GATTGACTTG CATGATCTTT TCGAGGGCGT GAGGGAGGTT CAGATGGTAC TTGATCTCCA CGGGTCCGTT GGTGGAGATG TCGATGGCTT

                                                                        Ad7 E2b 129K start//stop E2b pTP
8502  GCAAGAGGCC GCATCCCCGC GGCGCGACTA CGGTAC-CGC GCGGCGGGCG GTGGGCCGCG GGGTGTCCT TGGATGATGC AT--CTAAAA GCGGTGACGC
      *** * ** * *** **** *** **** * * * ** ** * * *   *  *   ***** *** * ** * * * * ***** ** * * ** ****** **
8339  GCAGGGTTCC GTGCCCCTTG GGCGCTACCA CCGTGCCCTT GTTTTTCCTT TTGGGCGGCG GTGGCTCTGT TGCTTCTTGC ATGTTTAGAA GCGGTGTCGA

              g             g
8599  GGGCGAGCCC CCGGAGGTAG GGGGGGGCTCC GGACCCGCCG GGAGAGGGGG CAGGGGCACG TCGGCGCCGC GCGCGGGCAG GAGCTGGTGC TGCGCGCGTA
      ***** ** * ** ** ** ** ****** ****** ***** * *  **** * * ** *** *** ***** ** * ***** *** ** * * ** **  ** ** *  * *
8439  GGGCGCGCAC CGGGCGGCAG GGGCGGCTCG GGACCCGGCG GCATGGCTGG CAGTGGTACG TCGGCACCGC GCGCGGGTAG GTTCTGGTAC TGCGCCCTGA

                                                                                             a
8699  GGGTTGCTGGC GAACGCGACG ACGCGGCGGT TGATCTCCTG AATCTGGCGC CTCTGCGTGA AGACGACGGG CCCGGTGAGC TTGAGCCTGA AAGAGAGTTC
      *  ** ** ********* ********** *** ***** *** ***** *** ** *  ** ** ** ****** **** ****** *** * *****  **
8539  GAAGACTCGC ATGCGCGACG ACGCGGCGGT TGACATCCTG GATCTGACGC CTCTGGGTGA AAGCTACCGG CCCCGTGAGC TTGAACCTGA AAGAGAGTTC
```

Table 10.1 (Continued)

```
                                                                             t
8799 GACAGAATCA ATTTCGGTGT CGTTGACGGC GGCCTGGCGC AAAATCTCCT GCACGTCTCC TGAGTTGTCT TGATAGGCGA TCTCGGCCAT GAACTGCTCG
     ********** ** ***** * ********** *** ** *   * ** ** * ******* **  ******** ** ******* ********** **********
8639 AACACAGAATCA ATCTCGGTAT CGTTGACGGC GGCTTGCCTA AGGATTTCTT GCACGTCGCC AGAGTTGTCC TGGTAGGCGA TCTCGGCCAT GAACTGCTCG


                                                              g
8899 ATCTCTTCCT CCTGGAGATC TCCGCGTCCG GCTCGCTCCA CGGTGGCGGC GAGGTCGTTG GAAATGCGGG CCATGAGCTG CGAGAAGGCG TTGAGGCCTC
     ********** ********** ****** ** **** *** * ********** ** ***** * ***** ** ***** ** * ****** **
8739 ATCTCTTCCT CTTGGAGATC TCCGCGGCCC GCTCGCTCGA CGGTGGCCGC GAGGTCGTTG GAGATGCGCC CAATGAGTTG AGAGAAAGCA TTCATGCCCG


8999 CCTCGTTCCA GACGCGGCTG TAGACCACGC CCCCTTCGGC ATCGCGGGCG CGCATGACCA CCTGCGCGAG ATTGAGCTCC ACGTGCCGGG CGAAGACGGC
     ********** ********** ******** **** *** *** * *** ********** **** ***** ********** ***** **** ****** **
8839 CCTCGTTCCA GACGCGGCTG TAGACCACAG CCCCCACGGG ATCTCTCGCG CGCATGACCA CCTGGGCGAG GTTGAGCTCC ACGTGGCGGG TGAAGACCGC


9099 GTAGTTTCGC AGGCGCTGAA AGAGGTAGTT GAGGGTGGTG GCGGTGTGTT CTGCCACGAA GAAGTACATA ACCCAGCGTC GCAACGTGGA TTCGTTGATA
     ***** * ******** * * ******** *** ****** *** **** * * *  ***** *** ***** * *** **** ** ** *** *** *
8939 ATAGTTGCAT AGGCGCTGGA AAAGGTAGTT GAGTGTGGTG GCGATGTGCT CGGTGACGAA GAAATACATG ATCCATCGTC TCAGCGGCAT CTCGCTGACA


9199 TCCCCCAAGG CCTCAAGGCG CTCCATGGCC TCGTAGAAGT CCACGGCGAA GTTGAAAAAC TGGGAGTTGC GCGCCGACAC GGTTAACTCC TCCTCCAGAA
     ** **** * ** ***** ********** ********** ****** ** ***** ** ******* ** **** ***** ** ****** ** ******
9039 TCGCCCAGCG CTTCCAAGCG CTCCATGGCC TCGTAGAAGT TCACGGCAAA GTTGAAAAAC TGGGAGTTAC GCGCGGACAC GGTCAACTCC TCTTCCAGAA


                                                                   ^^^                      Ad2 ins: ttc
9299 GACGGATGAG CTCGGCGACA GTGTCGCGCA CCTCGCGCTC AAAGGCTACA GGGGCCTCTT CTTCTTCTTC AATCTCCTCT TCCATAAGGG CCTCCCCTTC
     ******* ** ***** * **** ***** ** **** ** * *  * ***** ** ******* ***** ** *  * ****
9139 GACGGATAAG TTCGGCGATG GTGGTGCGCA CCTCGCGCTC GAAAGCTCCT AGGAT----- -TTCTTCCTC AATCTCTTCT TCTTCCACTA ACATCTCTTC


9399 TTCTTCTTCT GGCGGCGGTG GGGGAGGGGG GACACGGCGG CGACGACGGC GCACCGGGAG GCGGTCGACA AAGCGCTCGA TCATCTCCCC GCGGCGACGG
     *****    * ** * * * * ******** ** ***** ** ** **** **** * ** ******* ** * ** * * * *** ** ****** ***
9233 CTCTTCAGGT GGGGCTGCAG GAGGAGGGGG AACGCGGCGA CGCCGGCGGC GCACGGGCAG ACGGTCGATG AATCTTTCAA TGACCTCTCC GCGGCGGCGG


                                                                                                            g
9499 CGCATGGTCT CGGTGACGGC GCGGCCGTTC TCGCGGGGGC GCAGTTGGAA GACGCCGCCC GTCATGTCCC GGTTATGGGT TGGCGGGGGG CTGCCATGCG
     ***** **** ********** ** ****** ** * *** * *** *** ****** ** *** **** * *** ** ** ** * *
9333 CGCATAGTCT CGGTGACGGC ACGACCGTTC TCCCTGGGTC TCAGAGTGAA GACGCCTCCG CGCATCTCCC TGAAGTGGTG ACTGGGAGGC TCTCCGTTGG


                              ┌─5' 3rd late leader
                              a
9599 GCAGGGATAC GGCGCTAACG ATGCATCTCA ACAATTGTTG TGTAGGTACT CCGCCGCCGA GGGACCTGAG CGAGTCCGCA TCGACCGGAT CGGAAAACCT
     ******* ** ***** * ****** * ****** ********* ****** ** * * ******** *  ** ** ** **** * ********
9433 GCAGGGACAC CGCGCTGATT ATGCATTTTA TCAATTGCCC CGTAGGTACT CC---GCGCA AGGACCTGAT TGTCTCAAGA TCCACGGGAT CTGAAAACCT


          3rd late leader 3' ┐
9699 CTCGAGAAAG GCGTCTAACC AGTCACAGTC GCAAGGTAGG CTGAGCACCG TGGCGGGCGG CAGCGGGCG- --------GC GGTCGGGGTT GTTTCT----
     **** ** ********** *** ** ** ********** ******** * * * **** * ***** * ********** ** ****
9530 TTCGACGAAA GCGTCTAACC AGTCGCAATC GCAAGGTAGG CTGAGCACTG TTTCTTGCGG GCGGGGGCGG CTAGACGCTC GGTCGGGGTT CTCTCTTTCT


9786 ---------- ---------- ---GGCGGAG GTGCTGCTGA TGATGTAATT AAAGTAGGCG GTCTTGAGAC GGCGGATGGT CGACAGAAGC ACCATGTCCT
                          * * * ******** ***** **** *** ***** ** ** **** ********** * ** *** **** *** *
9630 TCTCCTTCCC CCTCTTGCGA GGGTGAGACG ATGCTGCTGG TGATGAAATT AAAATAGGCA GTTTTAAGAC GGCGGATGGT GGCGAGGAGC ACCAAGTCTT


9863 TGGGTCCGGC CTGCTGAATG CGCAGGCGGT CGGCCATGCC CCAGGCTTCG TTTTGACATC GGCGCAGGTC TTTGTAGTAG TCTTGCATGA GCCTTTCTAC
     ********** ** ** *** ******** * ***** *** ** ** ** * ******* * *** ** *** ***** ********** * * *** **
9730 TGGGTCCGGC TTGTTGGATG CGCAGGCGAT GAGCCATCCC CCAAGCATCA TCCTGACATC TGGCCAGATC TTTATAGTAG TCTTGCATGA GTCGTTCCAC


                                                                  a
9963 CGGCACTTCT TCTTCTCCTT CCTCTTGTCC TGCATCTCTT GCATCTATCG CTGCGGCGGC GGCGGAGTTT GGCCGTAGGT GGCGCCCTCT TCCTCCCATG
     ********** ***** **                                               * * ** ** * **** **** ****
9830 GGGCACTTCT TCTTCGCC-- ---------- ---------- ---------- ---------- ---------- ---------- ----CGCCCT GCCATGCATG


                                  c
10063 CGTGTGACCC CGAAGCCCCT CATCGGCTGA AGCAGGGCTA GGTCGGCGAC AACGCGCTCG GCTAATATGG CCTGCTGCAC CTGCGTGAGG GTAGACTGGA
      ** **** ** ** ** **** * ** ** * * ** ** ** *** ** * ** *** * * ****  * ******** ** ***** ** *
9864 CGAGTGATCC CGAACCCGCG CATGGGCTGG ACAAGTGCCA GCTCCGCTAC AACCCTTTCG GCGAGGATGG CTTGCTGCAC CTGGGTGAGG GTGGCTTGAA


10163 AGTCATCCAT GTCCACAAAG CGGTGGTATG CGCCCGTGTT GATGGTGTAA GTGCAGTTGG CCATAACGGA CCAGTTAACG GTCTGGTGAC CCGGCTGCGA
      **** ** * ****** *** ******** * ** ***** *** ***** * ******** **** ** ** ****** ** ******** * * ** **
9964 AGTCGTCAAA GTCCACGAAG CGGTGGTAGG CCCCGGTGTT GATTGTGTAG GAGCAGTTGG CCATGACTGA CCAGTTGACT GTCTGGTGCC CAGGGCGCAC


                  t          g
10263 GAGCTCGGTG TACCTGAGAC GCGAGTAAGC CCTCGAGTCA AATACGTAGT CGTTGCAAGT CCGCACCAGG TACTGGTATC CCACCAAAAA GTGCGGCGGC
      ********** *** * ** * ******* ** * ** **** ** * **** * ******* ** ********* ******** * * * *** *** ****
10064 GAGCTCGGTG TACTTCAGGC GCGAGTATGC GCGCGTGTCA AAGATGTAAT CGTTGCAGGT GCGCACCAGG TACTGGTAGC CGATGAGAAA GTGTGGCGAT


                                                         g
10363 GGCTGGCGGT AGAGGGGCCA GCGTAGGGTG GCCGGGGCTC CGGGGGCGAG ATCTTCCAAC ATAAGGCGAT GATATCCGTA GATGTACCTG GACATCCAGG
      ********** * ******** ** ** ********** ********** ******* * *** * ** ***** ********** **********
10164 GGCTGGCGGT ACAGGGGCCA TCGCTCTGTA GCCGGGGCTC CGGGGGCGAG GTCTTCCAGC ATGAGGCGGT GGTAGCCGTA GATGTACCTG GACATCCAGG
```

Table 10.1 (Continued)

```
                                                                          start E2b pTP
10463  TGATGCCGGC GGCGGTGGTG GAGGCGCGCG GAAAGTCGCG GACGCGGTTC CAGATGTTGC GCAGCGGCAA AAAGTGCTCC ATGGTCGGGA CGCTCTGGCC
       **** ****  ********** ** ** ** * * ** *****  ********* ********** ********* ****  * * ***** ** * ** *******
10264  TGATACCGGA GGCGGTGGTG GATGCACGTG GGAACTCGCG CACGCGGTTC CAGATGTTGC GCAGCGGCAT GAAGTAGTTC ATGGTAGGCA CGGTCTGGCC

          g       t       g                                                     r 5' VA1
10563  GGTCAGGCGC GCGCAATCGT TGACGCTCT- -AGACCGTGC -AAAAGGAGA GCCTGTAAGC GGGCACTCTT CCGTGGTCTG GTGGATAAAT TCGCAAGGGT
       ** ******  ***** ** * ********** ****   *   **** ** ** * *** *** * * ****** *** * ** ** * * ****
10364  AGTGAGGCGC GCGCAGTCAT TGACGCTCTG TAGACACGGA GAAAACGAAA GCG-ATGAGC -GGCTCGACT CCGTGGCCTG GGGG---AAC GTGGACGGGT

                        a          g
10660  ATCATGGCGG ACGACCGGGG TTCGAGCCCC GT-------- ATCCGGC-CG --TCCGCCGT GATCCATGCG GTTACCGCC- ---------- CGCGTGTCGA
        * ****    *** ** ****** **     *** * ** ** **** ** ** *** * ** ** * *** ****
10459  TGGGTCGCGG TGTACCCCGG TTCGAGTCCA AAGCTAAGCA ATCACACTCG GATCGGCCG- GAGCC--GCG GCTAACGTGG TATTGGCTAT CCCGTCTCGA

                                  VA1 3' ⌐TTTT
10738  ACCCAGGTGT GCGACGT--- --CAGACAAC GGGGGAGTGC TCCTTTTG-- GCTTCCTTCC AGG-CGCG-G CGGCTGCTGC G-CTAGCTTT TTTGGCCACT
       *****      *****      *** ** ** *** *       ***** **** *** * * *  ** ** * *  *** * * ****** * **
10556  -CCCAGC--- -CGACGAATA TCCAGGGTAC GGAGTAGAGT CGTTTTTGCT GCTTTTTTCC TGGACGTGTG CCATTGCCAC GTCAAGCTTT A----CAAC-

                                             r 5' VA2
10828  GGCCGCGCGC AGCGTAAGCG GTTAGGCTGG AAAGCGAAAG CATTAAGTGG CTCGCTCCCT GTAG-CCGGA GGGTTATTTT CCAAGGGTTG AGTCGCGGGA
       ** * ** *  ** *  ** *       ** *           * ***** ***** *** **** * *** * * * * * ******* ** **** *
10646  ------GCTC AG--TTCTCG G----GCCG- ---------- ---TGAGTGG CTCGCGCCC- GTAGTCTGGA GAAT-CAGTC GCCAGGGTTG CGTTGCGGTA

                              g
10927  --CCCCCGGT TCGAGTCT-- ---CGG---- -ACCGGCCGG ACT--GCGGC GAACGGGGGT TTGCCTCCCC -GTCATG--C AAGACCCCGC TTGCAAATTC
       ******** ***** **    ***        * ******* * *** * * ** **** *** * *** *****    * ********** ** * *
10718  TGCCCCCGGT TCGAGCCTAA GCGCGGCTCG TATCGGCCGG TTTCGCGCAC AAGCGAGGGT TTGGCAGCCC AGTCATTTCC AAGACCCCGC CAGCCGACTT

           VA2 3' ⌐TTTTT                       r 5' main body L1 RNA
                                                |start L1 52,55K
11010  CTCCGGAAAC AGGGA-CGAG CCCCTTTTTT ------GCTT TT----CCCA GATGCATCCG GTGCTGCGGC AGATGCGCCC C--------- ---CCTCCTC
       **** *     **** **** *** ******   * ** **  ****  ******** ******** * ********** *         *** ***
10818  CTCCAGTTTA CGGGAGCGAG CCC-TTTTT TTTTTTGTTT TTGTCGCCCA GATGCATCCA GTGCTGCGAC AGATGCGCCC CCAGCAACAG GCCCCTTCTC

11087  AGCAGCGGCA AGAGCAAGAG CAGCGGCAGA CA
       **** * **  * * * *  *  *        *
10917  AGCAACAGCC ACAAAAGGCT CTTCTTGCTC CT
```

middle rows, Ad5–Ad7; between middle and bottom rows, Ad7–Ad12; above top row, Ad5–Ad12). Positions where all three DNAs have different nucleotides are denoted by a colon under the bottom row. Expression signals and RNA coordinates are shown.

Between coordinates 0.0 and 31.7, the Ad5 DNA sequence is 99% homologous with that of Ad2 (GINGERAS et al. 1982; SHINAGAWA and PADMANABHAN 1979; PERRICAUDET et al. 1979; ALESTRÖM et al. 1980, 1982b). Whenever an Ad2 nucleotide differs from the Ad5 residue in the corresponding position, it is printed in lower case above the sequences. Deletions (relative to Ad5) in the Ad2 sequence are marked by the symbol ˆ, and insertions are indicated by "ins Ad2:" followed by the extra Ad2 residues printed in lower case.

Comparisons of the Ad5, Ad7, and Ad12 E1 sequences have been published (VAN ORMONDT et al. 1980a; VAN ORMONDT and HESPER 1983). SUGISAKI et al. (1980), KIMURA et al. (1981), and BOS et al. (1981) compared Ad5 and Ad12 E1 sequences, while ENGLER and VAN BREE (1982) compared the IVa2 regions of Ad7 and Ad5, and ENGLER et al. (1983) the E2B regions of Ad7 and Ad2.

Note: The sequences compared are from the l-strand. Consequently, expression signals of IVa2 and E2B should be read in the complementary sequence with opposite polarity.

11 Comparison of the E2A DBP-Gene Sequences of Human Ad2, Ad5, and Ad12

The E2A sequences of Ad5 (Sect. 5; upper row) and Ad12 (Sect. 9; lower row) have been shifted to obtain maximum homology, as described by KRUIJER (1983) (Table 11.1). The resulting gaps have been filled in with dashes. Ad5–Ad12 homologies are indicated by asterisks between the sequences. Expression signals and RNA coordinates are shown. The overall homology of Ad5 and Ad12 in this region is 51%. Between coordinates 61 and 67, the Ad5 DNA sequence is 95% homologous with that of Ad2 (Sect. 4). Whenever an Ad2 nucleotide differs from the Ad5 residue in the corresponding position, it is printed in lower case above the sequences. Insertions (relative to Ad5) in the Ad2 sequence are marked by "ins Ad2:" followed by the extra Ad2 residues printed in lower case.

Table 11.1. Comparison of the E2A DBP-gene sequences of Ad5 and Ad12 (from the 1-strands)

```
       stop L3 23K              "AAUAAA" L3      "AAUAAA" E2a
           Ad2 ins: g┐                                        Ad2 ins: c┐
 621  TAAAAATAAT GTACTAGAGA CACTTTCAAT AAAGGCAAAT GCTTTTATTT GTACACTCTC GGGTGATTAT TTACCCCCAC CCTTGCCGTC TGCGCCGTTT  5
      ****      *  ****    **  *   *** *** **     ******* *   ***       *    *      * *    **** ** **
 178  TAAA--CG-T GTACACAATG CATTAATAAT AAAACCA--- --TTTTATTA G----CTCAT TGGAG----- -CAT----AA GCTTG--T-C TGTTTTA-TT  12

       stop E2a DBP
 721  AAAAATCAAA GGGGTTCTGC CGCGCATCGC TATGCGCCAC TGGCAGGGAC ACGTTGCGAT ACTGGTGTTT AGTGCTCCAC TTAAACTCAG GCACAACCAT
      ********** *  *       ** *    ** **         ******** * *** * **** ****  ** * * *** *
 252  AAAAATCAAA TGGCTCTTCG CGACAGTCGC CGTGGTTGGT GGGCAGGGAT ATGTTTCTGT ACTGCAAACG CTGATGCCAC TTGAATTCTG GAATAACAAG

 821  CCGCGG---C AGCTCGGTGA AGTTTTCACT CCACAGGCTG CGCACCATCA CCAACGCGTT TAGCAGGTCG GGCGCCGATA TCTTGAAGTC GCAGTTGGGG
      ** **      **   * * ***** * ****** * ***** * **  *** * * ** ** ** ** ********* *** ** ***
 352  CCTAGGGGGG GAGCCGTCAA AATTTTCTCC CCACAGCTGG CGCACAAGTT GCAGGGCGCC CATAACATCA GGAGCAGAAA TCTTGAAGTC GCAATTAGGG

 918  CCTCCGCCCT GCGCGCGCGA GTTGCGGATAC ACAGGGTTGC AGCACTGGAA CACTATCAGC GCCGGGTGGT GCACGCTGGC CAGCACGCTC TTGTCGGAGA
      ** * *      ******  ********  ** ** **      ****** **  **  *   ***  *   *      **** * *    ***** *
 452  CC---AGCAT TGCCGCGCGC ATTGCGATAA ACTGGATTTG CGCACTGAAA AACCAACAAA CACGGATACT TAATACTGGC TAACGCTCCA GGGTCGGTTA

                                                              t       a
1018  TCAGATCCGC GTCCAGGTCC TCCGCGTTGC TCAGGGCGAA CGGAGTCAAC TTTGGTAGCT GCCTTCCCAA AAAGGGCGCG TGCCCAGGCT TTGAGTTGCA
      *          ** ** ***  *** ***** * *** * **  ***** *   **   ** * * *  ****     *** *     * *** *        **
 549  CTTCGTTGAT ATCAATGTTA TCCACATTGC TGAGGTTAAA AGGAGTGATT TTACACAGTT GACGCCCCAT CCGTGGCAGG CCATCTTGCT TGTTTAAACA

                                   g                             g
1118  CTCGCACCGT AGTGGCATCA AAAGGTGACC GTGCCCGGTC TGGGCGTTAG GATACAGCGC CTGCATAAAA GCCTTGATCT GCTTAAAAGC CACCTGAGCC
      ***** **  * ****** *  ** *       *****       *  ** ** ** ** ******** ** *  ** ** ******* *  ******
 649  TTCGCAGCGC ACTGGCATAA GGAGACGTTT TTGCCCATGT CGCATGTGAG GGTAGTCGGC CAGCATAAAA GCTTCAATTT GCCTAAAAGC TATTTGAGCC

                                                              a
1218  TTTGCGCCTT CAGAGAAGAA CATGCCGCAA GACTTGCCGG AAAAACTGATT GGCCGGACAG GCCGCGTCGT GCACGCAGCA CCTTGCGTCG GTGTTGGAGA
      **  **** **** * ** ** ****** *  ***** **** * **   ***   *   *** * * * ****** * ** *** *** *
 749  TTCATTCCTT CAGAATAAAA CAAGCCGCAG GACTTTCCGG AGAAAGAATT ATTCCCGCCA CCAACATCAT GAAAACAGCA GCGGGCATCG TCGTTTTTAA

1318  TCTGCACCAC ATTTCGGCCC CACCGGTTCT TCACGATCTT GGCCTTGCTA GACTGCTCCT TCAGCGCGCG CTGCCCGTTT TCGCTCGTCA CATCCATTTC
      * ** * **** *** *** ** * ** *** *** ** *** **   * **** ** *** *** ** ** ***** ** ***** ** * *********
 849  TTTGAACTAC ATTACGCCCC CAGCGGTTTT GCGCCACCTT GGCTTTCGAG GGGTTCTCTT TCAACGCTCG TTGCCCACTT TCGCTGGTTA CATCCATTTC

                                                      c
1418  AATCACGTGC TCCTTATTTA TCATAATGCT TCCGTGTAGA CACTTAAGCT CGCCTTCGAT CTCAGCGCAG CGGTGCAGCC ACAACGCGCA GCCCGTGGGC
      * *** ** **  *       *       * *** ** **  ** ******* * *****      *** * ***  *** *** ***  * **  *** ** *****
 949  CACCAAATGC TCTTTGCGCA CCATCTCCAT TCCATGCAGG CATCTAAGCT CCCCTTCGCG CTCGGTACAC TTATGCTCCC ACACGCAGCA ACCGGTGGGT

         g          t
1518  TCGTGATGCT TGTAGGTCAC CTCTGCAAAC GACTGCAGGT ACGCCTGCAG GAATCGCCCC ATCATCGTCA CAAAGGTCTT GTTGCTGGTG AAGGTCAGCT
      **         * * *    **         * ** *** *  * **** * *   * * **** ** *** *** *  *   * ****** ** * *   ** *******
1049  TCCCAGGAAT TCTGTTGGAC ACCGGCATAA GCTTGCATAT ATCCTTGCAA AAAGCGTCCC ATGAGCTCCT GAAAGGTTTT TTGGGACGAA AAAGTCAGCT

                                         t                                        c           t
1618  GCAACCCGCG GTGCTCCTCG TTCAGCCAGG TCTTGCATAC GGCCGCCAGA GCTTCCACTT GGTCAGGCAG TAGTTTGAAG TTCGCCTTTA GATCGTTATC
      **** ***** *  ** ***  ** ***** * *  ******  *            *       * * * ** **** *     *** * **      **** ***
1149  GCAAACCGCG CTTTTCTTCG TTGAGCCATG TTGTGCATAT TTTCTTGTAC ACGCTGCCCT GATCCGGCAA AAAACGAAAG GTGGCGCGCT CGTCGTGATC
```

Table 11.1 (Continued)

```
                     a                                               gg               t         gc
1718  CACGTGGTAC TTGTCCATCA GCGCGCGCGC AGCCTCCATG CCCTTCTCCC ACGCAGACAC GATGCGCACA CTCAGCGGGT T---CATCAC CGTAAT----
      *** ****** ** ***** * **        *     ** ****** ** ** **** * ** ** ** *  ***   **   *** * *   * **    **
1249  CACATGGTAC TTTTCCATTA GCATAGCCAT GGCTTCCATG CCTTTTTCCC AAGCTGAAAC TAGGGGCTGG CTTGCCGGAT TGCGAACAAC AACAACATTC

           a         a         t                         c                                                  c
1811  --TTCACTTT CCGCTTCGCT GGGCTCTTCC TCTTCCTCTT GCGTCCGCAT ACCACGCGCC ACTGGGTCGT CTTCATTCAG CCGCCGCACT GTGCGCTTAC
      **** *** *  *****     * ** * *     ***     * ** *** * **** **  *   *   * **   * *   * *   *   *  **
1349  TTTTCATTTT C---GTCGCT ---------- -----GTTTT GAGCGGAAGC CTTCAAAACG TGTACCTGCC TGGTTTCCAT TTTTTGAAAA GACTGAGAAC

           c         g
1909  CTCCTTTGCC ATGCTTGATT AGCACCGGTG GGTTGCTGAA ACCCACCATT TGTAGCGCCA C------ATC TTCTCTTTCT TCCTCGCTGT CCACGATTAC
      * **      **** * **   * ** ** *  ******* ***** * *   ** *   *     **** *** ** **     * * *        c
1431  CGTCTGCATG ATGCATAATG CGGACGGGCG GCATGCTGAA ACCCATTACT CCTAAAACTG CTCTTGGTGG TTCTGCCTCT TCTTC---TT CTGCACT---

           g                             g                 t    a                           t
2003  CTCTGGTGAT GGCGGGCGCT CGGGCTTGGG AGAAGGGCGC TTCTTTTTCT TCTTGGGCGC AATGGCCAAA TCCGCCGCCG AGGTCGATGG CCGCGGGCTG
      ****** **  * **     * *      *        * ** *       *  ** *** * **** **
1525  CTCTGGGGAA AGAGG---TA TCGCAGCCAT AGA---TTTC TTGACTTTTT TCTTTGG--- ---------- ---------- ---------- ----------

                     a         c         t                 g         g                   g
2103  GGTGTGCGCG GCACCAGCGC GTCTTGTGAT GAGTCTTCCT CGTCCTCGGA CTCGATACGC CGCCTCATCC GCTTTTTTGG GGGCGCCCGG GGAGGCGGCG
                 * *       * *         **  ***** **   * *          *         * *   * *       ** *******
1576  ---------- -AGGTAAAGG CACAGCTTCC AGTTCTTCTT CGCTTTCGGA ATCCAG---- ---------- -AAAGTATCT GCCCATTTTT GGCGGCGGCG

           c                             t
2203  GCGACGGGGA CGGGGACGAC ACGTCCTCCA TGGTTGGGGG ACGTCGCGCC GCACCGGCGTC CGCGCTCGGG GGTGGTTTCG CGCTGCTCCT CTTCCCGACT
      **  * *                                                          *** ** ** **** ** * *** *  *      **
1650  GCTGAGCGCT ---------- ---------- ---------- ---------- ---------- -GCGGTCTGG GGTGCGCTCC CTCTGTGAGT GCTGATTGCT

           start E2a DBP                         start L4 100K
2303  GGCCATTTCC TTCTCCTATA GGCAGAAAAA GATCATGGAG TCAGTCG
      *******   *   ****  * **** * *** * ****  *     * *
1699  GGCCATTATT TAATCCT--A GGCAAAGAAA CA-CATGATG GATCTGG

      NUMBER OF MATCHES 1 - 2     895 (.51)
```

12 Comparison of the Right-terminal DNA Sequences of Human Ad2 and Ad5

The sequences of the right-terminal 3% of Ad2 Sect. 6 and Ad5 (STEENBERGH and SUSSENBACH 1979) show 97% homology (Table 12.1). The sequences (upper row Ad2; lower row Ad5) have been shifted to obtain an optimum fit; the resulting gaps have been filled in with dashes. The asteriks between the rows mark the positions where the Ad2 and Ad5 sequences differ. Some landmarks have been indicated.

Table 12.1. Comparison of Ad2 and Ad5 DNA 97–100% (from the 1-strand)

```
9227  CCATGACAAA AGAACCCACA CTGATTATGA CACGCATACT CGGAGCTATG CTAACCAGCG TAGCCCCTAT GTAAGCTT-G TTGCATGGGC GGCGATATAA  2
         *                                                                     *          *
      CCTTGACAAA AGAACCCACA CTGATTATGA CACGCATACT CGGAGCTATG CTAACCAGCG TAGCCCCGAT GTAAGCTTTG TTGCATGGGC GGCGATATAA  5

9326  AATGCAAGGT GCTGCTCAAA AAATCAGGCA AAGCCTCGCG CAAAAAAGCA AGCACATCGT AGTCATGCTC ATGCAGATAA AGGCAGGTAA GTTCCGGAAC
                                                        *                                            *
      AATGCAAGGT GCTGCTCAAA AAATCAGGCA AAGCCTCGCG CAAAAAAGAA AGCACATCGT AGTCATGCTC ATGCAGATAA AGGCAGGTAA GCTCCGGAAC

                                                start E4 region 2          E4 region 1 stop
9426  CACCACAGAA AAAGACACCA TTTTTCTCTC AAACATGTCT GCGGGTTCCT GCATTAAACA CAAAATAAAA TAACAAAAAA AAAACATTTA AACATTAGAA
                                                * *                                  ***
      CACCACAGAA AAAGACACCA TTTTTCTCTC AAACATGTCT GCGGGTTTCT GCAT-AAACA CAAAATAAAA TAACAAAAAA A---CATTTA AACATTAGAA

9526  GCCTGTCTTA CAACAGGAAA AACAACCCTT ATAAGCATAA GACGGACTAC GGCCATGCCG GCGTGACCGT AAAAAAACTG GTCACCGTGA TTAAAAAGCA
      GCCTGTCTTA CAACAGGAAA AACAACCCTT ATAAGCATAA GACGGACTAC GGCCATGCCG GCGTGACCGT AAAAAAACTG GTCACCGTGA TTAAAAAGCA

9626  CCACCGACAG TTCCTCGGTC ATGTCCGGAG TCATAATGTA AGACTCGGTA AACACATCAG GTTGGTTAAC ATCGGTCAGT GCTAAAAAGC GACCGAAATA
         *                                                             *  **
      CCACCGACAG CTCCTCGGTC ATGTCCGGAG TCATAATGTA AGACTCGGTA AACACATCAG GTTGATT--C ATCGGTCAGT GCTAAAAAGC GACCGAAATA
```

Table 12.1 (Continued)

```
9726   GCCCGGGGGA ATACATACCC GCAGGCGTAG AGACAACATT ACAGCCCCCA TAGGAGGTAT AACAAAATTA ATAGGAGAGA AAAACACATA AACACCTGAA
       GCCCGGGGGA ATACATACCC GCAGGCGTAG AGACAACATT ACAGCCCCCA TAGGAGGTAT AACAAAATTA ATAGGAGAGA AAAACACATA AACACCTGAA

                                                                              start E4 region 1
9826   AAACCCTCCT GCCTAGGCAA AATAGCACCC TCCCGCTCCA GAACAACATA CAGCGCTTCC ACAGCGGCAG CCATAACAGT CAGCCTTACC AGTAAAAAA-
                                                                         *            *                           *
       AAACCCTCCT GCCTAGGCAA AATAGCACCC TCCCGCTCCA GAACAACATA CAGCGCTTC- ACAGCGGCAG CC-TAACAGT CAGCCTTACC AGTAAAAAAG

                                                  cap E4 mRNA                              "TATA" E4
9925   ---ACCTATT AAAAAA-CAC CACTCGACAC GGCACCAGCT CAATCAGTCA CAGTGTAAAA A-GGGCCAAG TACAGAGCGA GTATATATAG GACTAAAAAA
       ***              *                                          ↓      *             *
       AAAACCTATT AAAAAAACAC CACTCGACAC GGCACCAGCT CAATCAGTCA CAGTGTAAAA AAGGGCCAAG TGCAGAGCGA GTATATATAG GACTAAAAAA

10020  TGACGTAACG GTTAAAGTCC ACAAAAAACA CCCAGAAAAC CGCACGCGAA CCTACGCCCA GAAACGAAAG CCAAAAAACC CACAACTTCC TCAAATCTTC
                                                                                                              *
       TGACGTAACG GTTAAAGTCC ACAAAAAACA CCCAGAAAAC CGCACGCGAA CCTACGCCCA GAAACGAAAG CCAAAAAACC CACAACTTCC TCAAATCGTC

                                                                                       end ITR
10120  ACTTCCGTTT TCCCACGATA CGTCACTTCC CATTTTAAAA AAACTACAAT TCCCAATACA TGCAAGTTAC TCCGCCCTAA AACCTACGTC ACCCGCCCCG
                         *      *                 *                                          ↓
       ACTTCCGTTT TCCCACGTTA CGTAACTTCC CATTTTAAGA AAACTACAAT TCCCAACACA TACAAGTTAC TCCGCCCTAA AACCTACGTC ACCCGCCCCG

                                                                     see  Section A
10220  TTCCCACGCC CCGCGCCACG TCACAAACTC CACCCCCTCA TTATCATATT GGCTTCAATC CAAAATAAGG TATATTATtG ATGATG    3'
       TTCCCACGCC CCGCGCCACG TCACAAACTC CACCCCCTCA TTATCATATT GGCTTCAATC CAAAATAAGG TATATTATTG ATGATG    3'
```

13   Predicted Amino Acid Compositions and Predicted and Observed Molecular Weights of Some Early and Late Adenovirus Proteins

Tables 13.1 and 13.2 see pages 138, 139.

Table 13.1. Early proteins

Amino acid	Ad5 E1A	Ad5 E1B "19K"	Ad5 E1B "60K"	Ad5 E2B "140K"	Ad5 E2B pTP	Ad5 E2A DBP
Phe	6	10	18	50	27	19
Leu	23	23	37	104	62	39
Ile	12	5	21	34	22	16
Met	8	2	15	19	19	17
Val	20	7	39	63	47	34
Ser	20	16	31	65	29	41
Pro	46	6	22	69	46	45
Thr	11	5	27	60	32	21
Ala	14	14	36	83	61	47
Tyr	5	2	10	41	21	6
His	11	4	13	27	12	16
Gln	8	11	12	41	31	21
Asn	7	5	27	32	26	23
Lys	3	9	21	47	4	34
Asp	18	7	22	69	34	24
Glu	32	18	36	68	54	45
Cys	12	3	27	23	6	13
Trp	–	8	6	21	8	6
Arg	18	14	37	81	76	37
Gly	15	7	39	59	36	25
MW						
Predicted:	31 849	20 614	55 998	120 395	74 652	59 12?
Observed:	40–58K	15–19K	55–65K	140K	87K	72K

Table 13.2. Late proteins

Amino acid	Ad5 IX	Ad5 IVa2	Ad5 agno-protein	Ad2 L3 VI	Ad2 L3 23K	Ad5 L3 hexon
Phe	3	11	4	6	14	45
Leu	16	50	18	18	17	75
Ile	3	22	4	9	6	35
Met	3	16	2	6	7	29
Val	10	19	17	18	8	55
Ser	22	24	5	25	20	64
Pro	8	39	7	26	14	59
Thr	13	19	7	14	11	67
Ala	22	33	16	17	14	69
Tyr	2	14	3	2	7	57
His	–	19	6	2	8	15
Gln	6	24	3	14	12	40
Asn	5	18	1	12	10	74
Lys	2	20	3	12	8	40
Asp	7	29	8	10	5	65
Glu	3	19	11	12	9	49
Cys	–	7	2	1	8	7
Trp	1	5	4	5	3	13
Arg	8	35	13	18	11	46
Gly	6	26	11	23	12	64
MW						
Predicted:	14 458	50 885	16 149	27 012	23 067	109 16?
Observed:	12–14K	50K	13.6K	27K	not observed	90–120K

2 co- otein	Ad2 E3 "14K"	Ad2 E3 "14.5K"	Ad2 E4 region 2	Ad2 E4 "11K"	Ad2 E4 "14K"
	3	7	8	5	11
	16	10	18	19	12
	6	15	7	11	6
	4	3	6	4	7
	7	8	16	9	19
	4	11	10	2	6
	5	15	9	1	9
	12	7	3	3	4
	4	10	10	8	10
	3	5	4	2	5
	3	2	4	6	2
	8	6	6	2	4
	4	6	2	4	4
	10	3	1	1	–
	5	5	8	7	4
	13	2	9	12	7
	5	5	2	3	1
	–	3	–	1	–
	9	4	8	8	8
	7	3	5	8	9
437	14 738	14 528	15 306	13 255	14 276
K	14K	14.5K	17K	11K	14K

d2 4 K	Ad2 L4 VIII	Ad2 L5 fiber
	9	17
	14	56
	14	32
	6	12
	10	33
	22	62
	20	34
	14	68
	19	37
	8	17
	5	5
	15	18
	10	47
	3	34
	9	29
	8	18
	–	3
	2	4
	17	10
	22	46
5 022	24 702	61 916
3K	26K	62K

Acknowledgments. The authors are grateful to Drs. PETTERSSON and PERRICAUDET for communicating unpblished data and to Drs. HAMM and STÜBER for making available the sequence data on adenoviruses in the EMBL Sequence Data Bank.

References

Ahmed CMI, Chanda RS, Stow ND, Zain BS (1982a) The sequence of 3′ termini of mRNAs from early region III of adenovirus 2. Gene 19:297–301

Ahmed CMI, Chanda RS, Stow ND, Zain BS (1982b) The nucleotide sequence of mRNA for the Mr 19,000 glycoprotein from early gene block III of adenovirus 2. Gene 20:339–346

Akusjärvi G, Pettersson U (1978a) Sequence analysis of adenovirus DNA: I. Nucleotide sequence at the carboxy-terminal end of the gene for adenovirus type 2 hexon. Virology 91:477–480

Akusjärvi G, Pettersson U (1978b) Nucleotide sequence at the junction between the coding region of the adenovirus 2 hexon messenger RNA and its leader sequence. Proc. Natl Acad Sci USA 75:5822–5826

Akusjärvi G, Pettersson U (1979a) Sequence analysis of adenovirus DNA: complete nucleotide sequence of the spliced 5′ non-coding region of adenovirus 2 hexon messenger RNA. Cell 16:841–850

Akusjärvi G, Pettersson U (1979b) Sequence analysis of adenovirus DNA. IV. The genomic sequences encoding the common tripartite leader of late adenovirus messenger RNA. J Mol Biol 134:143–158

Akusjärvi G, Persson H (1981a) Gene and mRNA for precursor polypeptide VI from adenovirus type 2. J Virol 38:469–482

Akusjärvi G, Persson H (1981b) Controls of RNA splicing and termination in the major late adenovirus transcription unit. Nature 292:420–426

Akusjärvi G, Mathews MB, Andersson P, Vennström B, Pettersson U (1980) Structure of genes for virus-associated RNA1 and RNA2 of adenovirus type 2. Proc Natl Acad Sci USA 77:2424–2428

Akusjärvi G, Zabielski J, Perricaudet M, Pettersson U (1981) The sequence of the 3′ non-coding region of the hexon mRNA discloses a novel adenovirus gene. Nucleic Acids Res 9:1–7

Aleström P, Akusjärvi G, Perricaudet M, Mathews MB, Klessig D, Pettersson U (1980) Sequence analysis of adenovirus DNA. VI. The nucleotide sequence of the gene for polypeptide IX from adenovirus type 2 and its unspliced messenger RNA. Cell 19:671–681

Aleström, P, Stenlund A, Li P, Pettersson U (1982a) A common sequence in the inverted terminal repetitions of human and avian adenoviruses. Gene 18:193–197

Aleström P, Akusjärvi G, Pettersson M, Pettersson U (1982b) DNA sequence analysis of the region encoding the terminal protein and the hypothetical N-gene product of adenovirus type 2. J Biol Chem 257:13492–13498

Arrand JR, Roberts RJ (1979) The nucleotide sequences at the termini of adenovirus-2 DNA. J Mol Biol 128:577–594

Baker CC, Ziff EB (1980) Biogenesis, structures, and sites of encoding of the 5′ termini of adenovirus-2 mRNAs. Cold Spring Harbor Symp Quant Biol 44:415–428

Baker CC, Ziff EB (1981) Promoters and heterogeneous 5′ termini of the messenger RNAs of adenovirus-2. J Mol Biol 149:189–221

Baker CC, Hérissé J, Courtois G, Galibert F, Ziff E (1979) Messenger RNA for the Ad2 DNA binding protein: DNA sequences encoding the first leader and heterogeneity at the mRNA 5′ end. Cell 18:569–580

Berk AJ, Sharp PA (1978) Structure of the adenovirus 2 early mRNAs. Cell 14:695–711

Bos JL, Polder LJ, Bernards R, Schrier PI, van den Elsen PJ, van der Eb AJ, van Ormondt H (1981) The 2.2 kb Elb mRNA of human Ad12 and Ad5 codes for two tumor antigens starting at different AUG triplets. Cell 27:121–131

Brinckmann U, Darai G, Flügel RM (1983) The nucleotide sequence of the inverted terminal repetition of the tree shrew adenovirus DNA. Gene 24:131–135

Byrd PJ, Chia W, Rigby PWJ, Gallimore PH (1982) Cloning of DNA fragments from the left end of the adenovirus type 12 genome: transformation by cloned early region 1. J Gen Virol 60:279–293

Chow LT, Broker TR, Lewis JB (1979) Complex splicing patterns of RNAs from the early regions of adenovirus 2. J Mol Biol 134:265–303

Dekker BMM, van Ormondt H (1984) The nucleotide sequence of fragment *Hin*dIII-C of human adenovirus type 5 DNA (map positions 17.1–31.7) Gene 27:115–120

Denisova TS, Makhov AM, Gibadulin RA (1982) Identification of simian adenovirus SA7P. Vopr Virusol N4:483–488

D'Halluin JC, Milleville M, Boulanger PA (1983) Restriction maps of human adenovirus types 2, 5 and 3 for *Bcl*I, *Cla*I, *Pvu*I and *Sph*I endonucleases. Gene 21:171–173

Dijkema R, Dekker BMM (1979) The inverted terminal repetition of the DNA of weakly oncogenic adenovirus type 7. Gene 8:7–15

Dijkema R, Dekker BMM, Van Ormondt H (1982) Gene organization of the transforming region of adenovirus type 7 DNA. Gene 18:143–156

Engler JA, van Bree MP (1982) The nucleotide sequence of the gene encoding protein IVa2 in human adenovirus type 7. Gene 19:71–80

Engler JA, Hoppe MS, van Bree MP (1983) The nucleotide sequence of the genes encoded in early region 2b of human adenovirus type 7. Gene 21:145–159

Fowlkes DM, Shenk T (1980) Transcriptional control regions of the adenovirus VAI RNA gene. Cell 22:405–423

Fraser N, Ziff E (1978) RNA structures near poly(A) of adenovirus-2 late messenger RNAs. J Mol Biol 124:27–51

Friefeld BR, Lichy JH, Hurwitz J, Horwitz MS (1983) Evidence for an altered adenovirus DNA polymerase in cells infected with the mutant H5ts149. Proc Natl Acad Sci USA 80:1589–1593

Galibert F, Hérissé J, Courtois G (1979) Nucleotide sequence of the *Eco*RI-F fragment of adenovirus 2 genome. Gene 6:1–22

Garon CF, Parr RP, Padmanabhan R, Roninson I, Garrison JW, Rose JA (1982) Structural characterization of the adenovirus 18 inverted terminal repetition. Virology 121:230–239

Gingeras TR, Sciaky D, Gelinas RE, Bing-Dong J, Yen CE, Kelly MM, Bullock PA, Parsons B, O'Neill KE, Roberts RJ (1982) Nucleotide sequences from the adenovirus genome J Biol Chem 257:13475–13491

Hérissé J, Courtois G, Galibert F (1980) Nucleotide sequence of the *Eco*RI D fragment adenovirus 2 genome. Nucleic Acids Res 8:2173–2192

Hérissé J, Galibert F (1981a) Nucleotide sequence of the *Eco*RI E fragment of adenovirus 2 genome. Nucleic Acids Res 9:1229–1240

Hérissé J, Rigolet M, Dupont de Dinechin S, Galibert F (1981b) Nucleotide sequence of adenovirus 2 DNA fragment encoding for the carboxylic region of the fiber protein and the entire E4 region. Nucleic Acids Res 9:4023–4042

Jörnvall H, Aleström P, Akusjärvi G, von Bahr-Lindström H, Philipson L, Pettersson U (1981) Order of the CNBr fragments in the adenovirus hexon protein. J Biol Chem 256:6204–6212

Kimura T, Sawada Y, Shinawawa M, Shimizu Y, Shiroki K, Shimojo H, Sugisaki H, Takanami M, Uemizu Y, Fujinaga K (1981) Nucleotide sequence of the transforming region Elb of adenovirus 12 DNA: structure and gene organization, and comparison with those of adenovirus type 5 DNA. Nuclei Acids Res 9:6571–6589

Kruijer W (1983) Nucleotide sequence analysis of wild type and mutant genes encoding adenovirus DNA-binding protein: relation between structure and function of the protein. PhD Thesis, Utrecht

Kruijer W, van Schaik FMA, Sussenbach JS (1980) Nucleotide sequence of a region of adenovirus 5 DNA encoding a hitherto unidentified gene. Nucleic Acids Res 8:6033–6042

Kruijer W, van Schaik FMA, Sussenbach JS (1981) Structure and organization of the gene coding for the DNA binding protein of adenovirus type 5. Nucleic Acids Res 9:4439–4457

Kruijer W, van Schaik FMA, Sussenbach JS (1982) Nucleotide sequence of the gene encoding adenovirus type 2 DNA binding protein. Nucleic Acids Res 10:4493–4500

Kruijer W, van Schaik FMA, Speijer JG, Sussenbach JS (1983) Structure and function of adenovirus DNA binding protein: comparison of the amino acid sequences of the Ad5 and Ad12 proteins derived from nucleotide sequence of the corresponding genes. Virology 128:140–153

Maat J, van Ormondt H (1979) The nucleotide sequence of the transforming *Hin*dIII-G fragment of adenovirus type 5 DNA. Gene 6:75–90

Oosterom-Dragon EA, Anderson CW (1983) Polypeptide structure and encoding location of the adenovirus serotype 2 late, non-structural 33K protein. J Virol 45:251–263

Perricaudet M, Akusjärvi G, Virtanen A, Pettersson U (1979) Structure of two spliced mRNAs from the transforming region of human subgroup C adenoviruses. Nature 281:694–696

Perricaudet M, Le Moullec JM, Pettersson U (1980a) The predicted structure of two adenovirus T antigens. Proc Natl Acad Sci USA 77:3778–3782

Perricaudet M, Le Moullec JM, Tiollais P, Pettersson U (1980b) Structure of two adenovirus type 12 transforming polypeptides and their evolutionary implications. Nature 288:174–176

Persson H, Mathisen B, Philipson L, Pettersson U (1979) A maturation protein in adenovirus morphogenesis. Virology 93:198–208

Persson H, Jörnvall H, Zabielski J (1980) Multiple RNA species for the precursor to an adenovirus encoded glycoprotein: identification and structure of the signal sequence. Proc Natl Acad Sci USA 77:6349–6353

Shinagawa M, Padmanabhan R (1979) Nucleotide sequence at the inverted repetition of adenovirus type 2 DNA. Biochem Biophys Res Commun 87:671–678

Shinagawa M, Padmanabhan R (1980) Comparative sequence analysis of the inverted terminal repetitions from different adenoviruses. Proc Natl Acad Sci USA 77:3831–3835

Shinagawa M, Padmanabhan RV, Padmanabhan R (1980) The nucleotide sequence of the right-hand terminal SmaI-K fragment of adenovirus type 2 DNA. Gene 9:99–114

Shinagawa M, Ishiyama T, Padmanabhan R, Fujinaga K, Kamada M, Sato G (1983) Comparative sequence analysis of the inverted terminal repetition in the genomes of animal and avian adenoviruses. Virology 125:491–495

Smart JE, Stillman BW (1982) Adenovirus terminal protein precursor. Partial amino acid sequence and the site of covalent linkage to virus DNA. J Biol Chem 257:13499–12506

Stålhandske P, Persson H, Perricaudet M, Philipson L, Pettersson U (1983) Structure of three spliced mRNAs from region E3 of adenovirus type 2. Gene 22:157–165

Steenbergh PH, Sussenbach JS (1979) The nucleotide sequence of the right-hand terminus of adenovirus type 5 DNA: implications for the mechanism of DNA replication. Gene 6:307–318

Stetenbergh PH, Maat J, van Ormondt H, Sussenbach JS (1977) The nucleotide sequence at the termini of adenovirus type DNA. Nucleic Acids Res 4:4371–4389

Stillman BW, Topp WC, Engler JA (1982) Conserved sequences at the origin of adenovirus DNA replication. J Virol 44:530–537

Sugisaki H, Sugimoto K, Takanami M, Shiroki K, Saito I, Shimojo H, Sawada Y, Uemizu Y, Uesugi S, Fujinaga K (1980) Structure and gene organization in the transforming HindIII-G fragment of Ad12. Cell 20:777–786

Sung MT, Cao TM, Coleman RT, Budelier KA (1983) Gene and protein sequences of adenovirus protein VII, a hybrid basic chromosomal protein. Proc Natl Acad Sci USA 80:2902–2906

Temple M, Antoine G, Delius H, Stahl S, Winnacker EL (1981) Replication of mouse adenovirus strain FL DNA. Virology 109:1–12

Tolun A, Aleström P, Pettersson U (1979) Sequence of inverted terminal repetitions from different adenoviruses: demonstration of conserved sequences and homology between SA7 termini and SV40 DNA. Cell 17:705–713

Tooze J (1981) The molecular biology of tumor viruses. 2nd edn, part 2, DNA tumor viruses (revised). Cold Spring Harbor Laboratory, Cold Spring Harbor, NY

van Beveren CP, Maat J, Dekker BMM, van Ormondt H (1981) The nucleotide sequence of the gene for protein IVa2 and of the 5′ leader segment of the major late mRNAs of adenovirus type 5. Gene 16:179–189

van Ormondt H, Hesper B (1983) Comparison of the nucleotide sequences of early region E1b DNA of adenovirus types 12, 7 and 5 (subgroups A, B and C). Gene 21:217–226

van Ormondt H, Maat J, Dijkema R (1980a) Comparison of nucleotide sequences of the early E1a regions for subgroups A, B and C of human adenoviruses. Gene 12:63–76

van Ormondt H, Maat J, van Beveren CP (1980b) The nucleotide sequence of the transforming early region E1 of adenovirus type 5 DNA. Gene 11:299–309

Virtanen A, Pettersson U (1983) The molecular structure of the 9S mRNAs from early region 1A of adenovirus serotype 2. J Mol Biol 165:496–99

Virtanen A, Aleström P, Persson H, Katze MG, Pettersson U (1982a) An adenovirus agnogene. Nucleic Acids Res 10:2539–2548

Virtanen A, Pettersson U, Perricaudet M, Le Moullec JM, Tiollais P, Perricaudet M (1982b) Different mRNA from the transforming region of highly oncogenic and non-oncogenic human adenoviruses. Nature 295:705–707

Zain S, Roberts RJ (1979) Sequences from the beginning of the fiber messenger RNA of adenovirus 2. J Mol Biol 131:341–352

Zain S, Sambrook J, Roberts RJ, Keller W, Fried M, Dunn AR (1979) Nucleotide sequence analysis of the leader segments in a cloned copy of adenovirus 2 fiber mRNA. Cell 16:851–861

The Adenovirus Early Proteins

A.J. LEVINE

1 Introduction

The adenovirus early proteins are defined as those proteins encoded by the virus that are synthesized prior to and in the absence of viral DNA replication. The functions of these early viral proteins provide new insights into the mechanisms of gene regulation and DNA replication in higher eukaryotic cells. These adenovirus proteins regulate transcription in both a positive (BERK et al. 1979; JONES and SHENK 1979; ROSS et al. 1980a) and a negative (NEVINS and WINKLER 1980) fashion, as well as affecting the stability of viral mRNA (BABICH and NEVINS 1981). Some early proteins may be involved in RNA processing (KLESSIG and GRODZICKER 1979; SARNOW et al. 1982a) or RNA transport out of the nucleus. Other early proteins are required for viral DNA replication (VAN DER VLIET et al. 1975; CHALLBERG et al. 1980; STILLMAN et al. 1981; LICHY et al. 1981), specifying three distinct functions in this process. A subset of the early viral proteins are both necessary and sufficient for cellular transformation by this virus (SAMBROOK et al. 1975; GRAHAM et al. 1974, 1975, 1978; SHENK et al. 1979). Other early gene products can affect the frequency of transformation by adenovirus (GINSBERG et al. 1974; WILLIAMS et al. 1974; LOGAN et al. 1981). Finally, the host range of human adenoviruses can be extended by mutations in some early viral genes (KLESSIG and GRODZICKER 1979), implying that the

State University of New York at Stony Brook, School of Medicine, Department of Microbiology
Stony Brook, NY 11794, USA

Current Topics in Microbiology and Immunology, Vol. 110
© Springer-Verlag Berlin·Heidelberg 1984

Table 1. The adenovirus early proteins

Region	Coordinates (map units)	Transcripts (5′ 3′) (size)	Protein (MW)
E1A	1.3–4.6	r, 13S r, 12S r, 9S	53K, 44K 47K, 35K 28K
E1B	4.6–11.2	r, 22S r, 13S	58K 15–19K
E2A	61.7–66.6	l	72K
E2B	11 –31	l	87K, 105K
E3	76.6–86	r	gp19K, 13K, 14K, 15.5K
E4	91.3–99.0	l	11K, 25K (34K) 10K, 13K, 14K
Late genes expressed at early times			
IVa2	11.2–16	l	54K
L1	30.5–39.0	r	52K, 55K
Late leader	17 –22	r	13.5K, 13.6K (i-leader)
IX	9.8–11.2	r, 9S	12.5K

life cycle of the virus and its tissue pathology and disease patterns may vary with early gene function or alterations in such functions.

At least three classes of adenovirus early genes are now recognized, based upon their temporal appearance and regulation during virus infection (see Table 1): (1) The E1A gene products are termed immediate early gene functions. These genes are synthesized constitutively in infected cells shortly after infection. The E1A gene products are required to positively regulate the transcription of the (2) delayed early viral genes (E1B, E2A, E2B, E3, and E4 regions; Table 1) (BERK et al. 1979; JONES and SHENK 1979; NEVINS 1981). (3) Several viral genes which are predominantly transcribed at late times after infection (after DNA replication has begun) are also expressed at early times (IVa2, L1, late leader, and IX; Table 1). These immediate early, delayed early, and late gene products, all expressed at early times after infection, represent three differentially regulated classes of viral early genes. In addition, there is even differential regulation within the delayed early class of gene products. While most delayed early gene products are modulated down at late times (FLINT and SHARP 1976) the E2A gene product increases its levels along with and after viral DNA synthesis (VAN DER VLIET and LEVINE 1973). Thus an understanding of the regulation of the adenovirus early genes should contribute to the growing base of knowledge in eukaryotic gene expression.

At present there are some 25 early adenovirus proteins that have been identified by one means or another (see Table 1). While some of these gene products are essential for transcription (BERK et al. 1979; JONES and SHENK 1979) or DNA replication (VAN DER VLIET et al. 1975), other viral gene products appear to be dispensable when adenovirus in grown in tissue culture cells (JONES and SHENK 1978). The possibility remains that these "nonessential" proteins are retained by the virus for replication in its natural host. A protein could mediate an interaction with the immune system, leading to persistence of the virus in the body, by modulating down acute infections that would normally damage the host. The E3 19K glycoprotein (ROSS and LEVINE 1979; PERSSON et al. 1979a, b) associated with membrane fractions of infected cells would be a good candidate for such a function. A better characterization of the functions of these early proteins may then lead to a clear understanding of the biology of these viruses in their natural hosts.

The goal of this review of the adenovirus early proteins will be to focus upon the structure and functions of these proteins, emphasizing their roles in gene regulation, DNA replication, and modulation of virus host cell interactions. These proteins may well be prototypes for cellular gene functions whose capabilities we can infer from the information derived from the study of virus replication and transformation.

2 Methods for Detection

Several approaches have been employed to detect and identify the adenovirus early proteins. Direct purification of viral encoded proteins from infected cell lysates has been employed to isolate the E2A DNA-binding protein (DBP; 72K) (VAN DER VLIET and LEVINE 1973; JENG et al. 1978), and an E3 14K protein (PERSSON et al. 1979a). Polyacrylamide gel electrophoresis of infected cell-specific proteins (RUSSELL and SHEKEL 1972; ANDERSON et al. 1973; CHIN and MAIZEL 1976) has also led to the identification of a number of putative early viral proteins (see TOOZE 1981). A more specific assignment of the map positions of the adenovirus proteins was obtained by selection of mRNAs with genomic DNA restriction fragments and in vitro translation of these mRNAs (SABORIO and OBERG 1976; LEWIS et al. 1976; HARTER and LEWIS 1978; HALBERT et al. 1979). This approach has the advantage of providing evidence for the viral origin of the protein (by mRNA hybrid selection) and assigning a map position to the early gene on the viral genome. Finally, serum from animals bearing adenovirus-induced tumors has provided a source of antibodies directed against several adenovirus early proteins (POPE and ROWE 1964; RUSSELL et al. 1967). In adenovirus tumors, as in transformed cells, the viral DNA is integrated into a host cell chromosome (DOERFLER et al. 1974; SAMBROOK et al. 1979). A portion of this viral genome is transcribed (FLINT and SHARP 1976; FLINT et al. 1976) and translated into proteins. These animals recognize the viral proteins as foreign and produce antibodies directed against them. For this reason, some of the early proteins have been termed tumor antigens or tumor associated antigens. Antibodies from tumor-bearing animals have thus been employed to identify and quantitate the levels of several early proteins (GILEAD et al. 1976; LEVINSON and LEVINE 1977a, b; JOHANSSON et al. 1978; VAN DER EB et al. 1979; ROSS et al. 1980a, b). More recently monoclonal antibodies have been prepared against several early viral proteins (SARNOW et al. 1982b; CEPKO et al. 1981; REICH et al. 1983).

Once a protein was identified, genomic map assignments were obtained either by hybrid selection of mRNA using a DNA restriction fragment or by employing mutants that altered the protein or its levels (VAN DER VLIET et al. 1975; ROSS et al. 1980a, b). Collectively these approaches have identified and mapped about 25 early adenovirus proteins. The functions of some of these proteins have been deduced in two principal ways: (a) the use of mutants that alter the function of a gene product (GINSBERG et al. 1974; WILLIAMS et al. 1974), and (b) the development of functional assays in vitro such as DNA replication (CHALLBERG and KELLY 1979; KAPLAN et al. 1979; STILLMAN 1981) or transcription (MANLEY et al. 1979; WEIL et al. 1979). These approaches have begun to provide some insight into the mechanism of action of a few adenovirus early proteins. In addition, an extensive genetic analysis of temperature-sensitive mutants in the E2A 72K DBP gene and second-site temperature-independent revertants at that locus (NICOLAS et al. 1981, 1982, 1983a, b; LOGAN et al. 1981) have provided a detailed map of the structure-function relationships for this protein. In some cases oligomeric protein complexes have been detected in infected or transformed cells between two early viral proteins (SARNOW et al. 1984) or a viral encoded protein and a cellular protein (SARNOW et al. 1982c). Protein-protein interactions of this type imply common functions or modes of action. Finally, the subcellular localization of some adenovirus early proteins (CHIN and MAIZEL 1976; SARNOW et al. 1982a; DOWNEY et al. 1983) have implied possible functions for these gene products. Taken together, these approaches are beginning to provide the outlines of how adenovirus replicates and can transform cells in culture.

3 Identification, Structure, and Function

Employing the methods described in the previous section, 25 adenovirus early proteins have been detected and mapped to locations on the viral genome (Table 1). The structure and functions of the immediate early and delayed early gene products will now be reviewed.

3.1 The E1 Region Proteins:
Replicative and Transforming Functions

The E1 region of adenovirus can be divided into two segments, termed E1A and E1B, based upon two distinct transcriptional units (CHOW et al. 1977, 1979; EVANS et al. 1977; BERK and SHARP 1978) and two well-defined genetic complementation groups (HARRISON et al. 1977; JONES and SHENK 1979; ROSS et al. 1980a). Two types of mutants have been obtained in the E1A and E1B complementation groups: (a) point mutations (HARRISON et al. 1977) and (b) deletion mutants (JONES and SHENK 1979). Both types of mutants are defective for virus replication in HeLa cells and are propagated in line 293 human cells (GRAHAM et al. 1978), which are transformed with adenovirus and express the E1A and E1B functions. These E1A and E1B mutants fail to transform cells in culture (GRAHAM et al. 1978; SHENK et al. 1979; Ho et al. 1982), indicating the need for both complementation groups for transformation. While the E1A and E1B loci are divided into two distinct transcription units and two complementation groups, RNA processing or splicing of the two primary transcripts (CHOW et al. 1979) produces five different E1A proteins and two distinct E1B proteins (Table 1). For clarity these proteins will be considered separately.

3.1.1 The E1A Proteins

The E1A 12S and 13S mRNAs each produce two proteins whose apparent molecular weights in SDS-polyacrylamide gels are 47K and 35K (12S) and 53K and 44K (13S) (HARTER and LEWIS 1978). The 53K and 47K proteins share the same N-terminal end and differ only in that the 53K protein is about 6K longer at the C-terminal end. The 44K and 35K proteins share the same C-terminal amino acid sequences but differ at their N-terminal, with the larger protein having extra (46 amino acids) coding sequences spliced out of the smaller protein's mRNA. A 9S mRNA from E1A produces a 28K protein (Table 1) that shares peptides with the 44K (13S) and 35K (12S) proteins, just as the 53K (13S) and 47K (12S) proteins have common peptides (HARTER and LEWIS 1978; LEWIS et al. 1979). All five proteins derived from the three E1A mRNA's are translated in the same reading frame (PERRICAUDET et al. 1979). Thus the three mRNAs from the E1A region produce two sets of related proteins, the 53K-47K set and the 44K-35K-28K set, and each set has common peptides. Just how two mRNAs (13S and 12S) can encode four proteins (47K and 35K from the 12S and 53K and 44K from the 13S mRNA) is not clear, given that internal mRNA AUG start sites are thought not to function in eukaryotic cells. Perhaps a single protein is produced from each mRNA and proteolysis at a specific site cleaves the proteins into two components. The nucleotide sequence in the E1A region has been determined (VAN ORMONDT et al. 1978; BOS et al. 1981), and the E1A proteins have been predicted to be quite rich in proline and glutamic acid residues. Five or six E1A gene products with very acidic isoelectric points have been detected by two-dimensional gel electrophoresis of infected cell extracts (HARTER and LEWIS 1978). The molecular weights of the E1A proteins as calculated from the nucleotide sequence are all smaller than the gene products detected in SDS-polyacrylamide gels. This may be expected from the unusually high proline content of the E1A proteins, which can cause alterations in the migration of proteins in this gel system.

The functions of these E1A proteins have been elucidated by employing point mutations and deletion mutants in the E1A genes (HARRISON et al. 1977; JONES and SHENK 1979; SOLNICK 1981; RICCIARDI et al. 1981). Viruses with defects in the E1A genes fail to transcribe the E1B, E2A, E2B, E3, E4, and L1 regions of the genome (BERK et al. 1979; SHENK et al. 1979; NEVINS 1981). The proteins derived from the 12S mRNA (47K and 35K) are either not involved in this positive regulation or are redundant, i.e., have duplicate functions with the 53K-44K proteins. A mutant (pm975) with a defective splice donor site in the 12S mRNA has no detectable phenotype in HeLa cells (MONTELL et al. 1982). The mechanisms mediating this E1A positive regulation of transcription are at present unclear. Interaction with RNA polymerase II or DNA nucleotide sequences and counteraction of a cellular repressor bound to the viral genome (LOGAN and SHENK 1982) all remain formal possibilities. The levels of E1A proteins in infected and transformed cells appears to be quite low. Both the E1A mRNAs and proteins have short half-lives (NEVINS 1981, 1982). Not all of the early gene transcription units appear to be equally dependent upon the E1A proteins, i.e., E2 and E3 are more tightly regulated by E1A proteins than are E1B and E4 transcripts. In addition, a high multiplicity of infection with E1A deletion mutants can lower the dependence of the other early gene regions upon E1A function. One E1A mutant (hr440; SOLNICK 1981; SOLNICK and ANDERSON 1981) fails to produce E2A and E3 mRNAs after infection, but synthesizes wild-type levels of the E1B 22S mRNA (makes the E1B 58K protein) and E4 mRNAs. These observations serve to emphasize the heterogeneity of the responses to the E1A gene products and/or mutant gene products. This heterogeneity must be accounted for in any explanation of the mechanism of action of these proteins.

3.1.2 The E1B Proteins

The E1B 22S mRNA (4.6–11.2 mu) encodes a 58K protein (GILEAD et al. 1976; LEVINSON and LEVINE 1977a, b; SCHRIER et al. 1979; LASSOM et al. 1979) and a 15K–19K protein. The 13S mRNA derived from E1B sequences appears to encode only the 15K–19K polypeptide (HALBERT et al. 1979) which has no methionine-containing peptides in common with the larger 58K protein (BOS et al. 1981). All of the sera derived from adenovirus-induced-tumor-bearing animals contain antibodies against the E1B 58K protein, which appears to be the principle or major viral tumor antigen (ROSS et al. 1980a, b). Two types of mutants, point mutations and deletion mutants, have been employed to study the E1B functions (ROSS et al. 1980a). A large deletion (2350 bp) across this region (dl313) produces a virus that fails to synthesize immunologically detectable 58K and 15K products. Similarly, a point mutant (hr7) synthesizes no detectable 58K and a reduced level of 15K (ROSS et al. 1980a). The hr7 mutant overproduces (176%–215% of wild-type levels) the E2 72K, E3 19K and E4 11K proteins at low multiplicities of infection (10 pfu/cell) but not at high multiplicities (100 pfu/cell). The dl313 mutant produces normal levels of the E3 19K and E4 11K proteins and reduced levels of the E2 72K protein at low multiplicities of infection (ROSS et al. 1980a). Apparently one or both E1B proteins can affect the levels of other early region gene products in an allele-specific manner and in a multiplicity dependent fashion. Mutants in the E1B 58K gene product also affect the levels of several late adenovirus gene products (T. Shenk, S.J. Flint, and J.F. Williams, personal communications), which could explain why there is an overproduction of some early viral proteins. The E1B mutants synthesize adenovirus DNA but in some cases appear to have a DNA delay or DNA-reduced phenotype (B.W. Stillman, personal communication). Although there is no clear-cut interpretation of the function of the E1B 58K protein at present, it appears to regulate the levels of some of the early and late proteins either directly or indirectly via transcription or RNA processing.

The E1B 58K protein can be found in a noncovalent association with a cellular protein termed p53 in virus-transformed mouse, rat, hamster, and human cells (line 293 cells) (SARNOW et al. 1982c). Monoclonal antibodies directed against the E1B 58K protein immunoprecipitate this tumor antigen and coimmunoprecipitate the associated cellular p53 protein (SARNOW et al. 1982b). Similarly, monoclonal antibodies directed against p53 coimmunoprecipitate the E1B 58K protein (SARNOW et al. 1982b, c). The E1B 58K–p53 complex is heterogeneous, sedimenting between 18S and 35S. It appears to be an oligomeric protein complex which contains all of the cellular p53 protein and some of the transformed-cell E1B 58K protein (some 58K protein is in a free form) (SARNOW et al. 1982c). In SV40-transformed cells, the SV40 large T antigen is found in an oligomeric protein complex with this same p53 cellular protein (LINZER and LEVINE 1979; LANE and CRAWFORD 1979). The identity of p53 in the SV40 T–p53 and E1B 58K–p53 complexes rests upon an immunological identity (tested with several p53 monoclonal antibodies) and similar peptide maps of p53 obtained from both SV40 T–p53 and E1B 58K–p53 complexes (SARNOW et al. 1982c). That both an SV40 T antigen and an adenovirus tumor antigen are found in a physical complex with the same cellular protein in their respective transformed cells suggests some common functions or modes of action. Like the phenotype of E1B 58K mutants, SV40 T antigen is involved with the regulation of transcription or viral gene expression (TEGTMEYER 1974).

Levels of p53 are elevated in a variety of transformed cells when compared to their nontransformed counterparts (LINZER et al. 1979; BENCHIMOL et al. 1982; THOMAS et al. 1983). This protein has been conserved over evolutionary time spans in that a homologous p53 protein (similar peptide maps and antigenic sites) has been detected in mouse, rat, monkey, and human cells (SIMMONS et al. 1980; MALTZMAN et al. 1980; THOMAS et al. 1983). p53 protein from nontransformed cells has a very short half-life (about 20 min), while p53 in SV40-transformed cells is complexed with T antigen and has a long half-life (greater than 24 h) (OREN et al. 1981). Temperature-sensitive mutants in the SV40 T antigen structural gene (A gene) regulate p53 levels in a temperature-dependent fashion, with the T–p53 complex not detectable at the nonpermissive temperature (LINZER et al. 1979). This has led to the idea that p53 levels in some transformed cells are regulated at the post-translational or protein stability level and the physical association of SV40 T antigen or E1B 58K protein with p53 stabilizes p53 and reduces its turnover or rate of proteolysis (OREN et al. 1981). In resting, nontransformed cells stimulated into growth by the addition of fresh serum, p53 mRNA and p53 protein levels increase five- to eightfold in the late G_1-early S phase (REICH and LEVINE 1984). When monoclonal antibodies directed against p53 are microinjected into the nucleus of such serum-stimulated cells, they reduce the percentage of cells that enter the S phase (MERCER et al. 1982). Microinjection of the SV40 large T antigen into cells (TJIAN et al. 1978) and adenovirus infection of hamster cells (Rossini et al. 1979) results in the stimulation of cellular DNA synthesis, where G_0-arrested cells now enter the S phase of the cell cycle. Taken together, these observations suggest that p53 and the SV40 large T antigen are involved in regulating events in the cell cycle, resulting in the cellular DNA replication associated with transformation. The SV40 T–p53 and E1B 58K–p53 complexes result in increased levels of p53 in the transformed cell. These higher levels could result in signals promoting the entry of those cells into the S phase. In this case transformed cells would continually signal (via high p53 levels) the cell to enter the S phase and divide under conditions where nontransformed cells rest in G_0.

During productive infection of HeLa cells, the E1B 58K protein is not found to be associated with the cellular p53 protein (Sarnow et al. 1982c). Instead, the E1B 58K protein is physically complexed with an E4 25K adenovirus encoded protein (Sarnow et al. 1984). Mutants in the E1B 58K gene (dl342) disrupt the association of E1B 58K–E4 25K in the complex. The E4 25K protein was identified and assigned to region E4, subregion 6 by amino acid sequence analysis of the E4 25K peptide and matching of this sequence with the predicted amino acid sequence derived from the nucleotide sequence of the E4 region (Herisse et al. 1981). Mutations in the E4 25K and E1B 58K genes have similar phenotypes, indicating that the E1B 58K–E4 25K complex could provide a common phenotype (D.N. Halbert and Shenk, personal communication) in these mutants. Since the E1B 58K protein is found in an oligomeric complex with either the p53 or E4 25K proteins in transformed cells or in lytically infected cells respectively, the function of the E4 25K protein may lend some clues to the function of p53 in normal cells.

The E1B 15K protein is synthesized from both the 22S and 13S mRNAs, but is translated in a different reading frame (two-nucleotide shift) than the E1B 58K protein. It has been suggested that both E1B 15K and E1B 58K proteins are synthesized from the 22S mRNA at very early times after infection, while the E1B 15K protein is produced in higher levels from the E1B 13S mRNA at slightly later times during infection (Bos et al. 1981). Relatively little is known about the function of this protein during productive infection, but mutants exclusively in the E1B 15K gene have recently been isolated (T. Shenk, personal communication), and their phenotype is presently under investigation.

3.1.3 The E1 Region and Transformation

The transformed phenotype is often defined by the procedures employed to select for transformants. These procedures include: (a) immortality or production of permanent cell lines from primary cell cultures, (b) cellular growth in low serum concentrations, (c) formation of cellular foci by cells that grow on top of each other, (d) growth in agar or methocel suspension cultures, and (e) the ability to form tumors in animals (syngeneic or immunosuppressed). DNA fragments from the E1A and E1B regions are both necessary and sufficient to obtain transformants that express the transformed phenotype (Graham et al. 1974; Gallimore et al. 1974). The E1A region genes alone appear to be able to immortalize primary cells which otherwise would have a limited life span (VAN DER EB et al. 1979; HOUWELING et al. 1980; VAN DEN ELSEN et al. 1982). The E1B 15K gene is required for the production of transformed cell foci when it is accompanied by the E1A gene products. The E1A functions do not only serve to promote the transcription of the E1B genes in this process (VAN DEN ELSEN et al. 1983). The E1B 15K gene product expressed by itself in a primary cell is ineffective in producing transformed foci. Therefore at least two distinct functions, the E1A and E1B 15K gene products, are required for a complete transformation event in cell culture (VAN DEN ELSEN et al. 1983; Logan and Shenk, manuscript in preparation). The E1B 58K gene function is required for the transformed phenotype of producing tumors in animals (BERNARDS et al. 1983). Thus the adenovirus E1 region can be divided into three portions, each corresponding to one or more parts of the transformed phenotype: (a) E1A immortalization of primary cells, (b) E1A–E1B 15K foci formation by cells, and (c) E1A–E1B 15K–E1B 58K tumorigenic potential of cells in animals. In the latter case the association of the E1B 58K protein with p53 protein suggests a regulation of cell division (growth) in the environment of an animal tissue, where nontransformed cells fail to replicate.

Recently, cold-sensitive mutants in both E1A and E1B functions have been isolated (Ho et al. 1982). Mutants in E1A are cold sensitive for both establishment and maintenance of the transformed phenotype. Cold-sensitive mutants in E1B functions are transformation defective at both permissive (38.5 °C) and nonpermissive (32.5 °C) temperatures, but are cold sensitive for virus replication in HeLa cells. The rare cold-sensitive E1B gene transformants that are able to be come established at 38.5 °C do show a cold-sensitive phenotype for the maintenance of transformation. Thus both E1A and E1B functions appear to be required and involved in the initiation, establishment, and maintenance of the transformed phenotype. The hr6 mutant in the E1b 58K gene is cold sensitive for the maintenance of the transformed phenotype (J.F. Williams, personal communication); this differs from conclusions reached in studies employing DNA fragments to transform cells in culture (VAN DEN ELSEN et al. 1983; BERNARDS et al. 1983). The reasons for this remain unclear.

3.2 The E2 Proteins: The DNA Replicative Transcription Unit

The E2 transcription unit initiates at about 75.2 map units at early times and at 72.0 map units at later times in infection (CHOW et al. 1979). Splicing of this leftward primary transcript produces mRNA derived from the E2A gene (61.4–66.6 map units) that synthesizes the DBP (VAN DER VLIET et al. 1975) and the E2B gene products (11–31 map units). The E2B gene products include an 87K protein that is the precursor of the 55K protein covalently bound to the 5' ends of each adenovirus DNA strand (ROBINSON et al. 1973; REKOSH et al. 1977; GALOS et al. 1979; STILLMAN et al. 1981). This protein is required for the initiation of viral DNA replication, where it presumably acts as a primer for new DNA strands via a deoxycytidylic acid residue bound to the 87K precursor protein (REKOSH et al. 1977; CHALLBERG et al. 1980; STILLMAN 1981). A second E2B-derived protein of about 105K appears to be an adenovirus-encoded DNA polymerase with properties distinct from the known cellular DNA polymerases (LICHY et al. 1982). These two proteins (E1B 87K, E1B 105K) map between 19 and 29 units on the genome. The IVa2 structural protein, prominently synthesized at late times after infection, is produced in small amounts (11–15 map units) at early times as part of the E2 transcription unit (Table 1) (GALOS et al. 1979; CHOW et al. 1979). The three E2 early proteins E2A 72K, E2B 87K, and E2B 105K are all required for viral DNA replication.

The E2A 72K DBP was first isolated and purified based upon its ability to bind to single-stranded DNA (VAN DER VLIET and LEVINE 1973). The protein binds poorly, if at all, to the double-stranded DNA helix, but it does bind to the ends of linear double-stranded DNA (FOWLKES et al. 1979). Viral DNA replication initiates at one or both ends of the viral genome (WINNACKER 1974; HORWITZ 1976; SUSSENBACH and KUJK 1977). Initiation is followed by polynucleotide chain propagation producing one double strand of DNA and displacing a single-template strand which is associated with the E2A 72K DBP (SUSSENBACH and VAN DER VLIET 1972; LECHNER and KELLY 1977). The DBP is composed of 529 amino acids (KRUIJER et al. 1981) as deduced from the nucleotide sequence of this gene. The DBP can be cleaved with mild chymotrypsin treatment into two structural domains; a 26K N-terminal fragment and a 44K C-terminal peptide (KLEIN et al. 1979). The 44K domain, but not the 26K fragment, binds to single-stranded DNA and is generated by proteolysis in crude extracts of adenovirus-infected cells (VAN DER VLIET and LEVINE 1973; LEVINSON and LEVINE 1977a). There is an asymmetric distribution of methionine and leucine residues in the 72K DBP, with the great majority of these amino acids clustered in the C-terminal 44K domain (KLEIN et al. 1979). The DPB is a phosphoprotein (LEVINSON et al. 1977b), and isoelectric focusing produces molecules with pI between 7.5 and 5.5, indicating a great deal of heterogeneity between DBP molecules. Amino acid analysis yields both phosphoserine and phosphotheronine residues (AXELROD 1978), 95% of which can be removed by alkaline phosphatase activity, i.e., phosphomonester linkages (KLEIN et al. 1979). After phosphatase treatment the majority of the DBP has a pI of 7.5, indicating that most of the molecular charge heterogeneity is due to the addition of phosphate residues (KLEIN et al. 1979). Based upon these changes in pI after alkaline phosphatase treatment, peptide maps of phosphoserine and threonine containing residues, and the phosphate content of the DBP, it is estimated that the DBP molecules contain between one and 11 phosphate residues (KLEIN et al. 1979). Nine or ten of these phosphorylation sites reside in the N-terminal 26K domain, and a purified nuclear protein kinase (of cellular origin) is capable of adding phosphates to most of these authentic sites in vitro (LEVINSON et al. 1976; KLEIN et al. 1979). The degree of phosphorylation of any DBP molecule in the N-terminal domain does have an effect upon the ability of the C-terminal domain to bind tightly to DNA, i.e., DBP bound to single-stranded DNA and eluted at high salt concentrations has less phosphate per molecule (KLEIN et al. 1979) then DBP eluted with lower salt concentrations.

Two temperature-sensitive mutants that map in the structural gene of the DBP (VAN DER VLIET et al. 1975; KRUIJER et al. 1982), H5ts125 and H5ts107

(ENSINGER and GINSBERG 1972; GINSBERG et al. 1974), have been isolated. Both contain a proline to serine change at amino acid residue 413, located in the C-terminal domain (KRUIJER et al. 1982). The H5ts125 DBP is thermolabile compared to the wild-type protein for binding to single-stranded DNA (VAN DER VLIET et al. 1975), consistent with the C-terminal domain DNA-binding function (KLEIN et al. 1979). Both temperature-sensitive mutants fail to synthesize viral DNA at the nonpermissive temperature and are blocked at the polynucleotide chain propagation step (HORWITZ 1978) and, possibly, the initiation step of DNA replication (VAN DER VLIET and SUSSENBACH 1975). Soluble extracts prepared from H5ts125-infected cells kept at the nonpermissive temperature fail to support the replication of adenovirus DNA in vitro. The addition of purified wild-type DBP to these extracts now permits adenovirus DNA replication in vitro (HORWITZ 1978), demonstrating an in vitro complementation of H5ts125 by wild-type DBP. Indeed, the addition of just the 44K C-terminal fragment of the DBP is sufficient to complement the H5ts125-defective protein (ARIGA et al. 1980) for DNA replication in vitro.

The H5ts125 and H5ts107 mutants of the DBP have several additional phenotypes. At the nonpermissive temperature the DBP is synthesized but is rapidly degraded (VAN DER VLIET et al. 1975), leading to lower levels of the DBP in H5ts125-infected cells kept at the nonpermissive temperature than in wild-type-infected cells. The lower levels of the DBP in infected cells appear to lead to an overproduction in the rate of synthesis of the DBP (CARTER and GINSBERG 1976; CARTER and BLANTON 1978; NICOLAS et al. 1982). Thus the DBP autoregulates its own production, but whether this occurs at the transcriptional level, RNA processing level, or translation level is presently unclear. Two second-site revertants of H5ts125 which produce stable DBPs and are temperature independent for replication in HeLa cells have been isolated (NICOLAS et al. 1981). These mutants, r(ts125)13 and r(ts125)28, overproduce (three- to fivefold) a stable DBP in HeLa cells when compared to wild-type virus (NICOLAS et al. 1982). Both of these autoregulatory mutants contain the primary-site mutation of H5ts125 (proline to serine at residue 413) and a second-site mutation (histidine to tyrosine) at amino acid residue 508 (out of 529 residues) (KRUIJER et al. 1983). The second-site mutation, in the C-terminal end of the protein, indicates an interaction occurs between residues 413 and 508, stabilizing the protein in a conformation that is no longer temperature dependent but now fails to autoregulate the levels of DBP in infected cells. Whatever the mechanism of autoregulation of the DBP, it must interact with cellular functions as well. r(ts125)13 has a faulty autoregulatory protein in HeLa cells (overproduces DBP), but produces wild-type levels of DBP in line 293 human cells and CV-1 monkey cells in culture (NICOLAS et al. 1982). Thus the faulty autoregulatory phenotype of r(ts125)13 is host-range dependent, which is most readily understood via DBP interactions with cellular functions that differ in HeLa and line 293 or CV-1 cells. Regulating the levels of DBP in adenovirus-infected cells may well be selectively advantageous. The ratio of virus produced by r(ts125)13 in line 293 cells (regulated) versus HeLa cells (unregulated) is about 10:1. In contrast, r(ts125)127 and r(ts125)110, which are primary-site or true revertants of H5ts125 (serine back to proline at residue 413) (NICOLAS et al. 1981; KRUIJER et al.

1983), produce ratios of titers on line 293: HeLa cells of 0.83:1 and 2.3:1 respectively (NICOLAS et al. 1982). Thus r(ts125)13 replicates five- to tenfold better when autoregulated (in line 293 cells) than when overproduced (in HeLa cells), compared to wild-type or true revertants which regulate DBP levels normally in both cell types.

The DBP also regulates the levels of E1 and E4 gene products found in virus-infected cells. The E4 genes appear to be controlled by DBP at the transcriptional level (NEVINS and WINKLER 1980). Whether the DBP interacts with RNA polymerase II, recognizes specific viral sequences in the E4 transcription unit, or acts upon E4 transcripts indirectly (i.e., interacting with RNA for example) remains unclear. The E1A and E1B gene products are also controlled by the DBP, but in this case the DBP appears to effect the stability of E1A and E1B mRNAs (BABICH and NEVINS 1981). Here RNA processing, transport out of the nucleus, or mRNA stability in the cytoplasm could all result in this phenotype.

That the DBP may be involved in RNA processing in some way has been suggested by the study of adenovirus host-range mutants that replicate in monkey cells (KLESSIG and GRODZICKER 1979). The human adenoviruses infect monkey cells and produce normal levels of early proteins, replicate their viral DNA, but synthesize reduced levels of some late viral structural proteins (i.e., fiber) (TOOZE 1981). Providing the C-terminal portion or domain of SV40 large T antigen, either in an adenovirus-SV40 recombinant virus (GRODZICKER et al. 1974, 1976) or by coinfecting monkey cells with adenovirus and SV40 (RABSON et al. 1964), complements or suppresses the defect in late adenovirus protein production in monkey cells. Exactly how the SV40 T antigen corrects the defect in adenovirus late functions in monkey cells remains unclear. There is a suggestion, however, that the fiber mRNA in adenovirus-infected monkey cells is not processed or spliced in the same manner that fiber mRNA is in human cells (CHOW et al. 1979). This altered RNA processing reaction could account for the low levels of late adenovirus proteins and poor virus production. KLESSIG and GRODZICKER (1979) have isolated adenovirus mutants that replicate normally (produce late proteins and virus) in monkey cells. These mutations map in the N-terminal domain of the DBP gene (KLESSIG and GRODZICKER 1979). H5hr404, which produces normal levels of adenovirus in monkey cells, has a histidine to tyrosine change at amino acid 103 (out of 529 amino acids) (KRUIJER et al. 1982). These mutants suggest two interesting possibilities: (a) a functional relationship between the adenovirus DBP and the SV40 large T antigen exists, and (b) the adenovirus DBP could be involved in processing adenovirus late mRNA.

An additional line of evidence demonstrates a functional relationship between the SV40 large T antigen and the adenovirus DBP. In monkey cells, adenovirus H5ts125 fails to synthesize adenovirus DNA at the nonpermissive temperature because of the defect in the DBP. If these monkey cells are infected first with SV40 and then H5ts125 at the nonpermissive temperature, then adenovirus DNA is replicated (44% as efficiently as at the permissive temperature) and infectious virus is produced (3% as efficiently as at the permissive temperature) (LEVINE et al. 1974; WILLIAMS et al. 1974; RABEK et al. 1981). SV40tsA mutants, defective in the large T antigen, fail to suppress the H5*ts*125 defect at the nonpermissive temperature in monkey cells, indicating that the large T antigen of SV40 is responsible for suppressing the H5*ts*125 (DBP) defect in the DBP (RABEK et al. 1981). Thus two lines of experimental evidence indicate a functional relationship between the SV40 large T antigen and the adenovirus DBP: (a) T antigen suppresses the H5*ts*125 phenotype for DNA replication, and (b) a mutant DBP (hr404) and SV40 T antigen both relieve the block in the production of adenovirus late gene functions in monkey cells.

Yet another example of the interactions between the viral DBP and cellular functions is documented by the host-range temperature-conditional mutants of the DBP gene (NICOLAS et al. 1981). Second-site revertants of H5*ts*125 and H5*ts*107 were isolated by growth and plaquing of these mutants in HeLa cells at the nonpermissive temperature. Among the temperature-independent revertants isolated (NICOLAS et al. 1981) were several viruses – r(*ts*107)202, r(*ts*107)197, r(*ts*107)177, and r(*ts*107)20 – which replicated and plaqued in a temperature-independent fashion in HeLa cells (selected for in this cell line) but were temperature sensitive for growth and plaquing in line 293 cells. Genetic recombination, marker rescue experiments (NICOLAS et al. 1983b), and nucleotide sequencing (KRUIJER et al. 1983) with these mutants demonstrated that the host-range temperature-conditional phenotype was due to second-site mutations in the DBP gene. R(*ts*107)177, r(*ts*107)197 and r(*ts*107)202 contained the primary-site mutation (H5*ts*107, proline to serine at residue 413) and a second-site mutation of glycine to aspartic acid at amino acid residue 353. r(ts107)20 also contained the same primary-site mutation, but had a second-site mutation of alanine to proline at residue 347 (KRUIJER et al. 1983). Thus the host-range temperature-conditional mutants contains a primary site mutation (H5*ts*107), that can be separated by recombination (NICOLAS et al. 1983b) from a secondary-site mutation (at residue 347 or 353) regenerating the temperature-sensitive phenotype of H5*ts*107 in HeLa cells. These host-range temperature-conditional mutants produce normal or wild-type levels of early viral proteins, viral DNA, and late virus proteins in line 293 cells at the nonpermissive temperature. The mutants fail to synthesize virus particles or infectious virus in line 293 cells at the nonpermissive temperature (NICOLAS et al. 1983a). These same mutants are temperature independent for the production of virus particles and infectious virus when grown in HeLa cells. These observations imply that the DBP is involved in late virus protein production or assembly of virions, or even possibily that the DBP is incorporated in virions and the host-range temperature-conditional mutants are defective in this step in line 293 cells at 39.5 °C (NICOLAS et al. 1983a). The host-range temperature-conditional mutants indicate, once again, an active interaction between the DBP and cellular components that vary between cell lines.

Temperature-sensitive mutants in the DBP gene transform rat cells (at 37 °C) in culture with about fivefold greater efficiency than wild-type virus (GINSBERG et al. 1974; WILLIAMS et al. 1974; LOGAN et al. 1981). The efficiency of transformation of rat cells in culture is multiplicity dependent, but H5*ts*107 transforms cells five times more efficiently than wild-type virus at all multiplicities between 10 and 1000 pfu/cell (LOGAN et al. 1981). Primary-site revertants of H5*ts*107 (true revertants) that restore proline at amino acid residue 413, decrease fivefold in their efficiency of transforming rat cells in culture (LOGAN et al. 1981). The host-range temperature-conditional mutants, like H5ts107, produce an unstable DBP in infected cells and have an increased efficiency of transformation in rat cells (LOGAN et al. 1981). Because the E1A and E1B functions are both sufficient for transformation of rat cells in culture (GRAHAM et al. 1974) it is perhaps surprising that the DBP can effect the frequency of transformation. At present there are two possible ways in which the DBP might exert its effects upon the number of transformed cells detected after adenovirus infection: (a) the DBP can alter the stability of E1A and E1B mRNA's directly (BABICH and NEVINS 1981); (b) the DBP autoregulates its own levels. If this autoregulation were at the transcriptional level, then the entire E2 transcript, E2A and E2B proteins, would be effected by the concentration of the DBP. In this manner the E2A 72K gene product could also regulate the E2B 87K and 105K proteins. The mutant H5ts36, (WILLIAMS et al. 1974) which maps in the E2B gene region, is known to fail to replicate viral DNA and fails to transform cells at the nonpermissive temperature (WILLIAMS et al. 1974). While outside the E1 region of the genome, H5ts36 can affect the frequency of transformation when virions are employed to transform rat cells. In this way, H5ts107 could overproduce the E2 transcript (E2A and E2B), resulting in an enhanced rate of synthesis of unstable DBP and a stable overproduction of the H5ts36 gene product, which is known to effect the frequency of transformation (WILLIAMS et al. 1974; LOGAN et al. 1981).

Table 2 summarizes the various phenotypes of the DBP mutants, their genetic map positions, alterations in amino acids, and location in the N-terminal

Table 2. Mapping and phenotype of DBP mutations

	Mutant	Amino acid residue (1–529), amino acid change	Phenotype			
			HeLa	Line 293	Monkey	Mouse
1	H5ts125 H5ts107	413, pro → ser	ts DNA replication	ts DNA replication	ts DNA replication No virus	absolute DNA negative
2	r(ts107)177 197 202	413, pro → ser 352, gly → asp	ts⁺	ts for virus production and reduced DNA replication assembly defect	No virus	–
	r(ts125)20	413, pro → ser 347, ala → pro				
3	r(ts125)13 28	413, pro → ser 508, his → tyr	DBP over-produced ts⁺	DBP not over-produced ts⁺	DBP not over-produced No virus	–
4	r(ts107)127	413, ser → pro true revertant	ts⁺	ts⁺	ts⁺, no virus	–
5	H5r404	103, his → tyr	ts⁺	–	Virus produced	–

26K or C-terminal 44K domains. The multiple levels of regulation by this protein (transcription, RNA processing, mRNA stability), its extensive host-range phenotypes indicating interactions with host cell functions, and the well-documented positions of second-site mutations make the DBP an ideal candidate for the study of the mechanisms of eukaryotic gene regulation. Furthermore, the functional relationships between the SV40 large T antigen and the adenovirus DBP suggest that some general principles will emerge from the study of proteins with multifunctional domains. Clearly the adenovirus DBP is one of the most intensively studied eukaryotic viral proteins, and yet we are just beginning to probe the mechanisms of action of this protein.

3.3 The E3 Proteins: Dispensable Genes?

The E3 region transcripts are both numerous and complex in their splicing patterns (FLINT 1982). At least four major and four minor transcripts have been described (BERK and SHARP 1978; CHOW et al. 1979; KITCHINGHAM and WESTPHAL 1980) which cover 76.6–86 map units (rightward transcripts) of the genome. Four E3 proteins are known to be translated from these mRNAs, with estimated molecular weights of 13K, 14K, 15.5K, and 19K (LEWIS et al. 1976; GREEN et al. 1979; ROSS et al. 1980a, b). The E3 19K protein is a glycoprotein (ROSS and LEVINE 1979a, b; PERSSON et al. 1980a) associated with the membrane fractions of infected cells (CHIN and MAIZEL 1976; PERSSON et al. 1980b). Deletion and substitution mutants in the adenovirus E3 region of the viral genome have been employed to map the E3 19K glycoprotein. The Ad2 dlP305 virus (deletion of 83–84 map units) produces a normal E3 19K glycoprotein as does the Ad2 ND-4 virus (deletion of 81.2–85.5 map units), while the Ad2 ND-1 virus (80.3–85.5 map units deleted from E3) failed to synthesize an E3 19K glycoprotein in infected cells (ROSS and LEVINE 1979). This deletion substitution analysis indicated that the coding region between 80.3 and 81.2 map units contained the structural gene for the E3 19K glycoprotein. The nucleotide sequence of the E3 region (HERISSE et al. 1980) has been determined and an open reading frame for the E3 19K protein has been localized between 79.9 and 81.2 map units. This E3 protein is produced by three different mRNAs derived from E3 genes (FLINT 1982) which specify a polypeptide of 159 amino acids (18 439 daltons) containing an N-terminal hydrophobic signal sequence of 18 amino acid residues (HERISSE et al. 1980). The function of the E3 19K glycoprotein, like all of the E3 proteins, appears to be dispensable to the virus for replication in cell culture. Deletion mutants that eliminate the entire E3 region of the virus (JONES and SHENK 1978) replicate normally in cell culture (in vitro). Philipson and his collaborators (PERSSON et al. 1979b) have demonstrated that cytotoxic T lymphocytes can recognize the E3 19K glycoprotein on the surface of infected or transformed cells and reject these cells via T-cell-mediated killing. This killing requires H-2 (major histocompatability antigen) identity between killer T cells and their targets, as has been demonstrated in other systems (ZINKERNAGEL and DOHERTY 1974). Furthermore, a ternary complex of the E3 19K glycoprotein, the 44K glycoprotein H-2 antigen, and the

11K beta-2-microglobulin, expected from these results, could be detected in the plasma membrane of adenovirus-infected and -transformed cells (PERSSON et al. 1979b). In transformed cells expressing the E3 19K glycoprotein this protein may then act as a tumor-specific transplantation antigen (TSTA), although experiments carried out by GALLIMORE and PARASKEVA (1979) demonstrate a major TSTA activity mapping in the E1 region of the viral genome.

These experiments may have a bearing upon the mechanisms of adenovirus persistence in humans (in vivo). Adenoviruses were first isolated (ROWE et al. 1953) by culturing human adenoids surgically removed from children. Thirty-three of 53 adenoid cultures produced adenovirus in vitro, indicating that adenoviruses persist in an infectious form in tissues even without apparent clinical symptoms. Viral persistence in the body requires that an equilibrium exist between controlled virus replication and host defenses, so that the host is not destroyed by the virus. Either the E3 19K glycoprotein or the E1 TSTA could mediate this equilibrium between virus replication and T-cell (killer-cell)-mediated death of infected cells in vivo. Thus the E3 19K glycoprotein may have a "function" in vivo of sparing its host and favoring persistence, but be dispensable or nonessential in vitro when virus is grown in cell culture in the absence of an immune system.

Little is known about the functions of the other E3 proteins (13K, 14K, and 15.5K). PERSSON et al. (1978) has purified the E3 14K protein to homogeneity and it is clearly distinct from the E3 19K glycoprotein. The E3 genomic region is a good example of the complexity of mRNA species generated by splicing and the redundant production of the same protein by multiple mRNAs. The meaning of these observations should become clearer as E3 protein functions are established.

3.4 The E4 Proteins: Moving in on the Unknown

The E4 region of the genome extends from 91.3 to 99.0 map units and is transcribed in the leftward direction. The complete nucleotide sequence of this region has been determined (HERISSE et al. 1981) and 9–14 transcripts have been detected and mapped to this early region (CHOW et al. 1979; KITCHINGHAM and WESTPHAL 1980). All three possible reading frames could give rise to proteins or portions of proteins (via spliced mRNA). Reading frame 1 contains continuous nucleotide sequences that could encode an 11K protein (E4 subregion 3) and a 13K protein (E4 subregion 4). Reading frame 2 has continuous sequences for two different 14K proteins (E4 subregions 1 and 2), a 34K protein (E4 subregion 6), and a 10K protein (E4 subregion 7). Reading frame 3 contains an open reading frame for a 6K protein (E4 subregion 5) or portion of a protein derived from a spliced mRNA. Thus there are seven subregions with nucleotide sequences containing open reading frames from 6K to 34K in size (proteins), and these subregions are found in all three possible reading frames. Only subregion 4 and 6 sequences overlap, but they are read in different frames (1 and 2). It remains possible that combinations of these polypeptides are joined via splicing of the mRNAs to produce multiple sets of proteins. Hybrid selection of mRNAs with E4 DNA followed by RNA in vitro translation has detected 11K, 17K, 19K, 21K, and 24K proteins (LEWIS et al. 1976). Two proteins from E4, an E4 subregion 3 11K protein (SARNOW et al. 1982a; DOWNEY et al. 1983) and the E4 subregion 6 34K protein (SARNOW et al. 1983), have been studied in some detail.

The E4 11K protein detected in infected cells can be isolated in two forms, one with a pI of 5.4 and a second with a pI of 5.6 (SARNOW et al. 1982a). The 11K pI-5.4 protein is tightly associated with the nuclear matrix fraction (BEREZNEY and COFFEY 1975) of the infected cell. A role for the nuclear matrix in DNA replication (PARDOLL et al. 1980; BUCKLER-WHITE et al. 1980) and in adenovirus RNA processing (MARIMAN et al. 1982) has been suggested by several experiments. The fact that only the more acidic form of the E4 11K protein is associated with the nuclear matrix may suggest a method of regulating the association of protein with this structural (the nuclear matrix) element in the nucleus of a cell.

The E4 11K proteins from different human adenovirus serotypes are immunologically conserved (SARNOW et al. 1982a). Antibodies against the Ad2 E4 11K protein immunoprecipitate the Ad2 (group C), Ad12 (group A), Ad3 (group B), Ad9 (group D), and Ad4 (group E) homologous proteins. This is the only known adenovirus early protein that shows such a broad group-specific immunological conservation. The only other adenovirus protein with similar human adenovirus group specificity is the structural protein termed the hexon antigen. Similarly, the nucleotide sequence of the E4 11K protein gene from Ad2 and Ad5 shows only four base pair changes (out of 348 base pairs) and one amino acid change (out of 116 amino acids) (SARNOW et al. 1982a). Such conservation usually implies an important role for the protein during infection. A structural association with the cellular nuclear matrix might be selected for and preserved as an example.

Ad5 dl341 is a mutant in the E4 11K gene with a single base pair deletion resulting in a frame-shift mutation which terminates three amino acid codons after the deletion. This mutation could produce a 6K N-terminal fragment of the E4 11K protein. However, no immunologically detectable 11K or 6K protein was found in infected cells (SARNOW et al. 1982a). Ad5 dl341 is a viable mutant, replicating as well as wild-type virus in HeLa and WI38 cells in culture. This indicates either that the E4 11K protein is not essential for virus replication in cell culture, or that the 6K fragment functions, even though this cannot be detected with antibodies directed against the 11K protein. It also remains possible that other E4 proteins provide a redundant function for E4 11K (SARNOW et al. 1982a).

The E4 11K protein was shown to be encoded by a gene in E4 subregion 3 by mapping Ad5 dl341 to region E4 and by matching the amino acid positions of two methionines and seven leucines in the first 35 amino acids (N-terminal) of the E4 11K protein with the predicted amino acid sequence deduced from the nucleotide sequence of E4 subregion 3 (SARNOW et al. 1982a).

The E4 subregion 6 34K protein has been isolated and shown to have an apparent molecular weight in SDS-polyacrylamide gels of 25K (SARNOW et al. 1983). The positions of the methionine residues in two different tryptic peptides of the 25K protein were determined by amino acid sequencing and matched to the nucleotide sequence prediction of amino acid sequences for E4 subregion 6 (SARNOW et al. 1983). This E4 25K protein is found in a physical association or complex with the E1B 58K protein, as discussed in Sect. 3.1. The mutant Ad5 dl342 deletes one base in the E1B 58K gene and produces a frame shift and chain termination 30 amino acids later (SARNOW et al. 1983). In this mutant, the E1B 58K fragment is not immunologically detected and no complex with the E4 25K protein is produced. The phenotypes of this mutant and other E1B 58K mutants are the same as mutants in the E4 25K gene, indicating common functions for these two proteins found in a complex. Viruses with mutations in either the E1B 58K or E4 25K genes are defective (two logs lower virus titer) for replication in cell culture. It appears that the E1B 58K–E4 25K complex is involved in regulating the levels of early and late proteins, possibly at the RNA processing level, or protein modification steps. Further work on the function of this complex will provide interesting clues to how the virus regulates its own gene expression.

Little or nothing is known about the other E4 proteins, except that several additional deletion mutants in E4 have no defect for replication of the virus in cell culture. The possible role of these E4 proteins, as well as of the E3 region proteins, in virus replication in animals needs to be investigated.

4 Conclusions

To date about 25 early adenoviral proteins have been detected (Table 1). They fall into three groups with regard to their temporal regulation: (a) immediate early proteins (E1A) which are required to turn on the transcription of (b) the delayed early proteins (E1B, E2, E3, and E4), and (c) proteins synthesized at early times that are expressed in considerably higher levels at late times (E2, IVa2, the L1 proteins, the i-leader proteins, and protein IX) (see Table 1). The E1 genes and gene products are involved in a positive regulation of transcription (E1A) of the early genes and the regulation of the levels of early and late gene expression (E1B). This early region is both necessary and sufficient for transformation of cells in culture, but transformation frequencies can be affected by the E2 gene products as well. It may be suggested from these observations that viral gene products designed to optimally regulate the levels of other viral functions, can also act upon cellular genes, resulting in a transformed phenotype. The E2 gene products which are optimized to replicate viral DNA can affect the efficiency of transformation events. The single-strand DNA binding protein (E2A), DNA terminal protein (E2B) and DNA polymerase (E2B) compose the known E2 protein group. Studies with SV40 large T antigen, which is also required for cellular transformation, show that it too is involved in viral DNA replication (TEGTMEYER 1974) and the regulation of the levels of viral gene products (ALWINE et al. 1977). These analogies between the transforming genes of SV40 and adenovirus continue with the observation that both the SV40 large T antigen and the E1B 58K adenovirus gene product are physically associated with the same cellular protein, p53, in SV40- or adenovirus-transformed cells. Furthermore, the SV40 large T antigen suppresses an E2A temperature-sensitive mutation in the DBP, permitting adenovirus DNA replication under nonpermissive conditions, and allows adenovirus late gene products to be properly produced in monkey cells. These interrelationships between the SV40 and adenovirus transforming genes and gene products suggest some common or related functions and a unity in the mechanisms involved in cellular transformation.

Both the biochemical and genetic evidence point out the close interrelationships between viral and cellular proteins and functions. The E1B 58K–p53 complex and the various host-range phenotypes of the DBP mutants suggest that viral proteins must interact with cellular functions in both infected and transformed cells. Alternate forms of these oligomeric protein complexes, such as the E1B 58K–E4 25K association in productively infected cells and the E1B 58K–p53 complex in transformed cells, may help us to begin to understand the different possible fates of a virus infection, i.e., productive vs. transforming. The ability of viral proteins such as the DBP to interact with cellular functions certainly helps to explain the host-range limitations and productivity of a virus against different backgrounds.

The detection of a number of nonessential adenovirus early gene functions in cell culture (E3 and some E4 proteins) presents an interesting possibility. Because some of these proteins, such as the E4 11K protein, are conserved over evolutionary epochs, they may well have vital functions in the natural host or other tissues of an animal. The identification of such functions which operate in vivo but are not required in vitro (cell culture) opens up a new area of research and inquiry.

It is already clear that viruses provide a very favorable system for studying biological processes. The extensive and often complicated types of gene regulation operative during adenovirus infections will provide general principles for better understanding these cellular processes. Examples of positive (E1A) and negative (E2A DBP at the E4 region genes) control of transcription, RNA processing (E1B, E2A), mRNA stability (E2A DBP and E1 mRNA), translational controls (VA RNAs), protein stability (E1A proteins), protein modification (E2A, E4 11K), and association with different cellular compartments (E4 11K) are all part of the processes observed in adenovirus-infected cells. In the past 30 years the ground work has been laid, so that it is now possible to ask questions that should provide detailed answers concerning the mechanisms underlying the regulation of gene expression. The adenovirus system will surely continue to be one of the most productive contributors to this field of research.

References

Alwine JC, Reed SI, Stark GR (1977) Characterization of the autoregulation of simian virus 40 gene A. J Virol 24:22–32
Anderson CW, Baum PR, Gesteland RF (1973) Processing of adenovirus 2-induced proteins. J Virol 12:241–252

Ariga H, Klein H, Levine AJ, Horwitz MS (1980) A cleavage product of the adenovirus DNA binding protein is activie in DNA replication in vitro. Virology 101:307–310

Axelrod N (1978) Phosphoproteins of adenovirus 2. Virology 87:366–383

Babich A, Nevins JR (1981) The stability of early adenoviral mRNA is controlled by the viral 73Kd DNA binding protein. Cell 26:371–379

Benchimol S, Pim D, Crawford LV (1982) Radioimmune-assay of the cellular protein p53 in mouse and human cell lines. EMBO J 1:1–8

Berezney R, Coffey DS (1975) Nuclear protein matrix: association with newly synthesized DNA. Science 189:291–293

Berk AJ, Sharp PA (1978) Structure of the adenovirus 2 early mRNAs. Cell 14:695–711

Berk AJ, Lee F, Harrison T, Williams J, Sharp PA (1979) A pre-early Ad5 gene product regulates synthesis of early viral mRNAs. Cell 17:935–944

Bernards R, Schrier PI, Bos JL, Van der Eb A (1983) Role of adenovirus types 5 and 12 early region 1b tumor antigens in oncogenic transformation. Virology 127:45–54

Bos JL, Polder LJ, Bernards R, Schrier PI, Van den Elsen PJ, Van der Eb AJ, Van Ormondt H (1981) The 2.2Kb E1B mRNA of human ad12 and Ad5 codes for two tumor antigens starting at different AUG triplets. Cell 27:121–131

Buckler-White AJ, Humphrey GW, Piget V (1980) Association of polyoma T-antigen and DNA with the nuclear matrix from lytically infected 3T6 cells. Cell 22:37–46

Carter TH, Ginsberg HS (1976) Viral transcription in KB cells infected by temperature sensitive early mutants of adenovirus type 5. J Virol 18:156–166

Carter TH, Blanton RA (1978) Possible role of the 72,000 dalton DNA binding protein in regulation of Ad5 early gene expression. J Virol 25:664–674

Cepko CL, Changelian PS, Sharp PA (1981) Immunoprecipitation with two-dimensional pools as a hybridoma screening technique: production and characterization of monoclonal antibodies against adenovirus 2 proteins. Virology 11:385–401

Challberg M, Kelly TS (1979) Adenovirus DNA replication in vitro. Proc Natl Acad Sci USA 76:655–659

Challberg MD, Desidero SV, Kelly TJ (1980) Adenovirus DNA replication in vitro: characterization of a protein covalently linked to nascent DNA strands. Proc Natl Acad Sci USA 77:5105–5107

Chin WW, Maizel JV (1976) The polypeptides of adenovirus VIII. Further studies on early adenovirus polypeptides in vivo and localization of E2 and E2A to the cell plasma membrane. Virology 71:518–530

Chow LT, Roberts JM, Lewis JB, Broker TR (1977) A map of cytoplasmic RNA transcripts from lytic adenovirus type 2 determined by electron microscopy of RNA-DNA hybrids. Cell 11:819–836

Chow LT, Broker T, Lewis JB (1979) The complex splicing patterns of RNA from the early regions of Ad2. J Mol Biol 134:265–303

Doerfler W, Burger H, Ortin J, Fanning E, Brown DT, Westphal M, Winterhoff U, Weiser B, Schuck J (1974) Integration of adenovirus DNA into the cellular genome. Cold Spring Harbor Symp Quant Biol 39:505–522

Downey JF, Rowe DI, Bacchetti S, Graham FL, Bagley ST (1983) Mapping of a 14,000 dalton antigen to early region 4 of human adenovirus 5 genome. J Virol 45:514–523

Ensinger MJ, Ginsberg HS (1972) Selection and preliminary characterization of temperature sensitive mutants of type 5 adenovirus. Virology 10:328–339

Evans RM, Fraser N, Ziff E, Weber J, Wilson M, Darnell JE (1977) The initiation sites for RNA transcription in Ad2 DNA. Cell 12:733–739

Flint SJ (1982) Expression of adenoviral genetic information in productively infected cells. Biochem Biophys Acta 651:175–208

Flint SJ, Sharp PA (1976) Adenovirus transcription. V. Quantitation of viral RNA sequences in adenovirus 2 infected and transformed cells. J Mol Biol 106:749–771

Flint SJ, Sambrook J, Williams JF, Sharp PA (1976) Viral nucleic acid sequences in transformed cells. IV. A study of the sequences of Ad5 DNA and RNA in four lines of Ad5-transformed rodent cells using specific fragments of the viral genome. Virology 72:456–470

Fowlkes DML, Land ST, Linne T, Petterson U, Philipson L (1979) Interaction between the adenovirus DNA binding protein and double stranded DNA. J Mol Biol 132:163–180

Gallimore PH, Paraskeva C (1979) A study to determine the reasons for differences in the tumorigenicity of rat cell lines transformed by adenovirus 2 and adenovirus 12. Cold Spring Harbor Symp
Quant Biol 44:703–714

Gallimore PH, Sharp PA, Sambrook J (1974) Viral DNA in transformed cells. II. A study of the
sequences of adenovirus 2 DNA in nine lines of transformed rat cells using specific fragments
of the viral genome. J Mol Biol 89:49–72

Gallos RS, Williams J, Burger MH, Flint SJ (1979) Localization of additional early gene sequences
in the adenoviral chromosome. Cell 17:945–956

Gilead Z, Jeng YH, Wold WSM, Sugawara K, Rho HW, Harter ML, Green M (1976) Immunological
identification of two adenovirus induced early proteins possibly involved in cell transformation.
Nature 264:263–266

Ginsberg HS, Ensinger MS, Kauffman RS, Mayer AJ, Londholm U (1974) Cell transformation:
a study of regulation with types 5 and 12 adenovirus temperature-sensitive mutants. Cold Spring
Harbor Symp Quant Biol 39:412–426

Graham FG, Harrison TJ, Williams JF (1978) Defective transforming capacity of adenovirus type
5 host range mutants. Virology 86:10–21

Graham FL, Van der Eb AJ, Heyneker HL (1974) Size and location of the transforming regions
in human adenovirus type 5 DNA. Nature 251:687–691

Graham FL, Abrahams PJ, Mulder C, Heyneker HL, Warnaar SO, de Vrives FAJ, Fiers W, Van
der Eb AJ (1975) Studies on in vitro transformation by DNA and DNA fragments of human
adenoviruses and simian virus 40. Cold Spring Harbor Symp Quant Biol 39:637–650

Green M, Wold WSM, Brackmann K, Carlas MA (1979) Studies on early proteins and transformation
proteins of human adenoviruses. Cold Spring Harbor Symp Quant Biol 44:457–470

Grodzicker T, Anderson C, Sharp P, Sambrook J (1974) Conditional lethal mutants of adenovirus
2-simian virus 40 hybrids. I. Host range mutants of Ad2 + ND. J Virol 13:1237–1244

Grodzicker T, Lewis JB, Anderson CW (1976) Conditional lethal mutants of adenovirus type 2
simian virus 40 hybrids. II. Ad2 + ND1 host range mutants that synthesize fragments of the
Ad2 + ND1 30K protein. J Virol 19:559–568

Halbert DN, Spector DJ, Raskas HJ (1979) In vitro translation products specified by the transforming
region of adenovirus type 2. J Virol 31:621–629

Harrison T, Graham F, Williams J (1977) Host range mutants of adenovirus type 5 defective for
growth in HeLa cells. Virology 77:319–329

Harter M, Lewis J (1978) Adenovirus type 2 early proteins synthesized in vitro and in vivo: identification in infected cells of the 38,000 to 50,000 molecular weight proteins encoded by the left
end of the Ad2 genome. J Virol 26:736–744

Herisse J, Courtois G, Galibert F (1980) Nucleotide sequence of the EcoRI-D fragment of adenovirus
2 genome. Nucleic Acids Res 8:2173–2192

Herisse J, Rigalet M, Dupont R, de Dinectin C, Galibert F (1981) Nucleotide sequence of adenovirus
2 DNA encoding for carboxylic region of the fiber protein and the entire E4 region. Nucleic
Acids Res 9:4023–4042

Ho YS, Gallos R, Williams J (1982) Isolation of type 5 adenovirus mutants with a cold sensitive
host range phenotype: genetic evidence of an adenovirus maintenance function. Virology
122:109–124

Horwitz MS (1976) Bidirectional replication of adenovirus type 2 DNA. J Virol 18:307–314

Horwitz MS (1978) Temperature sensitive replication of H5ts125 adenovirus DNA in vitro. Proc
Natl Acad Sci USA 75:4291–4295

Houweling A, Van den Elsen PJ, Van der Eb AJ (1980) Partial transformation of primary rat
cells by the left most 4.5% fragment of adenovirus 5 DNA. Virology 105:537–550

Jeng YH, Wold WSM, Sugawara K, Green M (1978) Evidence for an adenovirus type 2 coded
early glycoprotein. J Virol 28:314–323

Johansson K, Persson H, Lewis AM, Pettersson U, Tibbetts C, Philipson L (1978) Viral DNA
sequences and gene products in hamster cells transformed by adenovirus type 2. J Virol
27:628–639

Jones N, Shenk T (1978) Isolation of deletion and substitution mutants of adenovirus type 5. Cell
13:181–197

Jones N, Shenk T (1979) An adenovirus type 5 early gene function regulates expression of other
early viral genes. Proc Natl Acad Sci USA 76:3665–3669

Kaplan M, Ariga H, Hurwitz J, Horwitz MS (1979) Complementation of the temperature sensitive defection H5ts125 adenovirus DNA replication in vitro. Proc Natl Acad Sci USA 76:5534–5537

Kitchingham GR, Westphal H (1980) The structure of Ad2 early nuclear and cytoplasmic RNAs. J Mol Biol 137:23–48

Klein H, Maltzman W, Levine AJ (1979) Structure-function relationships of the adenovirus DNA-binding protein. J Biol Chem 254:11051–11060

Klessig DF, Grodzicker T (1979) Mutations that allow human Ad2 and Ad5 to express late genes in monkey cells map in the viral gene encoding the 72Kd DNA binding protein. Cell 17:957–963

Kruijer W, Van Schark FAM, Sussenbach JS (1981) Structure and organization of the gene coding for the DNA binding protein of adenovirus type 5. Nucleic Acids Res 9:4439–4457

Kruijer W, Nicolas JC, Van Schark FAM, Sussenbach JS (1983) Structure and function of DNA binding proteins from revertants of adenovirus type 5 mutants with a temperature sensitive DNA replication. Virology 124:425–433

Lane DP, Crawford LV (1979) T antigen is bound to a host protein in SV40-transformed cells. Nature 278:261–263

Lassom NJ, Bagley ST, Graham FL (1979) Tumor antigens of human Ad5 in transformed cells and in cells infected with transformation defective host range mutants. Cell 18:781–791

Lechner RL, Kelly TJ (1977) The structure of replicating adenovirus 2 DNA molecules. Cell 12:1007–1015

Levine AJ, Van der Vliet PC, Rosenwirth B, Rabek J, Frenkel G, Ensinger M (1974) Adenovirus infected cell specific DNA binding proteins. Cold Spring Harbor Symp Quant Biol 39:559–568

Levinson AD, Levine AJ (1977a) The group C adenovirus tumor antigens: infected and transformed cells and a peptide map analysis. Cell 11:871–879

Levinson AD, Levine AJ (1977b) The isolation and identification of the adenovirus group C tumor antigens. Virology 76:1–11

Levinson AD, Levine AJ, Anderson S, Osborn N, Rosenwirth B, Weber K (1976) The relationship between group C adenovirus single-strand DNA binding proteins. Cell 7:575–584

Lewis JB, Atkins JF, Baum PR, Solem R, Gesteland RF, Anderson CW (1976) Location and identification of the genes for adenovirus type 2 early peptides. Cell 7:141–151

Lewis JB, Esche H, Smart JE, Stillman BW, Harter ML, Mathews MB (1979) Organization and expression of the left third of the genome of adenovirus. Cold Spring Harbor Symp Quant Biol 44:493–508

Lichy JH, Field J, Horwitz M, Hurwitz J (1982) Separation of the adenovirus terminal protein precursor from its associated DNA polymerase: role of both proteins in the initiation of adenovirus DNA replication. Proc Natl Acad Sci USA 79:5225–5229

Linzer DIH, Levine AJ (1979) Characterization of a 54K dalton cellular SV40 tumor antigen present in SV40 transformed cells and uninfected embryonal carcinoma cells. Cell 17:43–52

Linzer DIH, Maltman W, Levine AJ (1979) The SV 40 A-gene product is required for the production of a 54,000 MW cellular tumor antigen. Virology 98:308–318

Logan J, Shenk T (1983) The role of adenovirus E1A and E1B genes in transformation. In preparation

Logan J, Nicolas JC, Topp WC, Girard M, Shenk T, Levine AJ (1981) Transformation by adenovirus early region 2A temperature sensitive mutants and their revertants. Virology 115:419–422

Logan JS, Shenk T (1982) Transcriptional and translational control of adenovirus gene expression. Microbiol Rev 46:377–383

Maltzman W, Oren M, Levine AJ (1981) The structural relationships between 54,000 MW cellular tumor antigens detected in viral and nonviral transformed cells. Virology 112:145–156

Manley JL, Sharp P, Gefter M (1979) RNA synthesis in isolated nuclei: in vitro mutation of adenovirus 2 major late m-RNA precursor. Proc Natl Acad Sci USA 76:160–164

Manley JL, Fire A, Cano A, Sharp PA, Gefter ML (1980) DNA dependent transcription of adenovirus genes in a soluble whole cell extract. Proc Natl Acad Sci USA 77:3855–3859

Mariman ECM, Van Elkelen CAG, Reinders RJ, Berns AJM, Van Venroij WJ (1982) Adenoviral heterogeneous nuclear RNA is associated with the host nuclear matrix during splicing. J Mol Biol 154:103–119

Mercer WE, Nelson D, DeLeo AB, Old LJ, Baserga R (1982) Microinjection of monoclonal antibody to protein p53 inhibits serum-induced DNA synthesis in 3T3 cells. Proc Natl Acad Sci USA 79:6309–6312

Montell C, Fisher E, Caruthers M, Berk AJ (1982) Resolving the functions of overlapping viral genes by site-specific mutagenesis at a mRNA splice site. Nature 295:380–384

Nevins J (1981) Mechanism of activation of early viral transcription by the adenovirus E1A gene product. Cell 26:213–220

Nevins J (1982) Induction of the synthesis of a 70,000 dalton mammalian heat shock protein by the adenovirus E1A gene product. Cell 29:913–919

Nevins J, Winkler J (1980) Regulation of early adenovirus transcription: a protein product of early region 2 specifically represses region 4 transcription. Proc Natl Acad Sci USA 77:1893–1897

Nicolas JC, Suarez F, Levine AJ, Girard M (1981) Temperature independent revertants of adenovirus H5ts125 and H5ts107 mutants in the DNA binding protein: isolation of a new class of host range temperature conditional revertants. Virology 108:521–524

Nicolas JC, Ingrand D, Sarnow P, Levine AJ (1982) A mutation in the adenovirus type 5 DNA binding protein that fails to autoregulate the production of the DNA binding protein. Virology 122:481–485

Nicolas JC, Young CSH, Girard M, Levine AJ (1983a) Detection, rescue and mapping of mutations in the adenovirus DNA binding protein gene. Proc Nat Acad Sci (USA) 80:1674–1677

Nicolas JC, Sarnow P, Girard M, Levine AJ (1983b) Host range temperature conditional mutants in the adenovirus DNA binding protein are defective in the assembly of infectious virus. Virology 125:228–239

Oren M, Maltzman W, Levine AJ (1981) Post-translational regulation of the 54K cellular tumor antigen in normal and transformed cells. Mol Cell Biol 1:101–110

Pardoll DM, Vogelstein B, Coffey DS (1980) A fixed site of DNA replication in eukaryotic cells. Cell 19:527–536

Perricaudet M, Akusjarvi G, Virtanen A, Pettersson U (1979) Structure of the two spliced mRNAs from the transforming region of human subgroup C adenovirus. Nature 281:694–696

Persson H, Oberg B, Philipson L (1978) Purification and characterization of an early protein (E14K) from adenovirus type 2 infected cells. J Virol 28:119–139

Persson H, Sigmus C, Philipson L (1979a) Purification and characterization of an early glycoprotein from adenovirus type 2-infected cells. J Virol 29:938–948

Persson H, Kvist S, Ostberg L, Petersson PA, Philipson L (1979b) Adenoviral early glycoprotein E3-19K and ts association with transplantation antigens. Cold Spring Harbor Symp Quant Biol 44:509–517

Pope JH, Rowe WP (1964) Immunofluorescent studies of adenovirus 12 tumors and of cells transformed or infected by adenoviruses. J Exp Med 120:577–584

Rabek JP, Zakian VA, Levine AJ (1981) The SV40 A gene product suppresses the adenovirus H5ts125 defect in DNA replication. Virology 109:290–302

Rabson AS, O'Connor GT, Berezesky IK, Paul FJ (1964) Enhancement of adenovirus growth in African green monkey kidney cells by SV40. Proc Soc Exp Biol Med 116:187–196

Reich N, Sarnow P, Du Prey and Levine AS (1983) Monoclonal Antibodies which recognize native and denatured forms of the Adenovirus DNA-Binding Protein. Virology, 128:480–484

Reich N, Levine AJ (1984) Regulation of p53 gene expression during cell growth and division. Nature, in press

Rekosh DMK, Russell WC, Bellet AJD, Robinson AJ (1977) Identification of a protein linked to the ends of adenovirus DNA. Cell 11:283–295

Ricciardi RL, Jones RL, Cepko CL, Sharp PA, Roberts BE (1981) Expression of early adenovirus genes requires a viral encoded acidic polypeptide. Proc Natl Acad Sci USA 78:6121–6125

Robinson AJ, Younghusband HB, Bellet AJD (1973) A circular DNA-protein complex from adenoviruses. Virology 56:54–69

Ross SR, Levine AJ (1979) The genomic map position of the adenovirus type 2 glycoprotein. Virology 99:427–430

Ross SR, Flint SJ, Levine AJ (1980a) Identification of the adenovirus early proteins and their genomic map positions. Virology 100:419–432

Ross S, Levine AJ, Galos R, Williams J, Shenk T (1980b) Early viral proteins in HeLa cells infected with adenovirus type 5 host range mutants. Virology 103:475–492

Rossini MS, Weinmann R, Baserga R (1979) DNA synthesis in a temperature sensitive mutant of the cell cycle by polyoma virus and adenovirus. Proc Natl Acad Sci USA 76:4441–4445

Rowe WP, Huebiner RJ, Gillmore LK, Parrott RH, Ward TG (1953) Isolation of a cytogenic agent from human adenoids undergoing spontaneous degeneration in tissue culture. Proc Soc Expt Biol Med 84:570–573

Russell WC, Shekel JJ (1972) The polypeptides of adenovirus infected cells. J Gen Virol 15:45–47

Russell WC, Hayashi K, Sanderson PJ, Pereira HG (1967) Adenovirus antigens: a study of their properties and sequential development in infection. J Gen Virol 1:495–507

Saborio JL, Oberg B (1976) In vivo and in vitro synthesis of adenovirus type 2 early proteins. J Virol 17:865–872

Sambrook J, Botchan M, Gallimore R, Ozanne B, Pettersson U, Williams JF, Sharp PA (1975) Viral DNA sequences in cells transformed by simian virus 40, adenovirus 2 and adenovirus type 5. Cold Spring Harbor Symp Quant Biol 39:615–632

Sambrook J, Greene R, Stringer J, Mitcheson T, Hu SL, Botchan M (1979) Analysis of the sites of integration of viral DNA sequences in rat cells transformed by adenovirus 2 and SV40. Cold Spring Harbor Symp Quant Biol 44:569–584

Sarnow P, Hearing P, Anderson CW, Reich N, Levine AJ (1982a) Identification and characterization of an immunologically conserved adenovirus early region 11,000 MW protein and its association with the nuclear matrix. J Mol Biol 102:565–583

Sarnow P, Sullivan CA, Levine AJ (1982b) A monoclonal antibody detecting the adenovirus 5 E1b-58Kd tumor antigen: characterization of the E1b-58Kd tumor antigen in adenovirus infected and transformed cells. Virology 34:650–657

Sarnow P, Ho YS, Williams J, Levine AJ (1982c) Adenovirus E1b-58Kd tumor antigen and SV40 large tumor antigen are physically associated with the name 54Kd cellular protein in transformed cells. Cell 28:387–394

Sarnow P, Hearing P, Anderson C, Halbert DH, Shenk T, Levine AJ (1984) Adenovirus E1b-58Kd tumor antigen is physically assiciated with aw E4-25Kd protein in adenovirus productively infected cells. J. Virol. 49:642–700

Schrier PI, Van der Elsen PJ, Hertoghs JJL, Van der Eb A (1979) Characterization of tumor antigens in cells transformed by fragments of adenovirus type 5 DNA. Virology 99:372–385

Shenk T, Jones N, Colby W, Fowlkes D (1979) Functional analysis of Ad5 host range deletion mutants defective for transformation of rat embryo cells. Cold Spring Harbor Symp Quant Biol 44:367–375

Simmons DT, Martin MA, Mora PT, Chang C (1980) Relationship among T antigens isolated from various lines in adenovirus infected and transformed cells. J Virol 34:650–657

Solnick D (1981) An adenovirus mutant defective in splicing RNA from early region 1A. Nature 291:508–510

Solnick D, Anderson MA (1982) Transformation deficient adenovirus mutant defective in expression of region 1A but not region 1B. J Virol 42:106–113

Stillman BW, Lewis JB, Chow L, Mathews NB, Smart JE (1981) Identification of the gene and mRNA for the adenovirus terminal protein precursor. Cell 23:497–508

Sussenbach JS, Van der Vliet PC (1972) Viral DNA synthesis in isolated nuclei from adenovirus-infected KB cells. FEBS Lett 21:7–14

Sussenbach JS, Kuizk MG (1977) Studies on the mechanism of replication of adenovirus DNA. V. The location of termini of replication. Virology 77:149–158

Tegtmeyer P (1974) Altered patterns of protein synthesis in infection by SV40 mutants. Cold Spring Harbor Symp Quant Biol 39:9–16

Tegtmeyer P, Rundell K, Collins JK (1977) Modification of simian virus 40 protein A. J Virol 21:647–656

Thomas R, Kaplan L, Reich N, Lane DP, Levine AJ (1983) Characterization of human p53 antigens employing primate-specific monoclonal antibodies. Virology 131:502–517

Tjian R, Fey G, Graessmann A (1978) Biological activity of purified SV40 T-antigen proteins. Proc Natl Acad Sci USA 75:1279–1283

Tooze J (1981) Molecular biology of tumor viruses, 2nd ede. Part 2, DNA tumor viruses. Cold Spring Harbor, New York

Van den Elsen PJ, De Pater S, Howweling A, Van der Veer J, Van der Eb AJ (1981) The relationship between region E1a and E1b of human adenoviruses in cell transformation. Gene 18:175–185

Van den Elsen P, Howweling A, Van der Eb A (1983) Expression of region E1b of human adenoviruses in the absence of a functional E1A region is not sufficient for complete transformation. Virology 128:377–390

Van der Eb AJ, Van Ormondt H, Schrier PI, Lupker JH, Jochenisen H, Van der Elsen PJ, De Leys RJ, Kratt J, Van Bevern CP, Dykema R, De Wood A (1979) Structure and function of the transforming genes of human adenoviruses and SV40. Cold Spring Harbor Symp Quant Biol 44:383–399

Van der Vliet PC, Levine AJ (1973) DNA binding proteins specific for cells infected by adenovirus. Nature (New Biol) 246:170–174

Van der Vliet PC, Sussenbach JS (1975) An adenovirus type 5 gene function required for initiation of viral DNA replication. Virology 67:415–427

Van der Vliet PC, Levine AJ, Ensinger MJ, Ginsberg HS (1975) Thermolabile DNA binding proteins from cells infected with a temperature sensitive mutant of adenovirus defective in DNA replication. J Virol 15:348–354

Van der Vliet PC, Landberg J, Janz HS (1977) Evidence for a function of the adenovirus DNA binding proteins in initiation of DNA synthesis as well as in elongation on nascent DNA chains. Virology 80:98–109

Van Ormondt H, Naat J, De Waard A, Van der Eb AJ (1978) The nucleotide sequence of the transforming HpaI-E fragment of Ad5 DNA. Gene 4:309–328

Weil A, Luse DL, Segall J, Roeder RG (1979) Selective and accurate initiation of transcription at the Ad2 major late promoter in a soluble system dependent upon purified RNA polymerase II. Cell 18:469–481

Williams JF, Young CH, Austin P (1974) Genetic analysis of human adenovirus type 5 in permissive and nonpermissive cells. Cold Spring Harbor Symp Quant Biol 39:427–438

Winnacker EL (1974) Origins and termini of adenovirus type 2 DNA replication. Cold Spring Harbor Symp Quant Biol 39:547–550

Zinkernagel RM, Doherty PC (1974) Restriction of in vitro T cell mediated cytoxicity in lymphocytes choriomeningitis within a synegeneic or semiallogeneic system. Nature 248:701–704

Molecular Biology of S16 (SA7) and Some Other Simian Adenoviruses

T.I. Tikchonenko[1]

The adenovirus family includes at present approximately 100 species divided into subgenera according to their natural hosts. Adopting the suggestion of the Simian Adenovirus Working Team (KALTER et al. 1980), simian adenoviruses comprise a subgenus which includes 20 previously described virus species.[2] Compared with human adenoviruses, simian adenoviruses have on the whole been studied much less, although theoretically and evolutionarily, relationships between members of all groups of primate adenoviruses seem to be of great interest.

1 Biological Properties

S16 is capable of transforming cells of newborn rats and hamsters and of inducing tumors in these rodent species (HULL et al. 1965; McALLISTER et al. 1969). We have derived a number of clones differing in some properties, the degree of oncogenicity among them (PONOMAREVA et al. 1983). As may be seen in Table 1, the highest tumorigenicity is found in a small-plaque clone MBI, whose

---

1 D.I. Ivanovsky, Institute of Virology, 16, Gamaleya Street, 123098 Moscow, USSR

2 All the simian viruses are designated according to the new nomenclature: S1 (old name SV1); S2 (CV11); S3 (SV15); S4 (SV17); S5 (SV20); S6 (SV23); S7 (SV25); S8 (SV30); S9 (SV31); S10 (SV32); S11 (SV33); S12 (SV34); S13 (SV36); S14 (SV37); S15 (SV38); S16 (SA7); S17 (SA17); S18 (SA18); S19 (AA153); S20 (V340)

Current Topics in Microbiology and Immunology, Vol. 110
© Springer-Verlag Berlin·Heidelberg 1984

Table 1. Characteristics of adenovirus S16 clones

Clone designation	Plaque size (mm)	Replication cycle (h)	Virus yield (log PFU/ml)	Tumorigenicity		
				Virus dose (log PFU/ hamster)	Time of tumor development (days)	Rate of induction (%)
KB230	3.5±0.5	12	9.7±0.5	7.5	30–45	100
KB230	3.5±0.5	12	9.7±0.5	6.5	52–120	44
MBI	0.45±0.05	n.d.	n.d.	5.0	32–35	100
MBI	0.45±0.05	n.d.	n.d.	3.2	25–45	100
K47	4–5	n.d.	n.d.	n.d.	n.d.	n.d.
S16	0.45±0.05	16	8.7±0.5	6.0	32–100	100
S16	0.45±0.05	16	8.7±0.5	5.0	32–100	75

n.d., not done

oncogenicity significantly exceeded that of the original wild-type virus. The large-plaque clone KB230 was considerably less oncogenic, although from their neutralization with antisera both clones were identical with the wild-type virus. At the same time, these clones differed in virus yields upon replication in susceptible cells. The other differences in clone properties are discussed below.

Characteristics of the tumorigenic activity of whole S16 virus and its intact and fragmented DNA are presented in Table 2. S16 virus has earned a reputation as one of the most strongly oncogenic viruses, and it produces first tumors as early as 20–30 days after inoculation of syngeneic baby hamsters or rats, the former species being much more sensitive to the tumorigenic effect of this virus. Subcutaneous inoculation of 3–5 µg DNA per newborn hamster also induces tumors, preliminary fragmentation of DNA, or isolation of an individual DNA fragment (C SalI) carrying the oncogene, markedly increasing the tumor genicity of the preparation (PONOMAREVA et al. 1979a). Most likely this effect is due to better integration into the cell genome of fragments of viral DNA lower in molecular weight than the intact genome. A similar degree of oncogenicity was found in S5 virus, while that of S15 was 4–5 times lower (T.I. Ponomareva unpublished data). Both with whole virus and with DNA, the tumors induced were undifferentiated sarcomas.

Transformation of rodent cells by S16 virus and its DNA occurs in a similar manner (PONOMAREVA et al. 1979a, b). In transformation of primary cultures of WAG rat kidney cells or rat embryo fibroblasts, the efficacy of transformation was on the average 1.2 foci/µg DNA. Transformation foci were groups of epithelium-like cells with increased refraction and a trend to multilayer growth. As in tumor induction, prefragmentation of DNA with restriction endonucleases enhances the transforming activity, although in this case the stimulating effect is less marked (PONOMAREVA et al. 1979b).

All lines of the transformed cells, as well as the lines derived from tumors, has a typical phenotype: they could be passaged indefinitely, grew in the medium with 2% serum, formed colonies in semisolid agar, showed a peculiar morphology, grew on glass with higher density, and finally, T and S antigens were identi-

Table 2. Tumorigenicity of S16, its DNA, and transformed cells

Preparation inoculated	Animal species and age (days)	Amount of preparation per animal	No. of tumor bearers and time of tumor appearance in days						Total	Rate (%)
			10–11	12–13	14–19	20–30	30–100	100		
Virus	H, 1–3	10^6 PFU	–	–	–	20/20	–	–	20/20	100
Virus	H, 14–28	10^8 PFU	–	–	–	20/20	–	–	20/20	100
Virus	R, 1–3									
Virus	R, 10	10^8 PFU	–	–	–	–	5/18	–	5/18	27
DNA, intact	H, 1–3	3–5 µg	–	–	–	–	6/34	–	6/34	17
DNA + R EcoRI	H, 1–3	3–5 µg	–	–	–	–	3/20	–	3/20	15
DNA + R BamHI	H, 1–3	3–5 µg	–	–	–	–	5/13	–	5/13	38
DNA + R SalI	H, 1–3	3–5 µg	–	–	–	–	5/16	–	5/16	31
C SalI fragment	H, 1–3	0.6 µg	–	–	–	–	7/11	–	7/11	64
R cells, S16 + HBV	R, 1–3	$1–15 \times 10^6$ cells	15/15	–	–	–	–	–	15/15	100
R cells, S16 412	R, 1–3	1.4×10^6 cells	–	–	–	8/8	–	–	8/8	100
R cells, S16 + HBV	H, 1–3	$5–10 \times 10^6$ cells	23/23	–	–	–	–	–	23/23	100
R cells, S16 + HBV	H, 1–3	1×10^4 cells	–	–	2/8	6/8	–	–	8/8	100
H cells D2, S16	H, 14–23	1×10^3 cells	–	–	–	–	2/14	–	2/14	14
H cells D2, S16	H, 1–3	1×10^6 cells	–	–	–	5/7	2/7	–	7/7	100
R cells, S16 + HBV	H, 14–28	$1–5 \times 10^6$ cells	3/8	–	–	–	–	–	3/8	–
R cells, S16 412	H, 1–3	$1–10 \times 10^6$ cells	–	–	–	–	–	–	0/42	0

H, Syrian hamsters or hamster cells; R, rats or rat cells; S16 + HBV, cells cotransformed by S16 and hepatitis B virus D2, tumor induced by S16 D2; 412, transformation by S16 412 fied in the cells of all lines (PONOMAREVA et al. 1983). When transformed cells were inoculated into animals of the same (rat-rat or hamster-hamster) or different (rat-hamster) species, tumors developed. Different lines varied considerably in their tumorigenicity. A high activity was found with line D2 derived from the tumor induced by inoculation of intact DNA to newborn hamsters. In this case a minimal dose producing tumors in hamsters was 10^3 cells per 3-day-old animal, whereas a minimal dose for other cell lines was 1–2 orders higher on average (PONOMAREVA et al. 1983).

The highest oncogenicity, however, was observed in the AH-2 cell line cotransformed simultaneously by S16 DNA and hepatitis B virus DNA (S16+ HBV; Table 2). Thus inoculation of cotransformed AH-2 cells to newborn rats in a dose of $1–15 \times 10^6$ cells per animal resulted in 100% induction of tumors developing very early (10–11 days). The minimal inoculum consisting of 100 AH2 cells was able to induce tumors in newborn rats. With control rat cells transformed by S16 alone (in this case, line 412) inoculated to syngeneic animals, tumors were also induced in 100%, but developed much later (24–30 days; Table 2). In the experiments of PANIGRAHY et al. (1976). S16-transformed rat cells in a dose of $1–10 \times 10^6$ induced no tumors at all in baby rats (observation period up to 97 days), although they induced tumors in 30% of newborn hamsters. Human Ad12-transformed rat cells behave in a similar manner. After transplantation of the cells to syngeneic animals, the earliest tumor appearance varied from 17–18 days (PARASKEVA and GALLIMORE 1980) to 28 days (FREEMAN et al. 1967). The greatest differences between the cell line cotransformed by S16 in the presence of HBV DNA and cell lines transformed by S16 alone are revealed by experiments where the cells are transplanted to animals of another species. S16+HBV cells efficiently induced tumors in 2-week-old hamsters, 40% of the tumors appearing as early as 10 days post injection. At the same time, inoculation of hamsters with rat cells transformed by S16 alone induced no tumors in any of 42 inoculated animals. Here our data differ from the results of PANIGRAHY et al. (1976) cited above. Inoculation of hamsters with syngeneic cells (for instance, line D2 from hamster tumor) induced tumors within 25–100 days (PONOMAREVA et al. 1983; POTEBNYA et al. 1983). Comparison of our own data and those from the literature (PANIGRAHY et al. 1976; FREEMAN et al. 1967) shows that our cotransformed line AH-2 has the highest oncogenicity among all known types of adenovirus-transformed cells. (We shall discuss later a possible effect of HBV genome on manifestation of oncogenicity.)

Analysis of a number of hamster and rat cell lines transformed by S16 virus or derived from virus-induced tumors allowed the comparison of integration of two strongly oncogenic adenoviruses, H12 and S16 (GARTEL et al. 1983). DOERFLER et al. (1983) has demonstrated certain differences in integration of viral and cellular genomes between strongly oncogenic human Ad12 and nononcogenic Ad2 and Ad12. Unfortunately, at the time of our work Ad12 was the only strongly oncogenic adenovirus which had been studied in this respect. It was not clear, therefore, if the observed differences represented a general feature typical of the behavior of genomes of strongly oncogenic and nononcogenic viruses in transformed cells or if these differences were species specific. DOERFLER et al. (1980) assumed the difference in integration and persistence of DNA between Ad12 (persistence of complete genome and a large number of virus copies) and Ad2/Ad5 (persistence of only a part of virus genome and a smaller number of copies) to be explained by differences in the permissiveness of cells for these viruses. Thus rat cells are semipermissive for Ad2 (GALLIMORE 1974) and hamster cells are completely nonpermissive for Ad12 (FANNING and DOERFLER 1976). According to the hypothesis of DOERFLER et al. (1980), in semipermissive systems there is strong selection which operates against persistence of whole genomes of nononcogenic Ad2 and Ad5 adenoviruses in the transformed cells in that subsequent replication of virus genome and formation of virus or viral proteins could lead to the death of the cell. In Ad12-transformed nonpermissive cells, persistence and integration of intact adenovirus DNA can exert no damaging effect on the cell, which is conducive to persistence of a large number of copies of intact genome.

Hamster and rat cells are nonpermissive for S16 (ALSTEIN et al. 1976; PONO-MAREVA unpublished data) and therefore, according to Doerfler's hypothesis, our virus should have behaved like Ad12. In point of fact the situation proved to be more complicated. In two S16-transformed rat cell lines which we studied intact virus genomes were found, and in hamster cells transformed by the same virus, the S16 genome underwent deletion but in all cases was present in a small number of copies. In other words, in rat cells S16 behaved like the highly oncogenic Ad12, with the exception of a small number of copies, and in hamster cells like nononcogenic Ad2. It cannot be ruled out, however, that the danger of integration of the intact genome is conditioned not only by the permissiveness of cells for productive replication of adenovirus, but also by their capacity to support replication and partial expression of viral DNA. From this point of view it is important that although S16 virions are not produced in either rat or hamster cells, S16 DNA replicates in cells of the latter species (OGINO and TAKAHASHI 1970). There is no evidence as yet regarding the capacity of S16 DNA for replication in rat cells, but one may assume that replication or expression of S16 DNA in this system does not make persistence and integration of the intact viral genome dangerous for the survival of the transformed cells. Analysis of larger numbers of transformed rat and hamster cells is required for the final conclusion regarding the pattern of relationships between integration of adenovirus DNA and the capacity of the host cell to support replication of viral DNA or its expression.

2 Biochemical and Biophysical Properties of Virions

According to electron-microscopic studies of preparations obtained by negative staining and freeze etching, parameters of S16 virions are typical of adenoviruses (DUBICHEV et al. 1980). The capsid diameter and center-to-center distance in hexon were found to be 76 and 9.5 nm, respectively. The sedimentation constant of S16 virions ($S_{20,w}^0$) was 740S $\pm$ 15S. The diffusion constant ($D_{20,w}^0$) determined by laser-optic mixing spectroscopy (PUSEY et al. 1974) was $6.34 \pm 0.003 \times 10^8$ cm^2/sec (DUBICHEV et al. 1980). From the specific partial volume of DNA of 0.55 cm^3/g, mean partial volume of adenovirus protein 0.72 cm^3/g, and percent age DNA content of 11.8%. (DUBICHEV et al. 1979), the specific partial volume of S16 virions ($\hat{v}$) was found to be 0.7003 cm^3/g. From the above data the molecular weight of the virion of this adenovirus was calculated:

$$M = \frac{RTS^0_{20,w}}{P^0_{20,w}\, \omega(1 - w\rho_0)} = 185 \pm 10 \text{ Md}$$

This value is slightly lower than the 203.6 $\pm$ 10 Md found by us previously for nononcogenic human Ad6 (TIKCHONENKO et al. 1979). The hydrodynamic radius of the S16 particle calculated from the diffusion constant value (DUBICHEV et al. 1980) is 65 $\pm$ 1.5 nm, which is practically equal to half the distance between diametrally located fibrils (64 $\pm$ 1.5 nm) determined by electron microscopy (DU-BICHEV et al. 1980).

3 Physicochemical Characteristics of S16 DNA

Physical characteristics of the DNA of S16 and some other simian adenoviruses studied in our laboratory are presented in Table 2. On the whole, these data correspond to the existing concepts on the properties of a typical adenovirus DNA. The value of $S^0_{20,w}$ determined by us for S16 and a new genome variant S8N (SV30N) is slightly higher (30.5S) than that given by BURNETT et al. (1968, 1972). These differences are most likely due to aspects of experimental method (REINER et al. 1976). The values of molecular weights of DNA of all simian viruses studied (Table 3), calculated from both the results of electron microscopy and the hydrodynamic parameters of the molecule (DUBICHEV et al. 1979; DIMI-TROV et al. 1979; VILNIS et al. 1981) were found to coincide within the limits of methodical error. Our values of DNA molecular weight for S8N and S15 genomes differ significantly from those given by BURNETT et al. (1972) – 18.7 and 17.6 Md respectively.

GC content in DNA of different simian viruses determined by different methods was found to be approximately similar (57.8–59%). In this connection, noteworthy are the data on the existence of a certain correlation between the degree of oncogenicity and GC content in DNA. According to this correlation, known as the Green-Goodheart rule, in human adenoviruses GC content decreases with increasing degree of oncogenicity (PINA and GREEN 1965), whereas in simian adenoviruses this relationship is reversed (GOODHEART 1971). Among the simian adenoviruses listed in Table 4, S16 is strongly oncogenic and at the same time has the lowest content of GC, completely breaking this rule (see Table 2). We previously observed deviations from this relationship in DNA of nononcogenic human Ad6 (TIKCHONENKO et al. 1979). In those studies we demonstrated that the greatest deviations from the average GC content in DNA of adenoviruses were observed in the central and right regions. Therefore the impression is gained that the Green-Goodheart rule depends not on the primary structure of oncogene in the left part of the genome, but rather on its right and central parts (for references see TIKCHONENKO et al. 1981c). The latter cir-

Table 3. Physical characteristics of DNA of simian adenoviruses

Parameters	Adenovirus species	
	S16	S8N[c]
Buoyant density (ρ) g/cm^3	1.717 ± 0.001	1.7186 ± 0.001
CsCl and calculated GC (%)	57.6 ± 1	59.1 ± 1
Buoyant density (ρ) g/cm^3	1.229 ± 0.001	1.4295 ± 0.001
Cs$_2$SO$_4$ and calculated GC (%)	58.0 ± 3.0	60.0 ± 2.0
Melting temperature (°C) and calculated GC (%)	93.0 ± 0.5 57.7 ± 1.2	93.5 ± 0.1 58.9 ± 1.3
Average value of GC (%)	57.8	59.0
DNA length (μm) and molecular weight (Md)[a]	10.8 and 22.1 ± 0.4	10.4 and 21.5 ± 0.4
Sedimentation constant ($S_{20,w}^0$)	32.2 ± 0.7	31.6 ± 0.4
Intrinsic viscosity (dl/g)	92.0 ± 5.0	86.5 ± 5
Molecular weight (Md) by the equation of Sheraga, Mandelkern, and Flory[b] $\beta = 2.39$	22.5 ± 0.7	21.5 ± 0.8

[a] Molecular weight of DNA by length was calculated in comparison with the length of DNA of Col EI plasmid, which corresponded on the average to 2.06 Md/μm

[b] $M = \left[\dfrac{S_{20,w}^0 \cdot [\eta]^{1/3} \, \eta_0 \, N}{\beta(1 - \upsilon\rho_0)} \right]^{1/3}$

υ = specific partial volume of virion = 0.55 cm^3/g (REINERT et al. 1971)

[c] Due to an error in collection management, the S8N variant was previously studied and described under the name of S15 (SV38) (DIMITROV et al. 1978; DUBICHEV et al. 1979; VILNIS et al. 1981)

cumstance raises a question: how can these genome regions not necessary for the transforming and tumorigenic activity be associated with modulation of oncogenicity?

The most complete restriction map for currently known simian viruses has been drawn by us for DNA of wild-type S16 (Fig. 1). It contains 137 recognition sites for 16 enzymes in DNA of the wild-type and clone MBI and 10 additional recognition sites located in DNA of KB230 clone (see below). The restriction maps for DNA of some other simian adenoviruses available in the collection of our institute permitted accurate determination of species and identification of new variants differing in some properties from the prototype strains. Thus, a new variant S3ON was identified which had previously been described as SV38 (DIMITROV et al. 1979; VILNIS et al. 1981), as well as a new variant S16P, previously designated SV30 (DENISOVA and GIBADULIN 1982).

The nucleotide sequence in left-terminal repeat fragment determined for S16 (E.A. Skripkin, unpublished data) cloned in bacteria by means of GC connectors coincides with that described by TOLUN et al. (1979) with the exception of the initial eight nucleotides:

```
                        1 2 3 4 5 6 7 8 9 10
This study              5′ C T A T C T A T A T  .... 3′ OH
TOLUN et al. (1979)     5′ – – – – A T C A A T  .... 3′ OH
```

Table 4. Classification of simian adenoviruses

Species Peptido (kd)	Subgroup 1		Subgroup 2a		Subgroup 2b		Subgroup 3a			Subgroup 3b			Subgroup 4
	00, h1		00, h2		00, h2		02, h3			01, h3			02, h4
	S13	S4	S6	S14	S3	S5	S8	S2	S7	S11	S12	S15	S16
II	138	126	100	115	107 104	107 106	111 110	106 104	109 107 110	111	107 105	110 107 105	110 106
III	67	66	65.5	66	65	67	65.5	66	87	87	67	65.5	65.5
IIIa	66	56	65.2	64	59	65.5	65.2	64	67	86	66	65.2	65.2
IV	50	–	57	–	–	64.5	64	–	–	66	–	–	–
V	49.5	52	–	–	53 49.5	50.5	50.5	53	54	54	54	53	53
VI	25.5	26	26	26	30 27	31	30	29	29	29	29	29	29
VII	17.5	17.5	17.5	17	18	19.5	19	18	18	18	18	18	18

Oncogenicity, hemagglutination group (RAPOZA 1967)

00, Nononcogenic; 01, weakly oncogenic; 02, oncogenic
A multiple pattern of electrophoretic bands is indicated by two or three figures at one position in the table

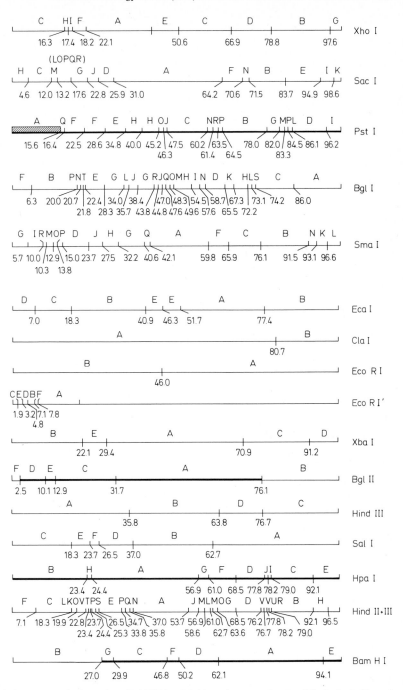

Fig. 1. Restriction maps of adenovirus S16 DNA. *Solid* bars in maps for *Bam*HI, *Pst*I, *Bgl*II, and *Hpa*I mark the fragments of the genome cloned in bacteria in plasmids. Restrictase designation is on the right. The oncogene position is marked by ▨. The size of the intact S16 genome is taken as 100%

Analysis of the data on the sequence of the left-terminal fragment in different adenoviruses (TOOZE 1980) showed the first eight nucleotides to manifest considerable variability even in different isolates of the same virus species. The S16 inverted repeats are the longest among other adenoviruses and consist of 192 nucleotides (E.A. Skripkin, unpublished data).

4 Cloning and Replication of S16 DNA

In most experiments studying the cell-adenovirus system, and in the analysis of the structural-functional organization of adenovirus genomes, individual fragments of viral DNA are used which are obtained by the action of enzymes – specific endonucleases. The problem of generating sufficiently pure isolated fragments of adenovirus DNAs in preparative amounts may be solved only with the help of recombinant plasmids carrying individual sequences of viral DNA. We created (see Fig. 1) recombinant plasmids containing all the internal fragments of *Bam*HI and *Bgl*II as well as complete sets of the *Pst*I and *Hpa*I fragments of S16 genome. At the same time, complete gene libraries of S5 and S8 were obtained. Both GC connectors and the linker method after removal of the terminal protein (NARODITSKY et al. 1983) were used for cloning of terminal fragments.

Of special interest are the plasmids carrying the left-terminal fragment of DNA with oncogene (10–12% of total genome). The recombinant plasmid carrying the A *Pst*I fragment of S16 DNA transforms rat embryo cells with formation of transformation foci and synthesis of virus-specific T antigen indistinguishable from that in the cells transformed by the left-terminal fragment of S16 genome not subjected to cloning in bacteria. We have also cloned oncogenes of simian viruses S5 and S8 (NARODITSKY et al. 1983).

The left-terminal part of S16 DNA with oncogene both isolated from viral DNA directly and after cloning in bacteria may be used in cotransformation experiments conducive to integration of heterogenous DNA. This effect was first described (TIKCHONENKO et al. 1981 b) in transformation of cells with a mixture of S16 DNA fragments obtained after hydrolysis by restriction endonucleases. The experiments of this kind demonstrated integration, along with the oncogene, of all the other adenovirus DNA fragments physically not connected with it. When heterogenous DNA such as pBR322 plasmid was added to the transforming mixture, it also integrated with the cell genome, although its frequency of integration was markedly lower than that of the oncogene and other fragments of adenovirus DNA. It is noteworthy that judging from the results of blotting experiments (TIKCHONENKO et al. 1981 b) and cloning of DNA of transformed and cotransformed cells (N.M. Chaplygina, unpublished results), all fragments of the mixture, including the heterogenous DNA, are integrated in close proximity to each other. The reasons for this phenomenon have not yet been elucidated, but in our case they are not associated with the presence of an excess of carrier DNA (see HANAHAN et al. 1980). The effect of cotransformation of heterogenous DNAs has also been described in conventional genetic transformation, for instance in the case of TK gene, but experiments of this kind require the use of special cells defective in the product of the transforming gene, in this case TK⁻ (BACCHETTI and GRAHAM 1978; MAITLAND and McDOU-GALL 1977; HANAHAN et al. 1980). The system of cotransformation based on the use of oncogenes seems to be much simpler. Recently, using this method, we cotransformed rat embryo cells with S16 encogene and human hepatitis B virus genome (POTEBNYA et al. 1983). Unlike conventional transformation by adenoviruses, S16 among them, cotransformation by S16 DNA hepatitis B virus genome produced transformed cells which grew poorly and continuous lines could heardly be derived from them. The cotransformed hepatitis B virus genome in the resulting continuous line AH-2 (Table 2) was detected in very small amounts in the first passages (approximately 0.1 genome/diploid cell genome), and in later passages disappeared from the cells completely (T.I. Kalinina, and A.L. Gartel, unpublished data). One gains an impression that the combined presence of some parts of S16 and hepatitis B genomes were incompatible with transformed cell viability, and that DNAs of the latter were rapidly eliminated. Nevertheless, rat cells cotransformed in this way had a very high degree of oncogenicity, which was unusual even for such a highly oncogenic virus as S16 (see above). The simultaneous lack of hepatitis B virus genome in AH-2 cells in late passages but retention of their abnormally high oncogenicity may be explained either by random selection of a record oncogenic line of transformed cells or by cocancerogenesis proceeding from the hit-and-run hypothesis. The latter seems quite probable for viruses of the type of hepatitis B virus which produce tumors (liver cirrhosis) but possess no oncogeneses of their own (DEINHARDT and OVERBY 1982). Studies on both the possibilities are under way.

An extract of green monkey kidney cells preinfected with adenoviruses was prepared for the study of S16 DNA replication in vitro using our modification of the method of CHALLBERG and KELLY (1979). In the presence of Mg^{2+}, ATP, and NTP the nuclear extract of adenovirus-infected cells can support replication of exogenous adenovirus matrix (MIROSHNICHENKO et al. 1982). The synthesis is semiconservative and occurs only on the matrix of the DNA-protein complex. The lack of replication in an extract from uninfected cells or on the free DNA matrix confirms the necessity of participation in replication of one or several proteins coded for by virus genome, primarily by its E2B region (STILLMAN et al. 1981; NAGATA et al. 1982). The results of examinations of the reaction products indicate that the newly synthesized polynucleotide chains of S16 are not bound covalently with the matrix and contain terminal protein. The replication system obtained from monkey kidney cells by a number of kinetic parameters and high nuclease activity differs from the system obtained from human infected cells described in the literature (CHALLBERG and KELLY 1979; REITER et al. 1980). Because of the abortive reproduction cycle of human adenoviruses in monkey cells, of great interest is the use of DNA-protein complexes of human adenoviruses of various serotypes as matrices for replication in our system. The DNA-protein complexes of Ad1 and Ad5 (group C) and Ad3 (group B) replicated effectively in our system in vitro. These experimental results and the data on normal initiation and rate of replication of human adenovirus DNA in simian cells in vivo (REICH et al. 1966; HASHIMOTO et al. 1973) indicate both great similarity in the mechanism of synthesis of human and simian adenovirus DNA and similar function of homologous parts of genome of different adenoviruses. Inverted terminal repeats of adenoviruses are known to contain two regions: AT-rich (the first 50–52 base pairs) and GC-rich (the next 50–100 base pairs). Human adenovirus DNA and S16 in positions 9–22 have a similar sequence of bases: 5′ ...ATAATATACCTTAT...3′. Three more regions have from three to six similar nucleotide pairs (TOOZE 1980; E.A. Skripkin, unpublished data). The sequence from the 5′ end to the 14th nucleotide in S16 is conservative and similar to human adenoviruses, Ad2 in particular (STILLMAN et al. 1982). Within the less conservative GC region, all human adenoviruses and S16 have the sequence GGGCGG at least once within a terminal repeat. Apparently the presence of homologous sequences in AT- and GC-rich domains permits human adenovirus DNA replication in extracts of monkey cells infected with S16. Similar data were recently obtained by STILLMAN et al. (1982) for DNA-protein complexes of human adenoviruses of different serotypes and a system from Ad2-infected HeLa cells. That such an assumption is justified is indirectly proved by our reverse experiment – replication of S16 DNA-protein complex in extracts from Ad1-infected HeLa cells (MIROSHNICHENKO et al. 1982).

5 Protein Component

5.1 Classification of Simian Adenoviruses by Protein

In general, virion proteins of simian adenoviruses are similar to those of human adenoviruses differing in size, serological specificity, and in a number of cases in the capacity for doubling of electrophoretic bands (see below). Thus, according to KHILKO et al. (1983), double or multiple bands are typical of polypeptide II and in some cases polypeptides V and VI of many simian viruses (Table 4). A similar picture was previously described for proteins V and VI of human Ad12 and Ad18 (WADELL 1979; TARODI et al. 1982). As this phenomenon is regularly reproducible in some human and simian viruses, it may serve a classification marker.

Based on the analysis of virion proteins V, VI, and VII, Table 4 presents classification of simian adenoviruses into six subgroups (1, 2a, 2b, 3a, 3b, and 4). At the same time, it shows characteristics of virion polypeptides II, III, IIIa, and IV (KHILKO et al. 1983). Previously, classification in the subgenus of simian viruses was based on serological and hemagglutinating properties of the virus and late and early virus proteins with due regard to oncogenicity (RAPOZA 1967; HULL et al. 1965; BURNETT et al. 1972). According to this classification, 16 virus species were divided into four subgroups, the fourth containing the only member, the strongly oncogenic S16, which is incapable of agglutinating red blood cells of rhesus monkeys and guinea pigs.

In our studies (KHILKO et al. 1981, 1983), we used for classification of 13 species of simian adenoviruses the simplest and most readily available method, i.e., polyacrylamide gel electrophoresis of virion proteins, successfully used previously by WADELL (1979) for classification of human adenoviruses. Human and simian adenoviruses were found to be similar in the general pattern of interspecies variability of structural proteins (polypeptide size and capacity for doubling of electrophoretic bands). Most variable are capsid polypeptides II, III, and IIIa, and therefore the whole set of size of these proteins may be used for identification of virus species. At the same time, the set of sizes of internal polypeptides V, VI, and VII, characterized as in human adenoviruses by considerable conservatism, may be used to divide simian adenoviruses into six subgroups. Subgroup 4 containing S16 and its variant S16P by the set of sizes of internal proteins V–VII, is evidently close to the subgroup 3b but differs from it markedly by the lack of hemagglutination and by strong oncogenicity. At the same time, the subgroup 4 differs from other strongly oncogenic adenoviruses, S5 and S8 in to group 3a, in the sizes of all three internal proteins.

5.2 Hexon and Hexon Gene

Hexon size in different species of simian adenoviruses varies greatly, from the maximum of 138 kd for S13 to the minimum of 100 kd for S6 (Table 4). As stated above, however, along with such interspecies differences, polypeptide II of eight species is also characterized by differences in electrophoretic mobility leading to multiplicity of bands of this protein (Table 4 and Fig. 2). Multiple electrophoretic zones of hexon polypeptides do not result from artifact proteolysis, because an identical pattern of zone distribution is observed with hexons isolated from mature virions and from a pool of free excess hexons in late stages of infection (GRIGORIEV et al. 1983b). At the same time, diffferent clones of one virus, S16 in particular, are capable of producing individual variants of hexon polypeptide. Thus, uncloned populations of S16 of different origin (S16-I and S16-II) contain three or four electrophoretic zones of polypeptide II in different ratios (Fig. 2). Two major bands of S16-I and S16-II hexon have apparent sizes of 110 and 113 kd and 106 and 110 kd respectively, and minor bands of hexons of the same two populations have sizes of 106 and 108–113 kd respectively. In different S16 clones isolated in our studies the variety of hexon polypeptides decreased or even disappeared completely. Thus clone KB230 had the only band of polypeptide II with a molecular weight of 106 kd, and clone MBI, along with a major band of 113 kd, had one minor band with an apparent size of 110 kd. Only clone 47 had two hexon bands of equal intensity, with apparent sizes of 106 and 110 kd, remaining unchangeable upon repeated cloning (GRIGORIEV et al. 1983b). The tests of quantitative neutralization of infectivity of clones MBI and KB230 and original wild-type populations were found to be identical, indicating the similarity of species-(type-)specific antigenic determinants. At the same time, competitive radioimmunoassay revealed subtle differences between S16-I hexon and clone KB230, attesting to differences in subspecies-specific determinants (GRIGORIEV et al. 1983b). These

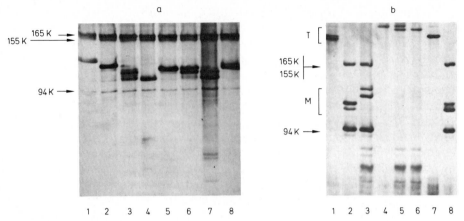

Fig. 2a, b. Electrophoresis of hexon of the wild type and clones and variants of S16
a Analysis of monomeric hexon polypeptides of different SI6 clones. Twelve percent polyacrylamide gel, staining with ammonia silver (KHILKO et al. 1983). Into each lane internal markers are added, their positions are indicated by *arrows:* subunits of *E. coli* RNA polymerase (155 and 165 kd) and phosphorylase A of rabbit kidney (94 kd). Lanes: *1,* H6 hexon; *2, E. coli β*-galactosidase; *3,* S16-II wild-type hexon; *4,* S16 clone KD230 hexon; *5,* S16 clone MBI hexon; *6,* S16-I wild-type hexon; *7,* S16 clone K47 hexon; *8,* S16 variant P hexon.
b Comparison of electrophoretic mobilities of monomeric and native trimeric hexon. Ten percent polyacrylamide gel. Lanes 2, 3, and 8 contain the same internal markers, as in **a**, indicated by *arrows.* Lanes *1, 2,* SI5 hexon; *4,* HI hexon; *6,* H5 hexon; *7, 8,* wild-type SI6-II hexon; *3, 5,* mixture of HI and H5 hexon. Before electrophoresis hexon preparations were incubated in the dissociation buffer (LAEMLI 1970) for 5 min at 100 °C (lanes *2, 3,* and *8*) or 20 °C (lanes *1, 4, 5, 6,* and *7*). The positions of monomeric (*M*) and trimeric (*T*) hexons are indicated by braces

differences corresponded to differences in oligopeptide maps of hexon in clones KB230 and MBI and differences in the physical map of the hexon region of the genome (VILNIS et al. 1981; LOPAREV et al. 1981).

The initiating triplet of gene II of S16 polypeptide is located at a distance of 60 base pairs to the right of the *Eca*I site and the terminating triplet at a distance of 70 nucleotides to the left of the *Sma*I site in the D *Bam*HI fragment (Fig. 1). Thus the hexon gene of this virus is located in the region corresponding to 50.8–59.0 units of the physical map (NARODITSKY et al. 1983). All the ten additional restriction sites present in clone KB230 DNA as compared with MBI clone were located in a small region corresponding to 52–59.6 units of the physical map, coinciding completely with the region of the hexon gene location. The heteroduplex analysis (Fig. 3) of two clone genomes by electron microscopy of hybrid molecules confirmed that the location of the heterology region corresponds to the location of the hexon gene (LOPAREV et al. 1981; MAKHOV et al. 1981). The oligopeptide maps of hexons of KB230 and MBI clones obtained with chemotrypsin indicated differences in the number and position in the map of at least six oligopeptides out of 50 spots found in the chemotryptic hydrolysate of MBI protein (TARASISHIN et al. 1981, 1982). From all these data it may be assumed that significant differences in the primary structure of the hexon polypeptide in some way affect the size of plaques formed

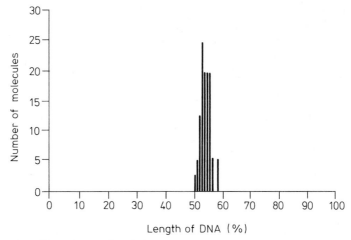

Fig. 3. Histogram of location of heterology regions in heteroduplex MBI/KB230 DNA, constructed according to the data of electron microscopy in 50% formamide. (Loparev et al. 1981a)

in the lytic infection induced by the two S16 clones. The mechanism of this phenomenon remains obscure.

Thus analysis of the data concerning hexons of different species and clones of adenoviruses convinces us that changes in the hexon structure occur widely in the virus population. Since hexon is the main adenovirus antigen responsible for induction of protective antibodies and virus neutralization by immune sera, this variability within the species should enhance the viability of the virus in its fight against the host immune system (Tooze 1980).

However, the multiplicity of hexon polypeptides found even in the preparations of a well-cloned virus, for example S16 clone K47 in Table 1, is due not only to multiple variants of the hexon gene, but also to the features of the post-translation processing of hexon and/or splicing and translation of its mRNA (Khilko et al 1981, 1983; Chaika et al. 1983). Although the formation of hexon protein seems not to be associated with widely known types of modification such as proteolysis, phosphorolysis, or glycosylation (Ginsberg 1979), there is still some indirect evidence in favor of some, as yet unknown, kind of modification of polypeptide II in the process of its maturation. Thus in the above-mentioned experiments by Khilko et al., only one species of polypeptide II was synthesized in cell-free translation in vitro of S16-I wild-type hexon mRNA or in pulse labeling in vivo, whereas after longer labeling in vivo multiple electrophoretic bands of hexon appeared characteristic of the protein component of the wild type (Chaika et al. 1983). Post-translation modification of unestablished nature could have been the cause of electrophoretic multiplicity of bromyanide polypeptides of human Ad2 hexon in the experiments of von Barr-Lindstrom et al. (1982). It is possible that such modification, occurring in the infected cell and absent in protein synthesis systems in vitro, is one of the reasons for the lack of trimer assembly from hexon polypeptides synthesized in a cell-free system (Cepko and Sharp 1982; Chaika et al. 1983). The postulated post-translation modification of the hexon structure could have occurred in parallel with the assembly of its trimer form or in its transport to the nucleus (CEPKO and SHARP 1982; GAMBKE and DEPPERT 1983). In any case, denaturation of hexon trimers to monomer polypeptides is irreversible (GRIGORIEV et al. 1983).

The indefinite or incomplete process of modification of hexon polypeptides is naturally manifested by the presence of bands with different electrophoretic mobility; in certain adenovirus clones (S16–K47) this feature is manifest at the level of phenotypic characteristic of the clone (GRIGORIEV et al. 1983). Despite the difference in the electrophoretic mobility of monomeric polypeptides II with different degrees or types of modification, upon their assembly into a trimer, trimeric hexons with either similar or different electrophoretic mobility may be formed (Fig. 2). The former variant is observed with S16-K47 clone, where in the presence of two types of monomeric polypeptide chains with apparent sizes 106 and 110 kd, only one kind of trimer hexon is formed. The latter circumstance may indicate that the parts of polypeptide II differing in their structure and conditioning the multiplicity of electrophoretic bands in the formation of capsomer happen to be in its internal regions and have no effect on the electrophoretic mobility of the trimer form. This is observed in S15 (KHILKO et al. 1981, 1983), where there are different types of trimer hexon and monomeric forms of polypeptide II differing in electrophoretic mobility. Thus the existence of two sources conducive to the multiplicity of electrophoretic forms of hexon polypeptides may be assumed from our own data and those from the literature.

5.3 Fiber

Fiber of human adenoviruses is known to contain type-specific, subgroup-specific, and intersubgroup-specific antigenic determinants, the spectrum of the determinants in human adenoviruses of different subgroups differing considerably (NORRBY 1969; WADELL and NORRBY 1969). Radioimmunoassay (RIA) of the fiber of simian adenovirus S16 showed ^{125}I-labeled fiber to be effectively precipitated not only by the homologous serum, but also by serum to simian adenoviruses S5 and S15, as well as by 30–40% by antiserum to human Ad6

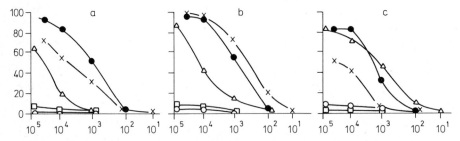

Fig. 4a–c. Competitive RIA of S16 fiber antigenic determinants. *Abscissa,* amount of protein (μg); *ordinate,* % competition. Conditions for RIA as described by TARASISHIN et al. (1982). In all cases ^{125}I-labeled S16 purified fiber was used. Competing preparations – disrupted virions: S16 (–●–●–); S5 (–x–x–); H6 (–o–o–). **a** S16 fiber – antiserum to S16 fiber (dilution 1:10000); **b** S16 fiber – antiserum to S5 (dilution 1:1000); **c** S16 fiber – antiserum to H6 (dilution 1:100)

(TARASISHIN et al. 1983). A detailed analysis of these cross-reacting antigenic determinants of S16 was performed by means of competitive RIA. The data presented in Fig. 4 indicate the presence in the fiber of this virus of the type-specific (Fig. 4a), intersubgroup-specific (Fig. 4b), and group-specific (Fig. 4c) antigenic determinants. Of special interest is the detection in S16 fiber of the most conservative group-specific antigenic determinant common for human and simian adenoviruses. The content of some antigenic determinants in S16 fiber is different: the content of type-specific antigenic determinants is highest and that of group-specific antigenic determinants is lowest.

5.4 Terminal Protein

This protein covalently bound to the 5′ phosphate group of human adeno virus DNA, is also present in simian adenoviruses S5 and S16 (DYACHENKO et al. 1981). The molecular weight of the terminal protein (55 kd) and the peptide maps of these proteins in simian adenoviruses examined were found to be similar to those of human adenoviruses. The similarity of terminal protein in human and simian adenoviruses once again confirms the high degree of conservatism of the 55-kd polypeptide due to the role ascribed to terminal proteins in the process of adenovirus DNA replication (CARUSSI 1977; REKOSH 1981; GREEN et al. 1979).

According to our data, terminal protein covalently bound to S16 DNA not only enhances the infectivity of isolated DNA preparations, but also inhibits their transforming and tumorigenic activity (PONOMAREVA et al. 1979a, b; GOLDBERG and PONOMAREVA 1981). This inhibiting effect was found not to be associated with either a decreased permeability of cell membrane for DNA-terminal protein complex as compared with free deproteinized DNA in transfection experiments (GRAHAM and VAN DER EB 1973) or the presence of any inhibitor in preparations of DNA with terminal protein (TIKCHONENKO et al. 1981c). A mixture of equal amounts of free DNA and DNA-terminal protein complex induced the same number of transformation foci as the equal amount of the former preparation. Thus the inhibiting effect of the terminal protein on the transforming and tumorigenic action of adenovirus DNA most likely occurs by the cys-mechanism associated with difficult integration of viral DNA in which the 5′-end is blocked by terminal protein. The inhibition was observed even when transformation was done by the left-terminal fragment of S16 DNA in which terminal protein blocks only one end of the polynucleotide chain (TIKCHONENKO et al. 1981c).

6 Summary

Three individual clones isolated from the original population of S16 adenovirus differ in plaque size, lytic cycle, virus yield, primary structure and processing of hexon, and degree of oncogenicity. The features of transformation and induction of tumors by S16 virions and intact and fragmented DNA are described. In transformed hamster cells the S16 genome undergoes deletion like nononcogenic human viruses, and in transformed rat cells intact virus genomes are found, as with strongly oncogenic human Ad12, but in both cell species the genome is present in a small number of virus copies. A convenient system of cotransformation providing for integration of heterogenous DNAs into cell genome has been developed on the basis of S16 oncogene.

A cell-free system has been derived from S16-infected green monkey cell nuclei, providing conditions for in vitro replication of simian and human adenovirus genomes complexed with terminal protein.

The biochemical, biophysical, and physicochemical parameters of S16 virions, DNA, and proteins are described. A system of classification of simian adenoviruses is proposed on the basis of electrophoretic mobility of virion proteins of 13 simian adenoviruses under study. The factors determining the phenomenon of multiplicity of electrophoretic bands of hexon protein have been studied. Data on the immunochemistry and biochemistry of fiber and terminal protein are presented, and inhibition by the latter protein in complex with DNA of the transforming and tumorigenic activity of DNA is described.

References

Alstein AD, Sarycheva DF, Dodonova NN (1967) Transforming activity of green monkey SA7 (C8) adenovirus in tissue culture. Science 158:1455–1456

Bacchetti S, Graham FL (1978) Transcription of viral sequences in cell transformed by adenovirus 5. Virology 89:347–359

Burnett JP, Harrington JA (1968) Simian adenovirus SA7 DNA: chemical, physical and biological studies. Proc Natl Acad Sci USA 60:1023–1029

Burnet JP, Mayne N, Butler LK, Harrington JA (1972) Chemical and physical relationship of oncogenic and non-oncogenic simian adenovirus DNA. J Gen Virol 17:245–253

Carusi EA (1977) Evidence for blocked 5' termini in human ad enovirus DNA. Virology 76:380–390

Cepko CL, Sharp PA (1982) Assembly of adenovirus major capsid protein is mediated by a nonvirion protein. Cell 31:407–415

Chaika OV, Khilko SN, Grigoriev VG, Komarov YuS, Ponomareva TI, Tikchonenko TI (1983) Physical, chemical and immunochemical properties of in vitro synthesized structural proteins of simian adenovirus S16 (SA7) (in Russian) A Biokhymia (USSR) (in press)

Challberg MD, Kelly TJ (1979) Adenovirus DNA replication in vitro. Proc Nat Acatl Sci USA 76:655–659

Deinhardt F, Overby LR (eds) (1982) Abstracts of the 2nd international Max V. Pettenkofer symposium on viral hepatitis. 19–22 October 1982, München

Denisova TS, Gibadulin RA (1982) Detailed study of the simian adenovirus SA7P genome and identification of its sequence in transformed cells (in Russian) 5:589–595

Dimitrov DH, Dubichev AG, Naroditsky BS, Dreizin RS, Tikchonenko TI (1979) Physicochemical properties and restriction maps of simian adenovirus type 38 DNA. J Gen Virol 44:69–80

Doerfler W, Stabel S, Ibelgaufts H, Sutter D, Neumann R, Groneber J, Schmidtmann KH, Deuring R, Winterhoff U (1980) Selectivity in integration sites of adenoviral DNA. Cold Spring Harbor Symp Quant Biol 44:551–564

Doerfler W, Gahlmann R, Stabel S, Deuring R, Lichtenberg U, Schulz M, Eick D, Leisten R (1983) On the Mechanism of Recombination Between Adenoviral and Cellular DNAs: The Structure of Junction Sites. In: Curr. Top. in Microbiology and Immunology, Vol. 109. Springer Berlin Heidelberg New York Tokyo

Dubichev AG, Dimitrov DH, Parfenov NN, Grigoriev VG, Tikchonenko TI (1979) Physico-chemical properties of adenovirus 38 type DNA (in Russian). Vopr Virusol 2:115–118

Dubichev AG, Parfenov NN, Chaplygina NM, Grigoriev VG, Dreizin RS, Tikchonenko TI (1980) Physical characteristics of simian adenovirus SA7 (in Russian). Vopr Virusol 2:180–183

Dyachenko NS, Goldberg EZ, Tarasishin LA, Naroditsky BS, Tikchonenko TI (1981) Oligopeptide mapping of terminal proteins of simian adenoviruses. In: Zhdanov VM (ed) (in Russian) Viruses of cancer and leukosis. Academy of Medical Sciences, Moscow, p 127–128

Fanning E, Doerfler W (1976) Intracellular forms of adenovirus DNA. V. Viral DNA sequences in hamster cells abortively infected and transformed with human adenovirus type 12. J Virol 20:373–383

Freeman AF, Black PH, Wolford R, Huebner RJ (1967) Adenovirus type 12 rat embryo transformation system. J Virol 1:362–367

Gallimore PH (1974) Interactions of adenovirus type 2 with rat embryo cells. Permissiveness, transformation and in vitro characteristics of adenovirus transformed rat embryo cells. J Gen Virol 25:263–273

Gambke C, Deppert W (1983) Specific complex of the late nonstructural 100,000-dalton protein with newly synthesized hexon in adenovirus type 2 – infected cells. Virology 124:1–12

Gartel AL, Chaplygina NM, Ponomareva TI, Tunnikov GI, Dreizin RS, Tikchonenko TI (1983) Analysis of sequences of simian adenovirus SA7 (C8) DNA in transformed rat cells and hamster tumour cells. J Gen Virol 64:1361–1366

Ginsberg HS (1979) Adenovirus structural proteins. In: Fraenkel-Conrat H, Wagner R (eds) Comprehensive virology. Plenum, New York, pp 409–457

Goldberg EZ, Ponomareva TI (1981) Some properties of the terminal-protein DNA complex of simian adenovirus SA7. In: Zhdanov VM (ed) Viruses of cancer and leukosis. Academy of Medical Sciences, Moscow, p 3–4 (in Russian)

Goodheart CR (1971) DNA density of oncogenic and nononcogenic simian adenoviruses. Virology 44:645–648

Graham FL, Van der Eb AJ (1973) A new technique of the assay of infectivity of human adenovirus DNA. Virology 52:456–467

Green M, Brackmann K, Wold WS, Mockey JK (1979) Conserved primary sequences of the DNA terminal proteins of five different human adenovirus groups. Proc Natl Acad Sci USA 76:4380–4384

Grigoriev VG, Khilko SN, Tikchonenko TI (1983a) The condition of stability of quaternary structure and immunoreactivity of adenoviral hexon (in Russian). Mol Genet Microbiol Virusol (USSR) (in press)

Grigoriev VG, Khilko SN, Tarassishin LA, Loparev VN, Naroditsky BS, Ponomareva TI, Tikchonenko TI (1983b) Intraspecies multiplicity of hexon polypeptide size and structure in simian adenovirus S16 (SA7). J Gen Virol (in press)

Hanahan D, Lane D, Lipsick L, Wigler M, Botchan M (1980) Characteristics of SV40-plasmid recombinant and its movement into and out of the genome of a murine cell. Cell 21:127–139

Hashimoto K, Nakajiama K, Oda K, Shinojo H (1973) Complementation of translation defect for growth of human adenovirus type 2 in simian cells by a simian virus 40-induced factor. J Mol Biol 81:207–223

Hull RN, Johnson JS, Culbertson CB, Wright HW (1965) Oncogenicity of the simian adenoviruses. Science 150:1044–1046

Kalter SS, Ablashi D, Espana C, Heberling RL, Hull RN, Lennette EH, Malherbe HH, McConnel S, Yohn DS (1980) Simian virus nomenclature. Intervirol 13:317–330

Khilko SN, Grigoriev VG, Naroditsky BS, Zolotarskaya EE, Dreizin RS, Tikchonenko TI (1981) Analysis of structural proteins of simian and human adenoviruses (in Russian). Vopr Virusol 1:48–51

Khilko SN, Grigoriev VG, Gurov AV, Fedorinov VV, Tikchonenko TI (1983) These use of polyacrylamide gel electrophoresis of virion proteins to classify simian adenoviruses. J Virol Meth (in press)

Laemmly UK (19707 Cleavage of structural proteins during the assembly of the head of bacteriophage T4. Nature 207:680–685

Loparev VN, Zavizion BA, Grigoriev VG, Vichovic EM, Naroditsky BS, Machov AM (1981) Comparative structural analysis of genomes of two clones of highly oncogenic SA7 virus (in Russian).

188   T.I. Tikchonenko

In: Zhdanov VM (ed) Viruses of cancer leucoses. Academy of Medical Sciences, Moscow, pp 88–90

Maitland NJ, McDougall JK (1977) Biochemical transformation of mouse cells by fragments of herpes simplex virus DNA. Cell 11:233–241

Makhov AM, Manykin AA, Loparev VN, Naroditski BS, Klimenko SM (1981) Heteroduplex analysis of simian adenovirus genomes (in Russian). Thesis of the II Conference on electron microscopy. Kishinev, pp 148–149

McAllister RM, Riggs GL, Reed C, Macpherson T (1969) Transformation of rodent cells by simian adenovirus SA7. Proc Soc Exp Biol Med 131:1442–1445

Miroshnichenko OI, Naroditski BS, Ponomareva TI, Tikchonenko TI (1982) Synthesis of SA7 and Ad5 adenovirus DNAs in the nucleus extract of the green monkey cells (in Russian). Mol Biol 16:782–789

Nagata K, Guggenheimer RA, Enomoto T, Lichy JH, Hurwitz J (1982) Adenovirus DNA replication in vitro: identification on of a host factor that stimulates synthesis of the preterminal protein – dCMP complex. Proc Natl Acad Sci USA 79:21, 6438–6443

Naroditsky BS, Loparev VN, Miroshnichenko OI, Vilnis A, Potebnya GG, Tikchonenko TI, Ponomareva TI (1983) Cloning of terminal and internal fragments of some human and simian adenoviruses. (in Russian) Mol Gen Microbiol Virusol (in press)

Norrby E (1969) The structural and functional diversity of adenovirus capsid components. J Gen Virol 5:221–236

Ogino T, Takahashi M (1970) Infection of simian adenovirus SA7 in hamster kidney and embryo cells. Biken J 13:303–312

Panigraphy B, McCormick KJ, Trentin JJ (1976) In vitro transformation of rodent cells by simian adenovirus 7 and bovine adenovirus type 3. Am J Vet Res 37:1503–1504

Paraskeva C, Gallimore PH (1980) Tumorogenicity and in vitro characteristics of rat liver epithelial cells and their adenovirus-transformed derivatives. Int J Cancer 25:631–639

Pina V, Green H (1965) Biochemical studies on adenovirus multiplication. IX. Chemical and base composition analysis of 28 human adenoviruses. Proc Natl Acad Sci USA 54:547–551

Ponomareva TI, Grodnitskaya NA, Goldberg EZ, Chaplysina NM, Naroditsky BS, Tikchonenko TI (1979a) Biological activity of the intact and cleaved DNA of the simian adenovirus 7. Nucleic Acids Res 6:3119–3131

Ponomareva TI, Chaplygina NM, Naroditsky BS, Grodnitskaya NA, Dreizin RS, Tikchonenko TI (1979b) Transforming and tumorigenic activities of simian adenovirus SA7 DNA (in Russian). Bull Exp Biol Med 12:698–700

Ponomareva TI, Grodnitskaya NA, Tunnikov GI, Dreizin RS, Chaplygina NN, Naroditsky BS (1983) Transformation of rat cells by highly-oncogenic simian adenovirus SA7 and non-oncogenic human adenovirus Ad6 and analysis of established cell lines (in Russian). Vopr Virusol 3:337–341

Potebnya GP, Ponomareva TI, Struk VI, Naroditsky BS, Tikchonenko TI (1983) Biological properties of rodent cells transformed and cotransformed by SA7 simian virus under different conditions (in Russian). Vopr Virusol (in press)

Pusey PN, Koppel DE, Shafer DW, Camerini-Oteno RD, Koening SH (1974) Intensity fluctuation spectroscopy of laser light scattered by solutions of spherical viruses: R17, Qß, BCV, PM2, and T7. I. Light-scattering technique. Biochemistry 13:952–960

Rapoza NP (1967) A classification of simian adenoviruses based on hemagglutination. Am J Epidemiol 86:736–745

Reich PR, Baum SG, Rose JA, Rowe WP, Weismann S (1966) Nucleic acid homology studies on adenovirus type 7 – SV40 interactions. Proc Natl Acad Sci USA 55:336–341

Reinert KE, Strassburger J, Triebal M (1971) Molecular weights and hydrodynamic properties for homogeneous native DNA, derived from diffusion, sedimentation and viscosity measurements on polydisperse samples. Biopolymers 10:285–307

Reiter T, Futterer J, Weingartner B, Winnacker EL (1980) Initiation of adenovirus DNA replication. J Virol 35:662–671

Rekosh D (1981) Analysis of the DNA-terminal protein from different serotypes of human adenoviruses. J Virol 40:329–333

Stillman BW, Lewis JB, Show LT, Mattews MB, Smart JE (1981) Identification of the gene and mRNA for the adenovirus terminal protein precursor. Cell 23:497–508

Stillman BW, Topp WC, Engler JA (1982) Conserved sequences at the origin of adenovirus DNA replication. J Virol 44:530–537

Tarasishin LA, Khilko SN, Dyachenko NS, Naroditsky BS, Tikchonenko TI, Vanzak NP, Dreizin RS, Loparev VN (1981) The oligopeptide analysis of hexon of human adenoviruses 1, 2, 6 and simian adenovirus SA7 (in Russian). Vopr Virusol 5:574–580

Tarasishin LA, Dyachenko NS, Vanzak NP, Khilko SN (1982) Radioimmunology analysis of the simian adenovirus SA7 hexon (in Russian). Vopr Virusol 2:192–197

Tarasishin LA, Grigoriev VG, Khilko SN, Vanzak NP, Dyachenko NS (1983) Immunochemical analysis of the simian adenovirus fiber. Vopr Virusol (in press)

Tarodi B, Pusztai R, Beladi I (1982) Structural polypeptides of type 12 human adenovirus. J Gen Virol 62:379–383

Tikchonenko TI, Dubichev AG, Parfenov NN, Chaplygina NM, Dreizin RS, Zolotarskaya EZ (1979) Biophysical properties of virions of human adenovirus of the type 6 and its DNA. Arch Virol 62:117–130

Tikchonenko TI, Dubichev AG, Lybchenko YL, Kvitko NP, Chaplygina NM, Dreizin RS, Naroditsky BS (1981a) The distribution of guanine-cytosine pairs in adenovirus DNAs. J Gen Virol 54:425–429

Tikchonenko TI, Chaplygina NM, Kalinina TI, Gartel AL, Ponomareva TI, Naroditsky BS, Dreizin RS (1981b) Integration of foreign genome fragments into cell transformed or contransformed with fragmented adenoviral DNA. Gene 15:349–359

Tikchonenko TI, Chaplygina NM, Kalinin VN, Gartel AA, Kalinina TI, Ponomareva TI, Surkov VV (1981c) Interrelationship between the integration of viral genomes and cell transformation. In: SV40, polyoma and adenoviruses. The Imperial Cancer Research Fund Tumor Virus Meeting, Cambridge, p 210

Tolun A, Aleström P, Petterson U (1979) Sequence of inverted terminal repetitions from different adenoviruses: demonstration of conserved sequences and homology between SA7 termini and SV40 DNA. Cell 17:705–713

Tooze J (1980) Molecular biology of tumor viruses: DNA tumor viruses. Cold Spring Harbor Laboratory. Cold Spring Harbor

Tunnikov GI (1982) Comparative analysis of cell lines derived from tumors and transformed cells induced by SA7 and Ad6 adenoviruses (in Russian). Ph D. Thesis, Institute of Virology, Moscow

Tunnikov GI, Ponomareva TI, Dreizin RS, Karmysheva VY, Zolotarskaya EE, Chaplygina NM (1983) Analysis of cell lines derived from hamster tumors induced by SA7 virus and its DNA (in Russian). Vopr Virusol 5:607–610

Vilnis AE, Zavizion BA, Fedorinov VV, Naroditski BS, Tikchonenko TI (1981) Physical and functional mapping of SV30 and SV20 adenovirus DNA (in Russian). Latvijas PSR Zinatnu akademijas vestis 9:96–111

Von Bahr-Lindström H, Jornvall H, Althin S, Philipson L (1982) Structural differences between hexons from adenovirus types 2 and 5: Correlation with differences in size and immunological properties. Virology 118:353–362

Wadell G (1979) Classification of human adenoviruses by SDS-polyacrylamide gel electrophoresis of structural polypeptides. Intervirology 11:47–57

Wadell G, Norrby E (1969) Immunological and other biological characteristics of pentons of human adenoviruses. J Virol 4:671–680

Molecular Epidemiology of Human Adenoviruses

G. Wadell

1 Introduction

The initial experiments by Rowe and his colleagues that led to the discovery of adenoviruses also provided fundamental data on the prevalence of these agents. Surgically removed adenoids from 53 children in Washington, DC were explanted in tissue culture. After an observation period of 4 weeks, 33 of the cultures showed a slowly progressive cytopathic effect. The agent isolated from these cultures was appropriately designated the adenoid-degenerating (AD) agent (Rowe et al. 1953). An etiologic relation to acute respiratory disease (ARD) was also soon established for adenoviruses (Hilleman and Werner 1954). The two fundamental properties of human adenoviruses – the acute respiratory infection and the persistent infection of lymphatic tissue – were thus recognized at an early stage.

The expressed genetic variability within the adenovirus family has since been found to be wide. Adenoviruses have been isolated from most studied species of placental mammals, marsupials, birds, and amphibians (Wigand et al. 1982).

Department of Virology University of Umeå S-901 85 Umeå

Several adenovirus species (formerly termed serotypes) (WIGAND et al. 1982) have been recognized in each host. The actual number found mirrors the effort spent on collection and typing of isolates. In man, 31 species were identified by 1965 (PEREIRA et al. 1965), and to date 41 different species have been recognized (DEJONG et al. 1983a).

Definition of a species relies on the distinct antigenic determinants that are capable of inducing neutralizing antibodies (WIGAND et al. 1982). These are the mediators of host protection against reinfection. The species designation rests consequently on fundamental biological properties. The genome products carrying the antigenic determinants responsible for induction of neutralizing antibodies represent only a minor fraction of the viral genome. This implies that analysis of cross-reactions measured by serological techniques gives information on a few gene products only and is not necessarily representative of the relatedness of the viral genome. This point is illustrated by the cross-reaction between Ad12, Ad18, and Ad31 in neutralization tests and hemagglutination inhibition assays (HIERHOLZER et al. 1975b; WIGAND and KELLER 1978), although the DNA homology between these types is only 48–69% (GREEN et al. 1979). Ad 40 and Ad 41 cannot be distinguished by hemagglutination inhibition (DEJONG et al. 1983a), although they are members of different subgenera, F and G (UHNOO et al. 1983). Furthermore, Ad4 and Ad16, which are members of subgenera E and B, respectively cross-react in neutralization tests (NORRBY and WADELL 1969; WADELL 1979).

All adenovirus strains that have obtained the same species designation are not identical (ROWE et al. 1958; WADELL and VARSANYI 1978). It is therefore pertinent to discuss species designation versus the genome type concept.

DNA restriction site analysis or genome typing can be used to ascertain the genetic variation within the species [WADELL and VARSANYI 1978; WADELL et al. 1981a (Ad7); BRUCKOVA et al. 1980 (Ad5); WADELL and DEJONG 1980 (Ad19); WADELL et al. 1980a (Ad4); Fujinaga and Hierholzer, personal communication (Ad8)].

The genome type concept i.e., the identification of distinct viral entities by DNA restriction site analysis, offers a chance to follow the epidemiological distribution of these viruses in time and space and allows comparison of their pathogenic and other biological features. The distinct genome types within a defined adenovirus species originally identified by DNA restriction analysis can also be differentiated by the use of specific monoclonal antibodies (DEJONG, personal communication; Ad40 and Ad41). A similar distinction can be obtained using solid-phase immunoelectron microscopy (SPIEM) (SVENSSON and VON BONSDORFF 1982).

2 Classification of the 41 Human Adenoviruses into Seven Subgenera

Several parameters have been used to classify human adenoviruses into subgenera. ROSEN (1960) originally proposed three groups, I–III, based on different hemagglutination of rat and rhesus monkey erythrocytes. Although the portion of the genome coding for the receptor binding sites on the adenovirus fiber represents only a very limited portion of the total adenovirus genome, several other biological properties are shared by adenoviruses grouped together according to Rosen. An elaborate system for subdivision of the human adenovirus species on the basis of differential hemagglutination properties has been proposed (WADELL 1970; HIERHOLZER 1973).

HUEBNER (1967) suggested that human adenoviruses be divided into subgenera on the basis of their oncogenicity for newborn hamsters. Subgenera A and B comprise adenovirus species that are "highly" oncogenic and "weakly" oncogenic respectively. The nononcogenic adenoviruses that can transform rodent cells in vitro are divided into subgenera C and D on the basis of differences in the antigenicity of the T antigen (MC ALLISTER et al. 1969). This classification is compatible with subdivision of adenoviruses according to the GC content of their genomes, although members of subgenera C and D could not be distinguished by their GC content (PINA and GREEN 1968; GREEN 1970).

The polypeptides of the virion represent the main portion of products of the adenovirus genome (BROKER et al. 1982). With the rationale that internal polypeptides are expected to be evolutionarily conserved and offer means to classify adenoviruses, we have examined the polypeptide pattern of 41 human adenovirus species and found that they can be divided into seven subgenera (Table 1). This method was compatible with the previous methods for classification of human adenoviruses, and extended these as regards Ad4 and the newly identified, enteric Ad40 and Ad41 (WADELL 1979; WADELL et al. 1980a).

An ultimate classification of viruses in general should be based on nucleotide sequence differences between genomes of different viral entities. The DNA homology of adenoviruses has been studied by filter hybridization (GREEN 1970), heteroduplex mapping (GARON et al. 1973), and liquid hybridization (GREEN et al. 1979). This classification was in complete agreement with the data obtained by classification on the molecular weight of the internal structural polypeptides of the virion (WADELL 1979; WADELL et al. 1980a).

In view of distinct differences in GC content in DNA of adenoviruses belonging to subgenera A (47–49%), B (49–52%), and C, D, and E (57–59%), we analyzed the DNA restriction pattern obtained with an $SmaI$ endonuclease which cleaves DNA at 5′ CCC GGG.

The $SmaI$ DNA restriction patterns of the 41 human adenovirus species have been determined (Table 1, Fig. 1). The following points were noted: (a) The limited range of the number of $SmaI$ fragments of the adenovirus genomes was characteristic for each subgenus. (b) The restriction patterns of the genomes of adenoviruses belonging to the same subgenus displayed several comigrating restriction fragments. This was not the case for adenoviruses belonging to subgenus A, due to the heterogeneity of their genomes and the low number of $SmaI$ fragments which characterized this subgenus. (c) Use of up to ten different DNA restriction enzymes revealed that in pairwise comparisons of two members of the same subgenus, more than 50% of the DNA restriction fragments comigrated, whereas analogous pairwise comparison of the genomes of adenoviruses classified into two different subgenera revealed less than 10% comigrating DNA

Table 1. Properties of human adenovirus subgenera A to G

Sub-genus	Species	DNA			Apparent molecular weight of the major internal polypeptides			Hem-agglu-tination pattern[c]	Oncogenicity in newborn hamsters
		Homo-logy (%)[a]	G+C (%)	Number of *Sma*I frag-ments	V	VI	VII		
A	12, 18, 31	48–69 (8–20)	48	4–5	51 to 51.5K 46.5 to 48.5K[d]	25.5 to 26K	18K	IV	High (tumors in most animals in 4 months)
B[e]	3, 7, 11, 14 16, 21, 34, 35	89–94 (9–20)	51	8–10	53.5 to 54.5K	24K	18K	I	Weak (tumors in few animals in 4–18 months)
C	1, 2, 5, 6	99–100 (10–16)	58	10–12	48.5K	24K	18.5K	III	nil
D[e]	8, 9, 10, 13, 15, 17, 19, 20, 22, 23, 24, 25, 26, 27, 28, 29, 30, 32, 33, 36, 37, 38, 39	94–99 (4–17)	58	14–18	50 to 50.5K[f]	23.2K	18.2K	II	nil
E	4	(4–23)	58	16–19	48K	24.5K	18K	III	nil
F	40	n.d.	n.d.	9	46K	25.5K	17.2K	IV	nil
G	41	n.d.	n.d.	11–12	48.5K	25.5K	17.7K	IV	nil

n.d., not done

[a] Per cent homology within the subgenus. Figures in brackets: homology with members of other subgenera
[b] The restricted DNA fragments were analyzed on 0.8–1.2% agarose slab gels. DNA fragments smaller than 400 bp were not resolved
[c] I, Complete agglutination of monkey erythrocytes; II, complete agglutination of rat erythrocytes; III, partial agglutination of rat erythrocytes (fewer receptors); IV, agglutination of rat erythrocytes discernible only after addition of heterotypic antisera
[d] Polypeptide V of Ad31 was a single band of 48K
[e] Only DNA restriction and polypeptide analysis have been performed with Ad32 to Ad39
[f] Polypeptides V and VI of Ad8 showed apparent molecular weights of 45K and 22K respectively. Polypeptide V of Ad30 showed an apparent molecular weight of 48.5K

restriction fragments. This tentative rule is not valid for subgenus A, and subgenus B is divided into two clusters of DNA homology when the rule is applied.

This procedure for subdivision of adenoviruses and identification of newly identified adenovirus species has been of value in the designation and classification of the recently detected species [WIGAND et al. 1980 (Ad36); WADELL et al. 1981b (Ad37); HIERHOLZER et al. 1982 (Ad39); WADELL et al. 1980a (Ad40); UHNOO et al. 1983 (Ad41)]. The detailed information on homologies between

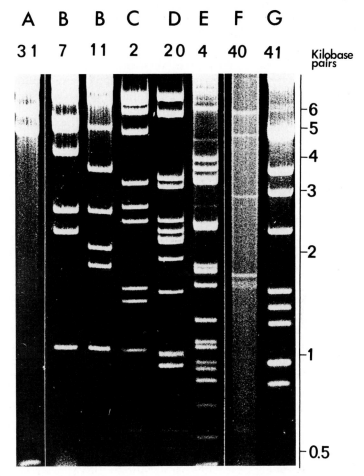

Fig. 1. DNA restriction patterns obtained after digestion of DNA from adenovirus species representing subgenera A to G with *Sma*I. The DNA fragments were separated by electrophoresis in 1.2% agarose slab gels

related genomes obtained by use of sequence specific endonucleases is second only to that from nucleotide sequence analysis.

A simplified dot-blot hybridization procedure for assigning adenovirus strains to the different subgenera has been suggested by SUZUKI et al. (1981).

3 Epidemiology of Human Adenoviruses

The global distribution of adenoviruses can be evaluated by analysis of the prevalence of antibodies and/or the frequency of isolation of adenovirus strains. Providing that an adenovirus infection results in a lifelong immunity that can be detected in extensive surveys for antibodies in different age-groups, screening for adenovirus-specific antibodies should give reliable information on the prevalence of adenovirus infection in different settings. It is pertinent to decide whether it is of interest to determine an immune response to adenoviruses in general or a species-specific immunity. Most mammalian adenoviruses share group-specific antigen that can be detected by complement fixation or enzyme-linked immunosorbent assay (ELISA). Naturally, species-specific assays have to be applied to obtain information on the prevalence of individual species.

Certain pitfalls have to be considered. The complement fixation test has frequently been used to assay prevalence of antibodies against adenoviruses, but complement-fixing antibodies usually need to be boosted if they are to persist for longer periods. Particularly in infants, the complement fixation reaction is highly inefficient in detecting an immune response to adenoviruses (Fox et al. 1977). It is our experience that ELISA should be preferred in detection of adenovirus group-specific antibodies. Serum neutralization assays are cumbersome but a most efficient means of detecting species-specific antibodies against a given adenovirus. This method is also efficient in screening the antibody response in infants (VAN DER VEEN 1963; Fox et al. 1977; KIDD et al. 1983).

Human adenoviruses cause eye disease and infections of the respiratory, gastrointestinal, and urinary tracts. Occasionally systemic infections, including spread to the CNS, are noted. Information on the contribution of human adenoviruses to viral respiratory disease is available in an extensive record of reports to the World Health Organization from 1967 to 1976 (WHO 1980). During this period adenoviruses accounted for 17771 of a total of 135702 reported isolations. Adenoviruses were second only to influenza A, which represented 28% of the reported isolates. Respiratory syncytial virus (RSV), parainfluenza viruses, *Mycoplasma pneumoniae,* and enteroviruses accounted for 12%, 10%, 10%, and 8% respectively.

A stratification of the reported adenovirus isolations by age revealed the following number of isolates per age-group: 3589 (<1 year); 6706 (1–4 years), 3027 (5–14 years); 1800 (15–24 years); 1117 (25–59 years) and 215 (>60 years).

This means that adenovirus isolations are reported at a rate second only to RSV from children below 14 years of age, 13592 adenovirus isolates versus 14694 isolates of RSV. There is, however, a clear distinction in age-dependent isolation frequency between the two virus groups. The majority of the RSV strains (8813) were isolated from 1-year-old children, whereas most of the adenovirus strains came from 1- to 4-year-old children (6706 isolates).

Acute respiratory diseases account for 20% of all deaths among children. The importance of adenoviruses in this context is not clear. As the highest mortality for this group of diseases is reported for infants below 1 year of age, RSV may have a higher impact than adenoviruses on mortality in this age-group.

The expressed genetic variability of adenoviruses is wide. It is therefore feasible to discuss the epidemiology and medical impact of the human adenoviruses as a function of their classification into subgenera. If not stated otherwise, all figures on isolation frequencies of human adenoviruses refer to the isolates typed and reported to WHO from 1967 to 1976 (WHO 1980). This record has been analyzed by ASSAD et al. (1974) and SCHMITZ et al. (1983).

3.1 Subgenus A

Ad12, Ad18, and Ad31 were infrequently reported representing only 144 strains of the 24184 reported typed adenovirus isolates. The members of subgenus A are distinguished from the other adenovirus species by three characteristics: (a) the majority of the isolates was obtained from infants (0–11 months old); (b) 91% of the reported isolates were recovered from stools; and (c) 60% of the children had gastrointestinal disease (SCHMITZ et al. 1983). It is difficult to evaluate a putative etiologic association to diarrhea in the absence of information on serological response in the children shedding adenoviruses of subgenus A. Infections with subgenus A members are relatively common. An extensive study on serum neutralization (SN) antibody prevalence in children in Rome revealed that the prevalence of antibodies against Ad31 and Ad18 was second only to that of those against the members of subgenus C and Ad3, whereas infections with Ad12 were less common (D'AMBROSIO et al. 1982).

The analysis of DNA restriction patterns is particularly advantageous in the identification of Ad12, Ad18, and Ad31, since they cross-react in both SN and hemagglutination inhibition (HI) assays (HIERHOLZER et al. 1975; WIGAND and KELLER 1978). It is highly likely that Ad31 isolates have frequently been mistyped as Ad12, since Ad31 was not described until 1965 (PEREIRA et al. 1965) and can be neutralized by sera against Ad12. This may also explain some of the heterogeneity within the Ad12 species demonstrated by GREEN et al. (1979).

3.2 Subgenus B

DNA restriction analysis of the eight species grouped into subgenus B clearly indicates that two clusters of DNA homology exist (Fig. 2) (WADELL et al. 1980a). The B:1 cluster contains Ad3, Ad7, Ad16, and Ad21, the B:2 cluster includes Ad11, Ad14, Ad34, and Ad35.

3.2.1 DNA Homology Cluster 1

3.2.1.1 Isolation Frequency

The members of the B:1 cluster are predominantly associated with respiratory infections. Ad3 and Ad7 account for 13% and 19.7% respectively of all adenovirus isolates typed and reported to WHO. Thus during the 10-year period covered by the WHO report, every third adenovirus isolate was reported as Ad3 or Ad7. Both species show an epidemic appearance (Fig. 3) (early literature on Ad7 reviewed in WADELL et al. 1980b, 1981a). Ad7 was the most frequently isolated adenovirus species during 1973 and 1974, when the number of Ad7 infections reported was three times as high as during the interepidemic years (SCHMITZ et al. 1983). In the WHO material, the peak incidences of Ad3 were less conspicuous. However, if the information is broken up on the number of isolates reported from each country, it is obvious that Ad3 can appear in epidemic patterns at 4- to 5-year intervals (Fig. 4).

Hind III

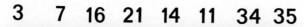

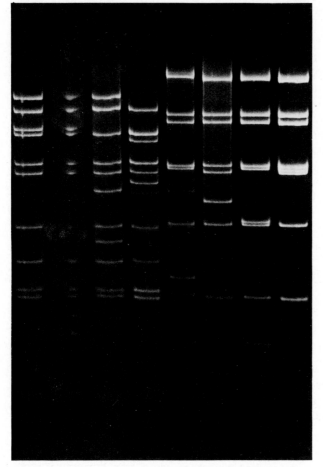

Fig. 2. Comparison of the genomes of adenovirus species belonging to subgenus B. Agarose slab electrophoresis was performed after restriction with *Hind*III

The age-specific incidence of adenovirus infections is usually presented for the following age groups: 0–11 months, 1–4 years, 5–14 years, and adults. Note that the information is presented as the number of isolates per population. The number of individuals in each stratum is naturally larger in the higher age groups, influencing the calculation of an age-specific incidence.

Both Ad3 and Ad7 are commonly isolated from all age groups up to 14 years but in particular from children below the age of 4. The number of reported Ad7 infections in adults is high – 18% of the total number of reported adenovirus infections. It is likely that reports from outbreaks among military recruits contribute to this figure.

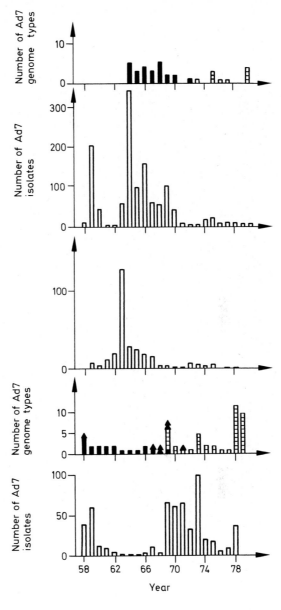

Ad7 (▼)   Ad7a (▲)   Ad7b (□)   Ad7c (■)

Fig. 3. The reported Ad7 isolates typed in Europe 1958 through 1978. Data presented from top to bottom, come from Sweden (Prof. Böttiger), the GDR (Prof. Starke), and the Netherlands (Dr. deJong). Ad7 strains from Sweden and from the Netherlands were genome-typed

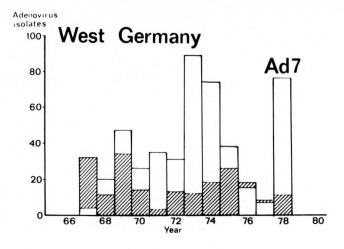

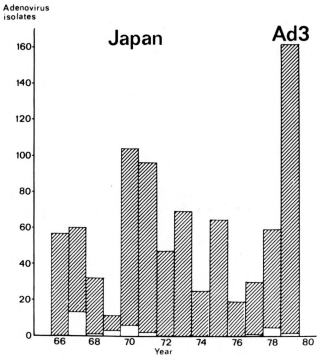

Fig. 4. Distribution of Ad3 and Ad7 strains isolated in West Germany (Dr. Knocke) and Japan (Dr. Kono) since 1966. Ad3 and Ad7 isolates are represented by *hatched* and *unfilled* columns respectively

3.2.1.2 Acquisition of Specific Immunity

Most studies of the prevalence of adenovirus antibodies have been performed with techniques that detect group-specific antibodies, such as complement fixation and ELISA. Species-specific immune response has been measured by SN or HI assays.

In an early study of Cleveland children, it was demonstrated that they acquired antibodies to Ad1 and Ad2 of subgenus C earlier than they were exposed to Ad3 and Ad7 (JORDAN et al. 1958). In the Netherlands Ad7-specific antibodies were detected in sera from umbilical cords, 4- to 5-year-old children, and adults in 40%, 15%, and 30% of cases, respectively (VAN DER VEEN 1963). In Japan, Ad7-specific antibodies were detected in 30% of children and in 50% of adult sera (TAI and GRAYSTON 1962). Ad3-specific antibodies were detected in 30% and 70% of the children and in 50% and 90% of the adults in the USA and Japan respectively (FOY and GRAYSTON 1976).

Antibody prevalence and the frequency of Ad7 isolations can be highly discordant. In Japan, 1628 adenovirus isolates were typed from 1966 to 1979. Only 2% of the adenovirus strains were typed as Ad7, whereas 52% of the isolates were typed as Ad3. All the Ad7 isolates in Japan were obtained from healthy carriers or from sporadic cases of pharyngoconjunctival fever (R. Kono, personal communication).

The incidence of Ad3 and Ad7 infections in Europe is exemplified by West Germany, where 1849 adenovirus isolates were typed and reported during the period 1967–1978. Ad3 and Ad7 accounted for 11% and 25%, respectively, of the total number of typed isolates (K.W. Knocke, personal communication).

It is obvious that the isolation frequency is influenced by the severity of the virus-associated disease prompting an isolation attempt and also by the tendency of the virus strain to cause persistent infections with shedding of infectious virus over extended periods, even years.

3.2.1.3 Molecular Epidemiology of Ad3 and Ad7

DNA restriction site analysis of the Ad7 isolates with BamHI, EcoRI, HpaI, HindIII, and SmaI revealed five Ad7 genome types; Ad7 prototype (BERGE et al. 1955), Ad7a, identified by ROWE et al. (1958), Ad7b, Ad7c (WADELL and VARSANYI 1978; WADELL et al. 1981a), and Ad7d, identified in China (Figs. 5, 6). A regional difference in the distribution of adenovirus genome types may, if they differ in virulence have contributed to the discordance between antibody prevalence and isolation frequency of Ad7 in Japan.

The distribution of the different Ad7 genome types obtained since 1958 has been analyzed in isolates from the different continents. In Europe a preponderance of the Ad7c and Ad7b genome types was noted. Only one Ad7 prototype strain and seven Ad7a strains were found among 123 Ad7 isolates. A longitudinal study on Ad7 strains collected in the Netherlands from 1958 to 1980 revealed that Ad7c circulated from 1958 to 1969, whereas Ad7b was not isolated until 1969 (WADELL et al. 1981a). A similar pattern was noted in Sweden, but Ad7b did not appear until 1972 (Fig. 3) (WADELL et al. 1981a).

A longitudinal study was also undertaken from 1958 to 1980 on Ad3 strains isolated in Sweden and the Netherlands. Only the Ad3 prototype was found in Europe, with the exception of two strains designated Ad3a isolated in 1963 and 1979 (Fig. 7).

The relative distribution of the Ad3 and Ad7 genome types has since then been analyzed in isolates from all continents, albeit so far in limited numbers. In Australia, the "European pattern" with a preponderance of the Ad3 proto-

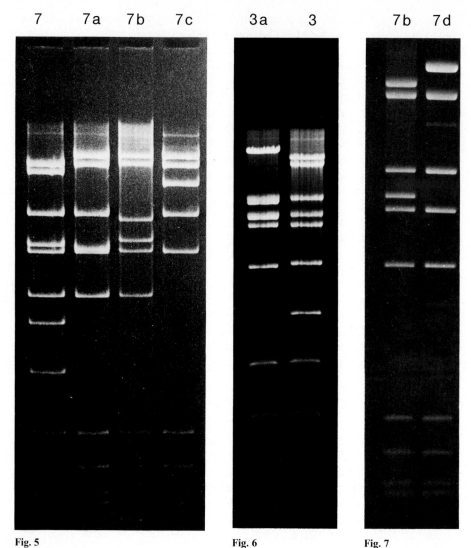

| 7 | 7a | 7b | 7c | 3a | 3 | 7b | 7d |

Fig. 5   **Fig. 6**   **Fig. 7**

Fig. 5. DNA restriction patterns of four Ad7 genome types obtained after cleavage with *Bam*HI. *Ad7* is the prototype strain Gomen

Fig. 6 and 7. DNA restriction patterns of the Ad3a, Ad3, Ad7b and Ad7d genome types obtained after cleavage with *Bam*HI

type and Ad7b was noted and the shift from Ad7c to Ad7b took place in 1975. The Ad7 prototype was detected in Australia as well as in Japan (Fig. 8).

    The Ad7 strains from USA were obtained from the Virus Watch program in Seattle, military recruits in San Francisco, and an outbreak of Ad7 infections in San Diego (STRAUBE et al. 1983). In China, a fifth Ad7 genome type, Ad7d, was identified that has not been found elsewhere. In South Africa, one Ad7b

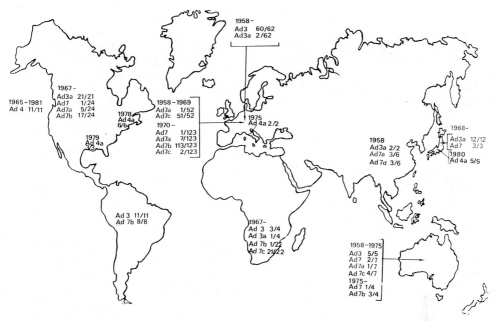

Fig. 8. The global distribution of Ad3, Ad7, and Ad4 genome types identified among wild-type isolates collected since 1958

strain was isolated in 1967 and Ad7c strains have been identified ever since. This means that Africa, China, and Japan are the only regions where Ad7b has not been detected in recent years.

Six of the 25 Ad7 and Ad7a strains were isolated from hosts without symptoms, whereas only two of the 142 Ad7b strains were shed from asymptomatic hosts. All the 88 Ad7c and the three Ad7d strains were isolated from sick persons. We suggest that the high prevalence of Ad7 antibodies in Japan and the exceedingly low incidence of reported Ad7 infections, which are sporadic and mild (R. Kono, personal communication), is due to an effective circulation of the Ad7 prototype, which is assumed to be of lower virulence than the Ad7b genome types.

DNA restriction analysis is indispensable in evaluation of the pathogenicity of Ad7 strains. A report on a fatal Ad7 pneumonia in a military recruit who died 15 days after administration of a live Ad7 vaccine illustrates an urgent need to genome-type the Ad7 strains from the index case and from contemporary isolates obtained from the basic training center in order to evaluate the pathogenicity of the live Ad7 vaccine (LOKER et al. 1974).

The Ad3a genome type was detected in both China and Japan; the only other region where it predominated was North America. The Ad3a isolates were obtained through the Virus Watch program in Seattle (Dr. Cooney) and from military recruits in San Francisco (Col. Smith). One additional Ad3a strain originated from a CSF isolate collected in Nova Scotia 1962. (FAULKNER and VAN ROOYEN 1962). Japan has the highest known prevalence of Ad3 infections in the world. Ad3a frequently causes clinical illness, and for this reason Ad3 is by far the most frequently isolated adenovirus species in Japan. It cannot be excluded that Ad3a was introduced to North America immigrants of Asiatic origin. It is pertinent to analyze the genome type of the adenovirus strains that have been reported to be associated with severe hyperlucent lung disease among Canadian Indian and Eskimo children of less than 2 years of age (SPI-GELBLATT and ROSENFELD 1983).

Ad21 can cause severe respiratory disease in children (LANG et al. 1969). The incidence is unknown but may be low. A study of SN antibody prevalence among Italian children (D'AMBROSIO et al. 1982) revealed that children aged 9–12 years displayed 7–20% antibody positivity when tested against Ad14, Ad21, Ad7 and Ad4. Such a low antibody prevalence could explain the out-breaks of respiratory disease among military recruits, that characterizes all these four adenovirus species. By 1976 Ad21 had been isolated from military recruits at all major U.S. Army basic training centers (TOP et al. 1976), prompting the introduction of a live enteric-coated Ad21 vaccine (TAKAFUJI et al. 1979).

3.2.2 DNA Homology Cluster 2

Ad11, Ad14, Ad34, and Ad35 account for less than 1% of all reported adenovi-rus isolates (SCHMITZ et al. 1983). There is a clear male preponderance among infected hosts. The prevalence of antibodies against Ad11 among Italian children is around 2% (D'AMBROSIO et al. 1982).

Ad11 can cause hemorrhagic cystitis (NUMAZAKI et al. 1968; MUFSON et al. 1973) and may be shed in urine after kidney transplantation with or without symptoms (LECATSAS et al. 1974), or during pregnancy (Gardner, personal com-munication). Ad34 and Ad35 were both originally isolated from renal transplant recipients (HIERHOLZER et al. 1975; STALDER et al. 1977). They were recently isolated from urine specimens from 10/10 AIDS patients (DEJONG et al. 1983b), which is remarkable in view of the fact that isolation reports on these two species are rare. Ad11, Ad34, and Ad35 are closely related on the genome level (Fig. 2) (WADELL et al. 1980a). They apparently form a group with a predilection for infections of the kidney and possibly of the urinary tract. Occa-sionally a kidney from a Ad11-seropositive donor can transmit Ad11 infection to the seronegative kidney transplant recipient (HARNETT et al. 1982). Ad14 is different, although falling within DNA homology cluster 2 and has been reported to cause outbreaks of respiratory disease among military recruits (VAN DER VEEN 1963).

3.3 Subgenus C

The subgenus C members account for 59% of all adenovirus isolates reported to WHO. Relative frequencies have been recorded of 25.4% for Ad2, 20.4% for Ad1, 11% for Ad5, and 2.4% for Ad6. They have been regarded as endemic adenoviruses but distinct epidemics do occur, although they do not show up in the WHO records where information from all reporting countries is a cumulated (SCHMITZ et al. 1983). BRUCKOVA et al. (1980) described an outbreak of a virulent Ad5a genome type in Czechoslovakia. Infections with subgenus C members are most frequent in children under the age of 4 years and rarely isolated among adults (SCHMITZ et al. 1983).

The prevalence of antibodies against three of the members of subgenus C is high but distinctly dependent on regional and social conditions. In Junior Village (Fox and HALL 1980) the antibody prevalence was 50% and 70% for Ad1 and Ad2 respectively by 2 years of age. The maximum antibody prevalence reached 80% for Ad1 and Ad2 and 50% for Ad5 in the 6–9 age-group. In Panama the HI antibody prevalence was 48%, 35%, and 27% for Ad2, Ad1, and Ad5 respectively in the 1–4 age group and 75%, 70% and 40% in a teenage group (Fox and HALL 1980).

In Stockholm a slow build-up of immunity was noted. The SN antibody prevalence for Ad2, Ad1, and Ad5 was 27%, 15%, and 8% respectively in the 1–3 age-group and 71%, 24%, and 27% respectively in the 9–12 age-group (STERNER 1962).

Estimation of the incidence of infection from isolation frequencies or antibody prevalence can be difficult, especially in the case of members of subgenus C. This problem was elegantly treated by Fox and COONEY in the Virus Watch program from New Orleans, New York, and Seattle (Fox et al. 1969, 1977). It was demonstrated that adenoviruses can be shed over periods up to 703 days. Adenovirus shedding was frequently intermittent, and reinfections may occur. Infants have been identified as the most frequent introducers of infection into the family, which is logical since infants are most susceptible to infection. These studies, which are the only elaborate, lucid analyses available, also demonstrated that 47–55% of all adenovirus infections resulted in no illness or in illness so slight that it escaped attention. Information on the contribution of adenovirus infection to illness was also gained, since 58% of the children infected with adenoviruses in Seattle were detected by serology alone. It was concluded that the true contribution of adenoviruses could be double that usually estimated on the basis of virus isolation alone. (Fox and HALL 1980). Clinical features of infections caused by the members of subgenus C are upper and lower respiratory tract disease and gastrointestinal illness (SCHMITZ et al. 1983). Furthermore, subgroup C members are the predominant causative agents in acute intussusception among children (NICOLAS et al. 1982).

An association of the subroup C members with the pertussis syndrome has been discussed. NELSON et al. (1975) reported that 39% of Bordetella-positive persons shed adenoviruses, compared to 14% shedding among Bordetella-negative persons ($p < 0.001$). Similar data were reported by KELLER et al. (1980). These observations may be evidence for reactivation of latent adenovirus infection by the Bordetella infection. A synergism between the adenovirus and the pertussis infection has also been proposed (KLENK et al. 1972). The role of adenoviruses in the pertussis syndrome is still not understood.

The mechanism of persistent infection which allows the prolonged shedding of the adenoviruses is not known. The demonstration of the frequent occurrence of Ad2 genome in tonsils from healthy children by DNA-DNA hybridization (EGGERS et al. 1978) is a thought-provoking follow-up to the original experiments of ROWE et al. (1953).

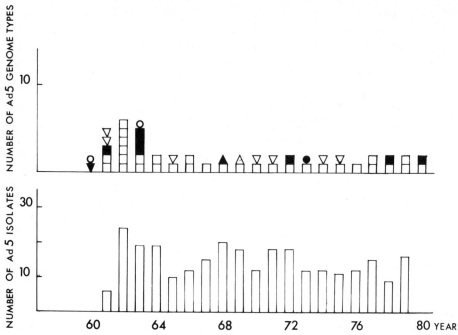

Fig. 9. Distribution of Ad5 isolates collected in the Netherlands since 1960 (Dr. deJong). Eight different genome types were identified after cleavage with *Bam*HI and *Eco*RI endonucleases

These observations may lead us to the tonsils or Peyer's patches as putative sources of the adenoviruses in the shedding children. Association with tonsils and adenoids appears to be unique to adenoviruses of subgenus C, although Ad6 is underrepresented (VAN DER VEEN and LAMBRIEX 1973).

Their high prevalence, their propensity to establish persistent infections, and their pronounced homology on the DNA level are all properties that facilitate recombination between members of subgenus C. Recombination has also been demonstrated experimentally by SAMBROOK et al. (1980).

We have, together with J.C. de Jong, performed a longitudinal study of Ad5 strains isolated in the Netherlands from 1958 to 1981. Restriction of DNA from 58 Ad5 virus strains by *Eco*RI and *Bam*HI has revealed eight different genome types (Fig. 9).

The Ad5 prototype was not isolated during this period in Holland. The Ad5a genome type (BRUCKOVA et al. 1980) accounted for 60% of all the isolates. Heterogeneity within Ad5 had previously been demonstrated by BRANDT et al. (1966), using the biological properties of a subtype of Ad5 which was identified by cross-reactivity in HI with Ad1. The pronounced variability of subgroup C members is not limited to Ad5, but has also been demonstrated for the other members of the subgroup (SAMBROOK et al. 1980); G. Wadell, unpublished observations). We therefore conclude that the expressed genetic variability within subgenus C is larger than within subgenus B, since five Ad7 genome types were identified among 258 Ad7 isolates.

3.4 Subgenus D

Subgenus D displays the largest expressed genetic variability, including more than half of all recognized human adenovirus species. However, infections with members of subgenus D are only infrequently reported to WHO; only 4.1% of all reported isolates belong to this subgenus (SCHMITZ et al. 1983). It has to be emphasized that the reporting system to WHO is strongly biased towards European and North American laboratories. The global situation for infections with members of subgenus D is consequently not adequately described.

Ad8 is the classical causative agent of epidemic keratoconjunctivitis (JAWETZ 1959) and accounts for half of all the reported isolates of members of subgroup D. Ad19 was originally isolated in 1955 but did not appear as a causative agent until 1973; it has since then contributed substantially to the adenovirus-associated cases of keratoconjunctivitis. In 1976 a new virus was identified, first as an intermediate strain (SCHAAP et al. 1980), then as a new adenovirus species, Ad37 (DEJONG et al. 1981; WADELL et al. 1981). This virus is associated with keratoconjunctivitis and is in some cases sexually transmitted.

A recent paper on the relative occurrence of Ad8, Ad19, and Ad37 in the USA clearly emphasizes that they are predominant pathogens of adenovirus associated eye disease in that country (KEMP et al. 1983).

The prevalence of antibodies against members of subgenus D is very low in Europe. In a study of SN antibodies among children in Rome, 2% or less had antibodies against Ad8 or Ad19 (D'AMBROSIO et al. 1983). Fifteen percent of adult Germans were immune to Ad19 (JUNG and WIGAND 1967).

In Zaire, however, the prevalence of antibodies against Ad19 is 85% (DESMYTER et al. 1974). It is furthermore clear that prevalence of antibodies against Ad8 is high in Taiwan and Japan, where Ad8 also appears in regular seasonal outbreaks (GRAYSTON et al. 1964). In Sapporo, adenoviruses were demonstrated to cause 39% of the viral infections of patients treated at an eye hospital in the period 1974–1979 (AOKI et al. 1981).

Molecular Epidemiology. At least two different genome types of Ad8 have been identified in Japan (FUJII et al. 1983). Their global distribution has not yet been acertained. The Ad19 prototype has not been found in isolates in Europe or in the United States, whereas the Ad19a genome type was originally detected in five patients from Holland and Belgium in 1973 and 1974 (WADELL and DEJONG 1981). Ad19a has now been demonstrated to occur among a number of isolates in the United States (KEMP et al. 1983). Several early Ad37 strains were at first misrepresented as Ad19 and later properly identified with the use of DNA restriction or homotypic sera in the SN reaction (KEMP et al. 1983). Subgenus D is characterized by numerous intermediate strains identified by the presence of SN and HI determinants from different species of human adenoviruses (WIGAND and FLIEDNER 1968). It should also be possible to distinguish these variants by means of restriction analyses. Ten different intermediate strains of subgenus D all showed unique restriction patterns (Wadell et al., unpublished).

3.5 Subgenus E

This subgenus accommodates only one human adenovirus species, Ad4. Ad4 is rarely isolated from children in Europe and the United States; it was isolated from four children out of 1800 with proven adenovirus disease (BRANDT et al. 1968). Ad4 has been a significant cause of outbreaks of respiratory disease among military recruits, prompting the development of a live Ad4 vaccine (TAKAFUJI et al. 1979). It accounts for 2.4% of the isolates reported to WHO with a preponderance of isolates obtained from adults only superseded by the members of subgenus D. Ad4 strains can be isolated from the respiratory tract, ocular specimens, stools, and urine (GUTEKUNST and HEGGIE 1964). There is a clear-cut difference in clinical picture between Ad3 and Ad4, causing conjunctivitis, and Ad8 and Ad19, causing more severe keratitis and preauricular lymphadenopathy (AOKI et al. 1982).

The prevalence of antibody against Ad4 in the Netherlands has been 50% in new borns, 25% among 4- to 5-year-olds (VAN DER VEEN 1963). The prevalence of Ad4-specific antibodies among adults is 30%, 50%, and 60% in the USA, Japan, and Taiwan respectively (FOY and GRAYSTON 1976).

DNA restriction analysis has revealed two genome types of Ad4: the Ad4 prototype and Ad4a (WADELL et al. 1980a). These two genome types are strikingly dissimilar; only 50% of the analyzed DNA restriction fragments comigrate (Fig. 10). All 15 Ad4 isolates recovered from military recruits in California from 1965 through 1981 were identidied as the Ad4 prototype. However, all 12 Ad4 strains from children in Japan were identified as the Ad4a genome type (Fig. 8).

It is of particular interest that Ad4a has been identified in three outbreaks of eye disease. Acute hemorrhagic conjunctivitis with a subconjunctival hemorrhage was observed in Rome in 1974 (MUZZI et al. 1975).

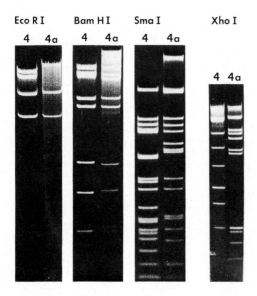

Fig. 10. The restriction patterns obtained after cleavage of the Ad4 prototype and Ad4a genome type with *Eco*RI, *Bam*HI, *Sma*I, and *Xho*I

In 1977 a 5-year-old boy died with disseminated Ad4 infection after treatment in an intensive care unit in Buffalo. A nosocomial outbreak of pharyngoconjunctival fever affecting 35 of his attendants and other personnel at the hospital resulted (FADEN et al. 1978). All 6 Ad4 strains were genome-typed as Ad4a (Fig. 8). A similar nosocomial outbreak of Ad4 conjunctivitis was reported from Chicago in 1981. In this case nine attendants to a patient with fatal Ad4 pneumonia developed conjunctivitis (LEWANDOWSKI and RUBENIS 1981). We have furthermore identified 3/3 eye isolates of Ad4 from Atlanta as Ad4a.

It was reported as early as 1964 (GRAYSTON et al. 1964) that Ad4 may cause conjunctivitis without respiratory symptoms. Outbreaks of Ad4-associated eye disease have recently been frequently described (TULL and HIGGINS 1980; AOKI et al. 1981, 1982). This may indicate a real increase in incidence. Only seven Ad4 strains associated with eye disease were reported to the WHO register from 1967 to 1976 (SCHMITZ et al. 1983). Furthermore, AOKI, reporting a consecutive study in a ophthalmology clinic in Sapporo, found no Ad4 strains from 1974 to 1977 and 33 Ad4 isolates in 1979 and 1980, Ad4 being second only to Ad8 as a cause of viral conjunctivitis. TULLO reports from Bristol 113 Ad4-associated cases of conjunctivitis during 7 months in 1978 (TULLO and HIGGINS 1980).

Ad4 is the adenovirus species that has been suggested to be most closely related to a putative common archetype of human adenoviruses (WADELL et al. 1980). This suggestion is based on the following reasoning: Subgenus E contains only one member, Ad4. Ad4 displays an immunological cross-reactivity on the hexon level with Ad16 of subgenus B (NORRBY and WADELL 1969) and also on the vertex capsomer level with several members of subgenus B (WADELL and NORRBY 1969). In addition, hyperimmune sera against Ad4 virion cross-react with exposed epitopes on the surface of virions of Ad40, a member of subgenus F (SVENSSON et al. 1983). Ad4 forms dodecons which are characteristic of members of subgenera B, D, and E only (NORRBY 1966; GELDERBLOM et al. 1967). The length of the Ad4 fiber is intermediate between members of subgenera C and D (WADELL et al. 1967; NORRBY 1969). The Ad4 fiber shows immunological cross-reactivity with fibers of members of both these subgenera (WADELL and NORRBY 1969). The hemagglutination properties of Ad4 are characteristic for members of subgenus C (WADELL 1969). The immunological reactivity of the tumor antigen originally justified a classification of Ad4 within subgenus B (HUEBNER 1967).

Furthermore, hyperimmune sera against members of subgenera A to E all cross-reacted with early antigens of Ad4, whereas early antigens of all other tested adenoviruses showed a restricted cross-reactivity (GERNA et al. 1982). Comparative DNA restriction analysis revealed that chimpanzee adenoviruses Pan 5, Pan 9, and Y 25 all showed similarity to Ad4 to such a degree that they could be classified within the human subgenus E (WADELL et al. 1980). The human adenoviruses can be classified into subgenera on the basis of the apparent molecular weight of the internal polypeptides of virions (WADELL 1979). Pan 5, Pan 9, and Y 25 are grouped within subgenus E also on the basis of this criterion (Wadell, unpublished).

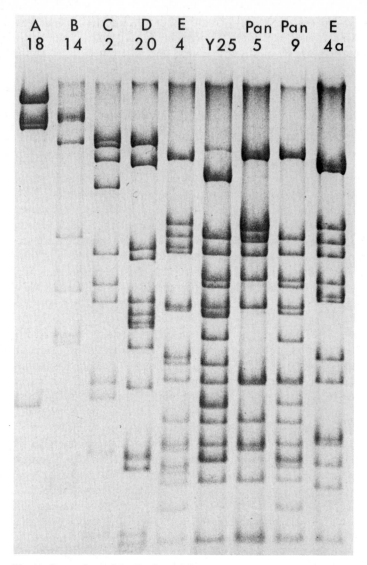

Fig. 11. Comparison of the *Sma*I restriction patterns of three chimpanzee adenoviruses, Y 25, Pan 5, and Pan 9, with adenovirus species representing the human subgenera A to E

If we expect that a common ancestor of human adenoviruses should display a wide cross-reactivity with the evolving species, then Ad4 is a potential candidate. If we then postulate a divergent evolution, a junior member of an adenovirus subgenus could be expected to show a lower degree of cross-reactivity with members of other subgenera. In the case of Ad4a this remains to be determined. It will be possible to determine if the suggested relation between Ad4 and other adenoviruses still holds true after comparison on the nucleotide level.

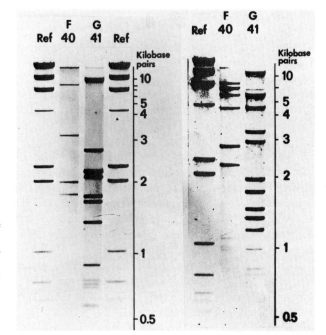

Fig. 12. Comparison of the *Hin*dIII and *Bgl*I restriction patterns of Ad40 (subgenus F) and Ad41 (subgenus G). Lambda DNA cleaved with *Hin*dIII and ØX 174 DNA cleaved with *Hinc*II were used as molecular weight references

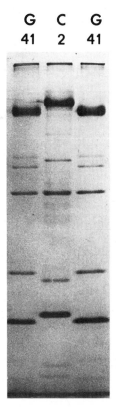

Fig. 13. SDS-polyacrylamide gel electrophoresis of virion polypeptide of Ad41 (subgenus G) and Ad2 (Subgenus C). The composition of separation gel was 15% acrylamide and 0.18% *bis*-acrylamide

3.6 Subgenera F and G

The enteric adenoviruses Ad 40 and Ad 41 are the only members of subgenera F and G respectively (Figs. 12 and 13). They were first demonstrated by FLEWETT et al. (1975), SCHOUB et al. (1975), and WHITE and STANCLIFF (1975) using electron microscopy. They are shed in large amounts – 10^{11} virus particles/g feces from children with diarrhea. They differ from all other adenoviruses in that they are fastidious and cannot be propagated in human embryonic kidney (HEK) cells and human diploid fibroblasts.

Ad41 undergoes complete replication in line 293 cells, an HEK cell line immortalized by transfection with Ad5 DNA containing the EIA and EIB regions (TAKIFF et al. 1981), but also in Hep2 and Chang conjunctiva cells, and some strains grow in tertiary cynomolgus cells (tCMK) (DEJONG et al. 1983).

Ad40 is efficiently replicated in primary to tertiary monkey kidney cells (DEJONG et al. 1983a) and grows in line 293 cells (DEJONG et al. 1983), but not in Hep2 or Chang conjunctiva cells.

Ad40 and Ad41 have been detected in stool specimens from Europe (JACOBSSON et al. 1979; JOHANSSON et al. 1980; KIDD et al. 1981; DEJONG et al. 1983), North America (RETTER et al. 1979; GARY et al. 1979), and Asia (DEJONG et al. 1983; Wadell, unpublished).

Around 50% of 6- to 8-year-old children from Africa, Asia, and Europe displayed SN antibodies to either Ad40 or Ad41, with no clear-cut difference in prevalence between the different populations (KIDD et al. 1983).

3.6.1 Clinical Features

An association between enteric adenoviruses and infantile diarrhea has been suggested (BRANDT et al. 1979), but also questioned (MADELEY et al. 1977). It was therefore pertinent to ascertain whether enteric adenoviruses had an etiological role in infantile diarrhea. A prospective study was performed 1981 in Uppsala (UHNOO et al. 1983). Almost all children (415) with diarrhea seeking treatment at the University Hospital were studied and 200 age- and season-matched healthy children were also examined. The sick children seroconverted and/or shed rotaviruses and adenoviruses in 45% and 13% of cases respectively, as compared with 3% and 1.5% in the control children. Infections with Ad40 and Ad41 respectively were identified in 15 and 19 of 49 children, whereas 15 children were infected with established human adenoviruses.

Paired serum specimens from 17 children shedding enteric adenoviruses were obtained and analyzed by the HI assay. Seroconversion was demonstrated in 70% of the serum pairs.

It was concluded that Ad40 and Ad41 are of etiologic importance in infantile diarrhea. Infections with Ad40 and Ad41 were frequently associated with diarrhea and/or vomiting. Diarrheas caused by Ad41 tended to become protracted. Infections with the established adenoviruses were associated with elevated temperature and respiratory symptoms to a higher degree than Ad40- and Ad41-associated infections (Table 2; UHNOO et al. 1983).

Table 2. Clinical findings in 49 diarrheic children excreting adenoviruses (UHNOO et al. 1983)

Clinical finding	Percentages with clinical finding		
	Ad40 (F)	Ad41 (G)	Established adenoviruses
	$(n=15)$	$(n=19)$	$(n=15)$
Vomiting	80	74	40
Fever			
37.9°–38.9°	33	26	14
>39°	27	11	73[a]
Total	60	37	87
Diarrhoea			
>8–10 times/day	60	37	20
>10 times/day	13	42	20
Total	100	94	40
Respiratory symptoms observed	27	11	73[a]

[a] $p<0.001$

4 Adenovirus Infections in the Immunocompromised Patient

The propensity of adenoviruses to cause persistent infections may create a health hazard to children with severe combined immunodeficiency (SCID), immuno-compromised individuals, and those with acquired immunodeficiency. After bone marrow transplantation, children with SCID may suffer from severe or lethal infections by adenoviruses of subgenera A, B:2, or C (Brigati, personal communication and SOUTH et al. 1982).

A prospective study on the etiology of the severe enteric infections in 78 bone marrow recipients (mean age 21 years) was performed from September 1980 to June 1981 in Baltimore by YOLKEN et al. (1982). Adenoviruses were found in 12 of the 31 cases in whom enteric pathogens could be identified. The mortality among infected and uninfected patients was 55% and 13%, respectively ($p<0.001$). The rate of graft versus host disease was higher in the infected patients, but the difference was not statistically significant. Six of the patients died within 11 days of their first positive stool culture for an enteric virus. Five of these six patients were infected with adenovirus. Unfortunately these adenovirus isolates were not typed, nor was any information on serologic response to adenoviruses presented.

A retrospective study of 15 immunocompromised patients in whom adeno-virus was isolated at the UCLA Center for Health Sciences during the period 1967–1978 was reported by ZAHRADNIK et al. (1980). All had high temperature (<39°), and pneumonia, elevated liver enzymes, and diarrhea were seen in 80%, 73%, and 33% respectively. Nine of the adenovirus-infected patients died. Ad4, the most common species, was isolated from five patients, all adults. Three of these five died during the acute illness. Ad4 was isolated from blood, buffy-coat, or urine in four of the five, indicating a disseminated infection. Adenovirus species of subgenus C were isolated from five patients, one adult and four teenagers or children. Three died during the acute illness. Ad7 and Ad11 infection subsides only very slowly. Ad11 was shed to urine over the course of 5 months. A prolonged shedding of Ad11 of similar length has been observed in a healthy woman during pregnancy and after delivery (Gardner, personal communication). It should again be pointed out that Ad11 is closely related to Ad34 and Ad35, which were recently isolated from 10/10 patients with AIDS (deJong et al. 1983b).

Teng has reported from Beijing that Ad3 and Ad7 infection following measles can cause very severe pneumonia, with 55% mortality among 6-month-old hospitalized children Teng (1960).

Adenovirus species subgenera A. B:2, and C, with predilections for persistent infections, should be expected to cause protracted infections in the immunocompromised host. Evidently members of the other subgenera may also be incriminated when the normal virus-host relation is disturbed. Information on the epidemiology of adenovirus infections in the immunocompromised host is, however, still scarce. The above-cited investigations suggest that adenovirus infections may substantially contribute to morbidity and mortality in these patients. There is consequently an urgent need for extensive prospective studies to ascertain the rate of primary or reactivated infections involving the different adenovirus species in the immunocompromised host.

5 Concluding Remarks

The collection of reports on adenovirus infections registered by WHO since 1967 and analyzed by Assad and Cockburn (1974) and Schmitz et al. (1983) is highly valuable, representing a source of information on the yearly frequency of adenovirus isolations, age and sex distribution, seasonal variation, occurrence in specimens from different body sites, association with clinical syndromes, and fatality.

The presentation of the yearly frequency of adenovirus isolations is based on cumulative information from the reporting laboratories. This may hide information on epidemic outbreaks in individual countries or limited regions. This point is best illustrated by the epidemiology of Ad3- and Ad7-associated infections. It is obvious that both Ad3 and Ad7 cause defined epidemic outbreaks (Fig. 3) in different countries. Ad7-associated outbreaks occurred in the Netherlands in 1958–1959 (Ad7c) and in Sweden in 1959; in the GDR in 1963, followed by a peak in Sweden in 1964; in the Netherlands in 1969 with a new genome type (Ad7b); in large outbreaks of Ad7b in England, the FRG, and the Netherlands in 1973 and 1974; and in a new peak of Ad7b infections in 1978 and 1979 in the same countries (Fig. 4; Wadell et al. 1980b).

It is obvious, but should be underlined, that it is not the occurrence of adenovirus but rather the frequency of adenovirus isolations that is reported to the WHO register.

It is evident that information on several different adenovirus entities (genome types) is by definition registered under one and the same adenovirus species. This may again obscure information on the nature of the adenovirus infection. This point is illustrated by Ad4, where a chance distribution of clinical symptoms in children and in adults was noted (SCHMITZ et al. 1983). This would not have been the case if information on the different Ad4 genome types had been registered. The adenovirus species within the same subgenus often show properties allowing general statements pertaining to the subgenus.

Subgenus A. The members frequently cause inapparent infections in infants. They are predominantly shed in stools and may cause diarrhea.

Subgenus B:1. The members may appear in epidemic outbreaks of conjunctivitis and or respiratory disease with fever. Ad7 appears in three epidemic patterns (WADELL et al. 1980b): (a) severe, at times fatal infections in children below the age of 2 years, usually in winter; (b) respiratory infection with favorable outcome among schoolchildren, with peak frequency during August and September; and (c) epidemic outbreaks of respiratory disease among military recruits. Ad3 has a lower tendency to cause respiratory disease among military recruits than Ad7, presumably due partly to a higher herd immunity against Ad3 among young adults (FOY and GRAYSTON 1976).

Subgenus B:2. With the exception of Ad14, members are characterized by a predilection for shedding via the urine. This may be protracted, and can occur with or without symptoms. Subgenus B:2 members are rarely isolated. A recent report on frequent shedding of Ad34 and Ad35 in AIDS patients (DEJONG et al. 1983b) heralds an upsurge of interest in these anonymous adenovirus species.

Subgenus C. Subgenus C viruses infect adenoids and tonsils persistently and are shed via stools over years. They are frequently associated with gastrointestinal disease, but serological confirmation is of particular importance to establish etiological relationships for the subgenus C members. They have a high incidence of infection in small children, with a preponderance in the winter months (SCHMITZ et al. 1983).

Subgenus D. Subgenus D members are characterized by severe eye infections, in particular among children in the southern hemisphere; infection of adults predominates in the northern hemisphere. Ad8 was the major cause of epidemic keratoconjunctivitis, in North America already in 1941, whereas the pathogenic Ad19a and Ad37 have appeared during the past 10 years. Shedding of subgenus D members via stool but not via the respiratory tract without symptoms is relatively common (BRANDT et al. 1968; SCHMITZ et al. 1983).

Subgenus E. Ad4 is the only human member, but several chimpanzee adenoviruses may also be classified into this subgenus. The two genome types Ad4 and Ad4a are markedly dissimilar on the genome level and may cause different syndromes. Ad4 is responsible for outbreaks of respiratory infections, predominantly among young adults, whereas Ad4a is a newly recognized agent causing conjunctivitis, frequently without respiratory symptoms.

Subgenera F and G. Ad40 and Ad41 are fastidious host-range-restricted adenoviruses which both grow in line 293 cells but not in HEK cells, an excellent substrate for the remaining 39 human adenovirus species. Ad40 and Ad41 each cause infantile diarrhea, each with unique clinical properties.

Adenovirus infections in the immunocompromised host should at last be given the consideration they have long merited.

The information gained on distribution and virulence, in particular of the Ad3, Ad4, Ad5, Ad7, Ad8, and Ad19 genome types, has demonstrated that DNA restriction endonucleases are indispensable tools in modern studies of the epidemiology of adenovirus infections.

Acknowledgments. I acknowledge the invaluable contribution of the following colleagues who shared their experience and adenovirus strains with us: M. Brůčková, Prague; C.H. v. Bonsdorf, Helsinki; C. Chany, Paris; Y. Chardonnet, Lyon; M. Cooney, Seattle; A. de Costa Linhares, Belem; J. deJong, Bilthoven; R. Faulkner, Halifax; L. Flugsrud, Oslo; S. Gardner, London; J. Hierholzer, Atlanta; T. Hovi, Helsinki; L. Irvine, Victoria; K.-F. Jen, Beijing; A. Kidd, London; R. Kono, Tokyo; M. Lagercrantz, Stockholm; G. Lecatsas, Pretoria; A. Mc Kenzie, Westmead; A. Nahmias, Atlanta; J. Nascimento, Rio de Janeiro; Y. Numazaki, Sendai; M. Pereira, London; S. Richmond, Bristol; M. Riepenhoff-Talty, Buffalo; M. Rosenbaum, Rockford; B. Schoub, Sandringham; C. Smith, San Francisco; R.N.P. Sutton, Manchester; M. Thompson, San Diego; M. Toth, Budapest; D. Tyrrell, Harrow; R. Wigand, Homburg; H. Willer, Hannover; S. Wolontis, Stockholm; G. Zissis, Brussels; I. Ørstavik, Oslo.

I am also grateful to Kristina Lindman, Assar Nording and Gunnar Sundell for skillful technical assistance and to Katrine Isaksson and Margaretha Lindström for excellent secreterial help.

The work performed in the author's laboratory was supported by grants from the Swedish Medical Research Council, the Swedish Agency for Research Cooperation with Developing Countries, and the World Health Organization.

References

Aoki K, Kato M, Ohtsuka H, Tokita H, Obara T, Ishii K, Nakazono N, Sawada H (1981) Clinical and etiological study of viral conjunctivitis during six years, 1974–1979, in Sapporo, Japan. Ber Dtsch Ophthalmol Ges 78:383–391

Aoki K, Kato M, Ohtsuka H, Ishii K, Nakazono N, Sawada H (1982) Clinical and aetiological study of adenoviral conjunctivitis with special reference to adenovirus types 4 and 19 infections. Br J Ophthalmol 66:776–780

Assad F, Cockburn WC (1974) A seven-year study of WHO viruslaboratory reports on respiratory viruses. Bull WHO 51:437–445

Bell JA, Huebner RJ, Rosen L, Rowe WP, Cole RM, Mastrota FM, Floyd TM, Chanock RM, Shvedoff RA (1961) Illness and microbial experiences of nursey children at Junior Village. Am J Hyg 74:267–292

Berge TO, England B, Mauris C (1955) Etiology of acute respiratory disease among service personnel at Fort Ord, California. Am J Hyg 62:283–294

Brandt CD, Wasserman FE, Fox JP (1966) The virus watch program IV. Recovery and comparison of two serological varieties of adenovirus type 5. Proc Soc Exp Biol Med 123:510–513

Brandt CD, Kim HW, Vargosko AJ, Jeffries BC, Arrobio JO, Rindge B, Parrott RH, Chanock RM (1968) Infections in 18.000 infants and children in a controlled study of respiratory tract disease. I. Adenovirus pathogenicity in relation to serologic type and illness syndrome. Am J Epidemiol 90:484–500

Brandt CD, Kim HW, Jeffries BC, Pyles G, Christmas EE, Reid JL, Chanock RM, Parrott RH (1972) Infections in 18,000 infants and children in a controlled study of respiratory tract disease. II. Variation in adenovirus infections by year and season. Am J Epidemiol 95:218–227

Brandt CD, Kim HW, Yolken RH, Kapikian AZ, Arrobio JO, Rodriguez WJ, Wyatt RO, Chanock RM, Parrott RH (1979) Comparative epidemiology of two rotavirus serotypes and other viral agents associated with pediatric gastroenteritis. Am J Epidemiol 110:243–254

Broker TR (1982) In: O'Brien SJ. Genetic maps. Natl Cancer Institute, Frederick, Maryland, p 74

Brůčková M, Wadell G, Sundell G, Syrůček L, Kunzová L (1980) An outbreak of respiratory disease due to a type 5 adenovirus identified as genome type 5a. Acta Virologica 24:161–165

D'Ambrosio E, Del Grosso N, Chicca A, Midulla M (1982) Neutralizing antibodies against 33 human adenoviruses in normal children in Rome. J Hygien Camb. 89:155–161

deJong JC, Wigand R, Wadell G, Keller D, Muzerie CJ, Wermenbol AG, Schaap GJ (1981) Adenovirus 37: identification and characterization of a medically important new adenovirus type of subgroup D. J Med Virol 7:105–118

deJong JC, Wigand R, Kidd AH, Wadell G, Kapsenberg JG, Muzerie CJ, Wermenbol AG, Firtzlaff RG (1983a) Candidate adenovirus 40 and 41: fastidious adenovirus from human infantile stool. J Med Virol 11:215–231

deJong PJ, Valderrama G, Spigland I, Horwitz MS (1983b) Adenovirus isolates from urine of patients with acquired immune deficiency syndrome. Lancet 1:1293–1296

Desmyter J, deJong JC, Slaterus KW, Verlaeckt H (1974) Kerato-conjunctivitis caused by adenovirus type 19. Br Med J 4:406

Eggers HJ, Doerfler W, Krämer B, Winterhoff U (1978) Persistence of adenovirus and adenovirus DNA in tonsillar tissue of man. Abst 4th Int Congress for Virology. The Hague August, 30-September, 6, 1978, p 219

Faden H, Gallagher M, Ogra P, McLaughlin S (1978) Nosocomial outbreak of pharyngoconjunctival fever due to adenovirus type 4. New York, Morb Mort Week Rep 27:49

Faulkner R, van Rooyen CE (1962) Adenovirus types 3 and 5 isolated from the cerebral fluid of children. Can Med Assoc J 87:1123

Flewett TH, Bryden AS, Davies H, Morris CA (1975) Epidemic viral enteritis in a long-stay children's ward. Lancet 1:4–5

Fox JP, Hall CE (1980) Viruses in families. PSG Littleton

Fox JP, Brandt CD, Wassermann FE, Hall CE, Spigland I, Kogon A, Elveback LR (1969) The virus watch program: a continuing surveillance of viral infections in metropolitan New York families. VI. Observations of adenovirus infections: virus excretion patterns, antibody response, efficiency of surveillance, patterns of infection, and relation to illness. Am J Epidemiol 89:25–50

Fox JP, Hall CE, Cooney MK (1977) The Seattle virus watch. VII. Observations on adenovirus infections. Am J Epidemiol 105:362–386

Foy HM, Grayston JT (1976) Adenoviruses. In: Evans AS (ed) Viral infections of humans. Epidemiology and control. Wiley, New York, pp 53–96

Fujii S, Nakazono N, Sawada H, Ishii K, Kato M, Aoki K, Ohtsuka H, Fujinaga K (1983) Restriction endonuclease cleavage analysis of adenovirus type 8: Two new subtypes from patients with epidemic keratoconjunctivitis in Sapporo, Japan. Jap J Med Sci Biol 36:307–313

Garon CF, Berry KW, Hierholzer JC, Rose JA (1973) Mapping of base sequence heterologies between genomes from different adenovirus serotypes. Virology 54:414–426

Gary GW Jr, Hierholzer JC, Black RE (1979) Characteristics of noncultivable adenoviruses associated with diarrhoea in infants: A new subgroup of human adenoviruses. J Clin Microbiol 10:96–103

Gelderblom H, Bauer H, Frank H, Wigand R (1967) The structure of group II adenoviruses. J Gen Virol 1:553

Gerna G, Cattaneo E, Grazia Revello M, Battaglia M (1982) Grouping of human adenoviruses by early antigen reactivity. J Infect Dis 145:678–682

Grayston JT, Yang YF, Johnston PB, Ko LS (1964) Epidemic keratoconjunctivitis on Taiwan: Etiological and clinical studies. Am J Trop Med Hyp Med 13:492–498

Green M (1970) Oncogenic viruses. Annu Rev Biochem 39:701–756

Green M, Mackey JK, Wold WSM, Rigden P (1979) Thirty-one human adenovirus serotypes (ad1–Ad31) from five groups (A–E) based upon DNA genome homologies. Virology 93:481–492

Gutekunst RR, Heggie AD (1961) Viremia and viruria in adenovirus infections: Detection in patients with rubella or rubelliform illness. N Engl J Med 264:374–378

Harnett GB, Bucens MR, Clay SJ, Sakev BM (1982) Acute haemorrhagic cystitis caused by adeno-virus type 11 in a recipient of a transplanted kidney. Med J Australia 1:565–567

Hierholzer J (1973) Further subgrouping of human adenoviruses by differential hemagglutination. J Infect Dis 128:541–550

Hierholzer JC, Atuk NO, Gwaltney JM (1975a) New human adenovirus isolated from a renal transplant recipient: description and characterization of candidate adenovirus type 34. J Clin Microbiol 1:366–376

Hierholzer JC, Gamble WC, Dowdle WR (1975b) Reference equine antisera to 33 human adenovirus types: homologous and heterologous titers. J Clin Microbiol 1:65–74

Hierholzer JC, Kemp MC, Gary GW, Spencer HC (1982) New human adenovirus associated with respiratory illness: candidate adenovirus type 39. J Clin Microbiology 16:15–21

Hilleman MR, Werner JH (1954) Recovery of new agents from patients with acute respiratory illness. Proc Soc Exp Biol Med 85:183–188

Huebner RJ (1967) Adenovirus-directed tumor and T antigens. In: Pollard M (ed) Perspectives in virology, vol 5. Academic, New York, pp 147–166

Jacobsson PÅ, Johansson ME, Wadell G (1979) Identification of an enteric adenovirus by immuno-electro-osmopheresis (IEOP) technique. J Med Virol 3:307–312

Jawetz E (1959) The story of shipyard eye. Br Med J 1:873–878

Johansson ME, Uhnoo I, Kidd AH, Madeley CR, Wadell G (1980) Direct identification of enteric adenovirus, a candidate new serotype associated with infantile gastroenteritis. J Clin Microbiol 12:95–100

Jordan WS, Badger GF, Dingle JH (1958) A study of illness in a group of Cleveland families. XV. Acquistion of type-specific adenovirus. Antibodies in the first five years of life: Implications for the use of adenovirus vaccine. N Engl J Med 258:1041–1044

Jung D, Wigand R (1967) Epidemiology of group II adenoviruses. Am J Epidemiol 85:311–319

Keller MA, Aftandelians R, Connor JD (1980) Etiology of pertussis syndrome. Pediatrics 66:50–55

Kemp MC, Hierholzer JC, Cabbradilla CP, Obijeski JF (1983) The changing etiology of epidemic keratoconjunctivitis: antigenic and restriction enzyme analyses of adenovirus types 19 and 37 isolated over a ten year period. 148:24–33

Kidd AH, Chrystie IL, Banatvala JE, Hawkins G (1981) Infection by fastidious enteric adenoviruses in childhood. Lancet 2:37–372

Kidd AH, Banatvala JE, de Jong JC (1983) Antibodies to fastidious faecal adenoviruses (species 40 and 41) in sera from children. J Med Virol 11:333–341

Klenk EL, Gaultney JV, Bass JW (1972) Bacteriologically proved pertussis and adenovirus infection. Am J Dis Child 124:203–207

Lang WR, Howden CW, Laws J, Burton JF (1969) Bronchopneumonia with serious sequelae in children with evidence of adenovirus type 21 infection. Br Med J 1:73

Lecatsas G, Prozesky OW, van Wyk J (1974) Adenovirus 11 associated with haemorrhagic cystitis after renal transplantations. S Afr Med J 48:1932

Lewandowski RA, Rubenis M (1981) Nosocomial conjunctivitis caused by adenovirus type 4. J Inf Dis 143:28–31

Loker EF, Hodges GR, Kelly DJ (1974) Fatal adenovirus pneumonia in a young adult associated with Ad7 vaccine administered 15 days earlier. Chest 66:197–199

McAllister RM, Nicolson MO, Reed G, Kern Jl, Gilden RV, Huebner RJ (1969) Transformation of rodent cells by adenovirus 19 and other group D adenoviruses. J Natl Cancer Inst 43:917–923

Mufson MA, Belshe RB, Horrigan TJ, Zollar IM (1973) Cause of acute hemorrhagic cystitis in children. Am J Dis Child 126:605–609

Muzzi A, Rocchi G, Lumbroso B, Tosato G, Barbieri F (1975) Acute hemorrhagic conjunctivitis during an epidemic outbreak of adenovirus-type-4 infection. Lancet 2:822–823

Nelson KE, Gavitt F, Batt MD, Kallick CA, Reddi KT, Levin S (1975) The role of adenoviruses in the pertussis syndrome. J Pediatr 86:335

Nicolas JC, Ingrand D, Fortier B, Bricout FA (1982) One year virological survey of acute intussuscep-tion in childhood. J Med Virol 9:267–271

Norrby E (1966) The relationship between the soluble antigen and the virion of adenovirus type 3. I. Morphological characteristics. Virology 8:236–248

Norrby E (1969) The structural and functional diversity of adenovirus capsid components. J Gen Virol 5:221–236

Norrby E, Wadell G (1969) Immunological relationships between hexons of certain human adenoviruses. J Virol 4:663–670

Numazaki Y, Shigeta S, Kumasaka T, Miyazawa T, Yamanaka M, Vano N, Takai S, Ishida N (1968) Acute hemorrhagic cystitis in children: isolation of adenovirus type 11. N Engl J Med 278:700–704

Pereira MS, Pereira HG, Clarke SKR (1965) Human adenovirus type 31. A new serotype with oncogenic properties. Lancet I:21–23

Piña M, Green M (1965) Biochemical studies on adenovirus multiplication. IX. Chemical and base composition analysis of 28 human adenoviruses. Proc Natl Acad Sci USA 54:547–551

Retter M, Middleton PI, Tam JS, Petric M (1979) Enteric adenovirus. Detection, replication and significance. J Clin Microbiol 10:574–578

Rosen L (1960) Hemagglutination-inhibition technique for typing adenovirus. Am J Hyg 71:120–128

Rowe WP, Huebner RJ, Gillmore LK, Parrot RH, Ward TG (1953) Isolation of a cytopathogenic agent from human adenoids undergoing spontaneous degeneration in tissue culture. Proc Soc Exp Biol Med 84:570

Rowe WP, Hartley JW, Huebner RJ (1958) Serotype composition of the adenovirus group. Proc Soc Exp Biol Med 97:465–470

Sambrook J, Sleigh M, Engler JA, Broker TR (1980) The evolution of the adenoviral genome. Ann NY Acad Sci 354:426–452

Schaap GJ, deJong JC, Van Bijsterveld OP, Beekhuis WH (1979) New intermediate adenovirus type causing conjunctivitis. Arch Ophthalmol 97:2336–2339

Schoub BD, Koornhof HL, Lecatsas G, Prozesky OW, Freiman I, Hartman E, Kassel H (1975) Virus in acute summer gastroenteritis in black infants. Lancet 1:1093–1094

Schmitz H, Wigand R, Heinrich W (1983) World-wide epidemiology of human adenovirus infections. Am J Epidemiol 117:455–466

Scott TM, Madeley CR, Cosgrove BP, Stanfield JP (1979) Stool viruses in babies in Glasgow 3. Community studies. J Hyg (Camb) 83:469–485

South MA, Dolen J, Beach DK, Mirkovic RR (1982) Fatal adenovirus hepatic necrosis in severe combined immune deficiency. Pediatr Infect Dis 6:416–419

Spigelblatt L, Rosenfeld R (1983) Hyperlucent lung: Long-term complication of adenovirus type 7 pneumonia. Can Med Ass J. 128:47–49

Stalder H, Hierholzer JC, Oxman MN (1977) New human adenovirus (candidate adenovirus type 35) causing fatal disseminated infection in a renal transplant recipient. J Clin Microbiol 6:257–265

Sterner G (1962) Adenovirus infection in childhood: an epidemiological and clinical survey among Swedish children. Acta Paediatr Scand [Suppl] 142:1–30

Straube RC, Thompson MA, van Dyke RB, Wadell G, Connor JD, Wingard D, Spector SA (1983) Adenovirus type 7b in children's hospital. J Infect Dis 147:814–819

Suzuki N, Ueno T, Yamashita T, Fujinaga K (1981) Grouping of adenoviruses and identification of restriction endonuclease cleavage pattern of adenovirus DNAs using infected cell DNA: simple and practical methods. Microbiol Immunol 25:1291–1301

Svensson L, von Bonsdorff CH (1982) Solid-phase immune electronmicroscopy (SPIEM) by use of protein A and its application for characterization of selected adenovirus serotypes. J Med Virol 10:243–253

Svensson L, Wadell G, Uhnoo I, Johansson M, v Bonsdorff CH (1983) Cross reactivity between enteric adenoviruses and adenovirus type 4: Analysis of epitopes by solid phase, immune electron microscopy. J Gen Virol 64:2517–2520

Tai FH, Grayston JT (1962) Adenovirus neutralizing antibodies in persons on Taiwan. Proc Soc Exp Biol Med 109:881–884

Takafuji ET, Gaydos JC, Allen RG, Top FH Jr (1979) Simultaneous administration of live, enteric-coated adenovirus types 4, 7 and 21 vaccines: safety and immunogenicity. J Infect Dis 140:48–53

Takiff HF, Strauss SE, Garon CF (1981) Propagation and in vitro studies of previously non-cultivatable enteric adenoviruses in 293 cells. Lancet 2:832–834

Teng C-H (1960) Adenovirus pneumonia epidemic among Peking infants and pre-school children in 1958. Chin Med J 80:331–339

Top FH Jr, Brandt WT, Russell PK (1976) Adenovirus ARD in basic combat trainees. In: research in biological and medical sciences: annual progress report 1975/1976. Walter Reed Army Inst of Research, Washington DC, p 462–465

Tullo AB, Higgins PG (1980) An outbreak of adenovirus type 4 conjunctivitis. Br J Ophtalmol 64:489–492

Uhnoo I, Wadell G, Svensson L, Johansson M (1983) Two new serotypes of adenoviruses causing infantile diarrhea. Dev Biol Stand 55:311–318

Van der Veen J (1963) The role of adenoviruses in respiratory disease. Am Rev Resp Dis 88:167–180

Van der Veen J, Lambriex M (1973) Relationship of adenovirus to lymphocytes in naturally infected human tonsils and adenoids. Infect. Immun 7:604–609

Wadell G (1969) Hemagglutination with adenovirus serotypes belonging to Rosen's subgroup II and III. Proc Soc Exp Biol Med 132:413–421

Wadell G (1970) Structural and biological properties of capsid components of human adenoviruses. Habilitation thesis. Karolinska Institute. Stockholm, pp 1–39

Wadell G (1979) Classification of human adenoviruses by SDS polyacrylamide gel electrophoresis of structural polypeptides. Intervirology 11:47–57

Wadell G, Norrby E (1969) Immunological and other biological characteristics of pentons of human adenoviruses. J Virol 4:671–680

Wadell G, Varsanyi TM (1978) Demonstration of three different subtypes of adenovirus typ 7 by DNA restriction site mapping. Infect Immun 21:238–246

Wadell G, deJong JC (1980) Use of restriction endonucleases for identification of a genome type of adenovirus 19 associated with kerato-conjunctivitis. Infect Immun 27:292–296

Wadell G, Norrby E, Schönning U (1967) Ultrastructure of soluble antigens and virion of adenovirus type 4. Arch Ges Virusforsch 21:234–242

Wadell G, Hammarskjöld M-L, Winberg G, Varsanyi T, Sundell G (1980a) Genetic variability of adenoviruses. Ann N Y Acad Sci 354:16–42

Wadell G, Varsanyi T, Lord A, Sutton RNP (1980b) Epidemic outbreaks of adenovirus 7 with special reference to the pathogenicity of adenovirus genome type 7b. Am J Epidemiol 112:619–628

Wadell G, deJong JC, Wolontis S (1981a) Molecular epidemiology of adenoviruses. Alternating appearance of two different genome types of adenovirus 7 during epidemic outbreaks in Europe 1958 to 1980. Infect Immun 34:368–372

Wadell G, Sundell G, deJong JC (1981b) Characterization of candidate adenovirus 37 by SDS polyacrylamide gel electrophoresis of virion polypeptides and DNA restriction site mapping. J Med Virol 7:119–125

White GPB, Stancliffe D (1975) Viruses and gastroenteritis. Lancet 2:703

Wigand R, Fliedner D (1968) Serologically intermediate adenovirus strains: a regular feature of group II adenoviruses. Arch Ges Virusforsch 24:235–256

Wigand R, Keller D (1978) Relationship of human adenoviruses 12, 18 and 31 as determined by hemagglutination inhibition. J Med Virol 2:137–142

Wigand R, Gelderblom H, Wadell G (1980) New human adenovirus (candidate adenovirus 36). A novel member of subgroup D. Arch Virol 64:225–233

Wigand R, Bartha A, Dreizin RS, Esche H, Ginsberg HS, Green M, Hierholzer JC, Kalter SS, McFerran JB, Pettersson U, Russell WC, Wadell G (1982) Adenoviridae: second report. Intervirology 18:169–176

World Health Organization (1980) Viral respiratory diseases. Technical report, series no. 642

Yolken RH, Bishop CA, Townsend TR, Bolyard EA, Bartlett J, Santos GW, Saral R (1982) Infectious gastroenteritis in bone-marrow-transplant recipients. N Engl J Med 306:1009–1012

Zahradnik JM, Spencer MJ, Porter DD (1980) Adenovirus infection in the immuno compromised patient. Am J Med 68:725–732

The In Vitro Replication of Adenovirus DNA

B.R. Friefeld[1], J.H. Lichy[2], J. Field[2], R.M. Gronostajski[2], R.A. Guggenheimer[2], M.D. Krevolin[3], K. Nagata[2], J. Hurwitz[2], and M.S. Horwitz[1, 3, 4]

1 Introduction

Adenovirus (Ad) DNA is a linear double-stranded molecule of approximately 36000 bp with a covalently bound 55-kilodalton (K) terminal protein (TP) linked to the 5′ terminus of each strand (Robinson et al. 1973; Rekosh et al. 1977; Carusi 1977). Ad DNA has inverted terminal repeats of about 100 bp with the exact length depending on the serotype (Steenbergh et al. 1977; Arrand and Roberts 1979; Shinagawa and Padmanabhan 1979). A highly conserved sequence extending from nucleotides 9 to 22 from either end of the molecule may serve as a recognition site for proteins involved in DNA replication (Shinagawa and Padmanabhan 1980; Tolun et al. 1979). In addition, the 5′-terminal dCMP residue is conserved in all serotypes sequenced. The TP is attached via a phosphodiester bond between a β-hydroxyl group of a serine

---

1 Departments of Cell Biology,
2 Developmental Biology and Cancer,
3 Microbiology and Immunology,
4 Pediatrics, Albert Einstein College of Medicine, Bronx, NY 10461, USA

Current Topics in Microbiology and Immunology, Vol. 110
© Springer-Verlag Berlin·Heidelberg 1984

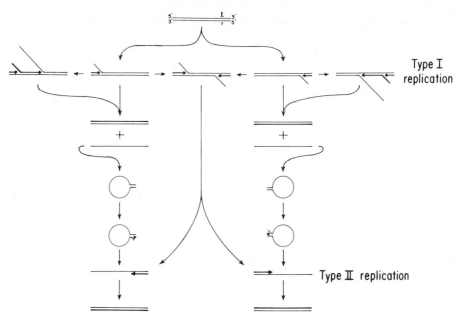

Fig. 1. Model for Ad2 DNA replication (see text for details). From LECHNER and KELLY 1977)

residue in the protein and the 5′-phosphate end of the DNA (DESIDERIO and KELLY 1981). The TP is synthesized as an 80K precursor (pTP) which is processed late in infection to the 55K form by an Ad-coded protease (CHALLBERG and KELLY 1981; STILLMAN 1981; LICHY et al. 1982b). Mapping of the TP by in vitro translation of mRNAs hybridized to restriction fragments of Ad DNA (STILLMAN et al. 1981) showed it to be a viral gene product encoded between map coordinates 11 and 30 in the E2B region. Subsequent determination of the DNA sequence of this region (ALESTROM et al. 1982), together with partial amino acid sequence studies of the TP (SMART and STILLMAN 1982) further localized the TP gene to an open reading frame between coordinates 28.4 and 23.2 on the leftward strand.

Since none of the known DNA polymerases can initiate DNA synthesis without a primer, the discovery of the TP suggested a novel priming mechanism for the replication of Ad DNA. REKOSH et al. (1977) proposed that the TP is a primer for DNA synthesis and that initiation occurred by linking the 5′ PO_4 of the first deoxynucleotide, dCMP, to the TP. The 3′-OH end of the dCMP would be free to serve as a primer for elongation by conventional addition of dNTPs. Proteins covalently linked to DNA are not unique to the adenovirus system but have been detected in association with replicative DNA of the parvovirus H1 (REVIE et al. 1979), hepatitis B virus (GERLICH and ROBINSON 1980), *Bacillus subtilis* phage φ29, RNA genomes of the picornaviruses poliovirus and encephaliomyocarditis virus (GOLINI et al. 1978), and some plant viruses (DAUBERT et al. 1978). The TP linked to the φ29 genome has been shown to be required for the initiation of replication in vivo by analysis of temperature sensitive (ts) mutants (MELLADO et al. 1980). In addition, the ϕ29 protein was shown to undergo the partial reactions characteristic of initiation via the protein priming mechanism, including the covalent addition of the first nucleotide in the chain to the protein and the elongation of the protein nucleotide intermediate (PÊNALVA and SALAS 1982). However, the functions of the covalently linked proteins in parvovirus H1, hepatitis B, and the picornaviruses are currently unknown.

Ad DNA replication initiates at either DNA terminus, but it is uncommon to have active replication forks at both ends. As the nascent DNA chain elongates continuously in the $5' \rightarrow 3'$ direction along one strand of the parental DNA, the other parental strand is displaced (type I replication of LECHNER and KELLY 1977). Replication of the displaced single strand (type II replication) then initiates at its 3' terminus and the nascent strand elongates until a full-length double-stranded DNA molecule has been formed (Fig. 1). For the replication of the displaced single strand (type II replication), it has been proposed that the two complementary ends of the single strand form a circular "duplex panhandle" structure (GARON et al. 1972, 1975; WOLFSON and DRESSLER 1972). Conceivably, the initiation of DNA replication within the double-stranded region of the 100-bp terminal repeat would be identical to the initiation of type I molecules (STEENBERGH et al. 1977; ARRAND and ROBERTS 1979), but subsequent elongation on single-stranded template would be different.

2 In vitro DNA Replication

The first cell extracts in which Ad DNA could replicate in vitro contained endogenous replicative intermediates which had been initiated in vivo (KAPLAN et al. 1977; ARENS and YAMASHITA 1978; BRISON et al. 1977). These intermediates were elongated to full-sized progeny DNA, but initiation of new rounds of replication did not occur. Such extracts failed to replicate exogenous Ad DNA templates. These endogenous systems yielded information on the role of the Ad DNA-binding protein (DBP) in elongation (HORWITZ 1978). However, these systems were heavily contaminated with cellular DNA polymerases (ABBOUD and HORWITZ 1979; VAN DER WERF et al. 1980), which obscured the presence of a viral coded DNA polymerase subsequently detected (ENOMOTO et al. 1981).

Many of the disadvantages of the endogenous systems were overcome by the development of an in vitro system capable of replicating exogenously added DNA (CHALLBERG and KELLY 1979a, b). The critical component of this system was a nuclear extract prepared from Ad-infected HeLa cells which had been treated with hydroxyurea 2 h post infection. The hydroxyurea treatment blocked viral DNA replication, but permitted the accumulation of proteins involved in replication. Extracts prepared 20–22 h after infection were nearly free of endogenous viral DNA, but contained proteins required for replication. DNA synthesis with this system required nuclear extract from Ad-infected cells, ATP, Mg^{++}, the four dNTPs, and Ad DNA covalently linked to the 55K TP (Ad

DNA-pro). No Ad DNA synthesis was detected in nuclear extracts from unin-
fected cells; less than 5% as much DNA synthesis was observed with deprotein-
ized Ad DNA as with Ad DNA-pro. Heterologous DNA templates such as
T7 and φX174 DNA also failed to replicate in this system (KAPLAN et al. 1979).
These observations suggested that the TP covalently linked to the parental
DNA is necessary for replication.

Characterization of this system indicated that in vitro replication closely
mimicked replication in vivo (CHALLBERG and KELLY 1979a, b; KAPLAN et al.
1979). Replication initiated specifically at DNA termini and the nascent DNA
chain could be elongated to lengths approximating full-sized Ad DNA. Replication in vitro retained the sensitivity to aphidicolin characteristic of Ad DNA
replication in vivo. In an electron microscopic study of the products of an
in vitro replication reaction, about 5% of the molecules observed were type
I replicative intermediates, indicating displacement synthesis similar to that observed in vivo. No type II molecules were unambiguously identified, suggesting
that replication of the displaced single strand did not account for a significant
fraction of the DNA synthesis detected in vitro (CHALLBERG and KELLY 1979b).

Replicative DNA synthesis was shown to be dependent upon the Ad DBP
(KAPLAN et al. 1979). Extracts prepared from the temperature-sensitive (ts)
DNA-negative Ad DBP mutant H5ts125 were active at 30° C but inactive at
38° C; activity could be restored at 38° C by the addition of wild-type Ad
DBP. The H5ts125 Ad DBP did not restore activity at the higher temperature,
nor did the E. coli DBP. The requirement for the Ad DBP provided additional
evidence that replicative DNA synthesis in vitro utilized the same enzymatic
pathways as in vivo replication.

Since the in vitro DNA replication system catalyzed initiation as well as
elongation, it became possible to study the properties of nascent DNA chains
soon after initiation. CHALLBERG et al. (1980) showed that terminal restriction
fragments of Ad DNA products synthesized in vitro were linked to protein
by demonstrating their aberrant migration in an agarose gel unless treated with
protease before electrophoresis. Similarly, HORWITZ and ARIGA (1981) observed
that all nascent DNA chains synthesized in a brief incubation were tightly
bound to protein as determined by binding to BND-cellulose under conditions
that retain only DNA-protein complexes (Fig. 2 and see below). These results
were consistent with the concept that the terminal protein served as a primer,
but did not rule out alternative mechanisms for attaching protein to the nascent
strand.

The infected nuclear extract used for the in vitro replication system of CHALL-
BERG and KELLY (1979a, b) was subsequently modified into a two-component
system dependent upon the addition of a cytoplasmic extract of Ad-infected
cells and a nuclear extract from uninfected HeLa cells with Ad DNA-pro as
template (IKEDA et al. 1981; LICHY et al. 1981). This modification simplified
further fractionation of Ad-encoded proteins from the infected cytosol extract
and host proteins from the uninfected nuclear extract. Subsequent studies were
directed towards purification of replication factors from these extracts and characterization of the various reactions involved in Ad DNA replication. Assays
were developed to study the initiation reaction, early elongation of nascent

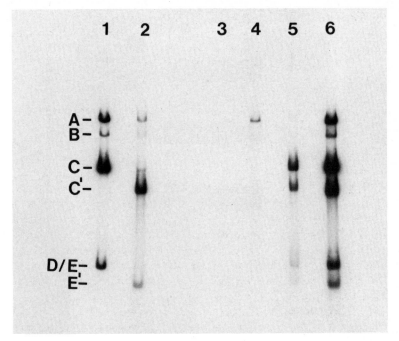

Fig. 2. Ad2 DNA synthesized in vitro is linked to protein. Five aliquots of Ad DNA-pro (0.15 µg in each) were digested with *Xba*I restriction endonuclease for 1 h. The DNA synthesis reaction was begun with the addition of uninfected HeLa nuclear extract, Ad2-infected cytoplasm, and the necessary nucleotides. After 180 min synthesis, one reaction was terminated by the addition of NaDodSO$_4$ and pronase. The four others were stopped by EDTA and pyrophosphate, pooled and processed for BND-cellulose column chromatography. Deproteinized double-stranded DNA was eluted with 1 M NaCl; single-stranded DNA was eluted with 1 M NaCl/2% caffeine. Single- and double-stranded DNA covalently linked to protein remained bound until eluted with 1% NaDodSO$_4$/ 8 M urea. *C* and *E* bands designate terminal fragments which contain the origins of Ad DNA replication; *C'* and *E'* bands represent displaced single strands produced during a second round of in vitro DNA replication. Lanes: *1* and *2*, electrophoresis of deproteinized DNAs eluted by 1 *M* NaCl and 1 *M* NaCl/2% caffeine respectively; *3–5*, DNAs recovered from the chromatography of DNA-protein samples eluted by 1 *M* NaCl (*3*), 1 *M* NaCl/2% caffeine (*4*), or 1% NaDodSO$_4$/8 *M* urea (*5*); *6*, intact sample treated with NaDodSO$_4$ and pronase without the BND-cellulose chromatography separation step. Reaction mixtures contained 25 m*M* Hepes (pH 7.5), 5 m*M* MgCl$_2$, 0.5 m*M* dithiothreitol, 0.05 m*M* dATP/dGTP/dCTP, 3.75 m*M* ATP, and 1.5 µ*M* (α^{32}P)-dTTP

DNA chains to the 26th nucleotide, and further elongation of the genome. The protein priming model previously discussed predicted that initiation of Ad DNA replication occurs by the covalent linkage of the first 5' deoxynucleotide, dCMP, to the 80K pTP, probably via the reaction: pTP + dCTP → pTP − dCMP + PPi. The product, pTP − dCMP, would then serve as the primer for further DNA elongation. This reaction was measured by the in vitro formation of a covalent complex between the 80K pTP and dCMP (LICHY et al. 1981; PINCUS et al. 1981).

The requirements for the formation of an 80K protein-deoxynucleotide complex are shown in Fig. 3. A cytoplasmic extract and a nuclear extract from Ad-infected HeLa cells were incubated in the presence of Ad DNA-pro, Ad

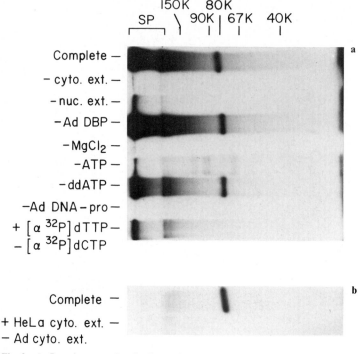

Fig. 3a, b. Requirements for the formation of an 80K-dCMP complex. In all cases, electrophoretic migration was from left to right. *SP,* spacer gel. The standards used were *E. coli* RNA polymerase (150K, 90K, and 40K) and bovine serum albumin (67K). **a** The complete system contained Ad DBP (2 µg), ddATP (40 µM), and crude nuclear extract (*nuc. ext.*) and cytoplasmic extract (*cyto. ext.*) from Ad2-infected HeLa cells. Incubation was for 120 min at 30° C. **b** The complete reaction contained aphidicolin (100 µM), crude nuclear extract from uninfected cells, and crude cytoplasmic extract from Ad2-infected cells. The *HeLa cyto. ext.,* was a crude cytoplasmic extract prepared from uninfected HeLa cells. Reaction mixtures contained 25 mM Hepes (pH 7.5), 5 mM MgCl₂, 2 mM dithiothreitol, 3 mM ATP, 0.15 µg Ad DNA-pro, and 0.5 µM (α³²P)-dCTP (200–800 Ci/ mmol). Reactions were stopped by the addition of 50 µl of 0.18 M sodium pyrophosphate/0.05 M EDTA and 25 µl of 50% (wt/vol) trichloroacetic acid. The mixture was centrifuged for 10 min, and the pellet was washed with ether, dissolved in 35 µl sample buffer, and processed for electrophoresis and autoradiography

DBP, ATP, ddATP, MgCl₂, and (α³²P)-dCTP. The reaction products were analyzed on an SDS-polyacrylamide gel and ³²P-labeled bands detected by autoradiography. A ³²P-labeled 80K product was shown to be pTP-dCMP (see below). This product was not detected when Ad DNA-pro, MgCl₂, or either the nuclear or cytoplasmic extract was omitted from the reaction. The omission of Ad DBP or of ddATP had no effect on the amount of product formed.

Synthesis of the 80K product specifically required dCTP. However, low levels of an 80K product were occasionally detected with (α³²P)-dATP and (α³²P)-dTTP, the second and third nucleotides from the 5′ terminus respectively, but not with (α³²P)-dGTP, which is not present until the 26th nucleotide from the 5′ terminus. The nature of the DNA requirement for synthesis of the 80K product resembled that found for in vitro DNA elongation (KAPLAN et al. 1979;

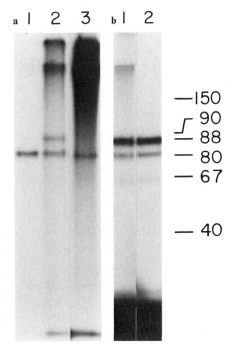

Fig. 4a, b. Requirement for formation of elongated protein-nucleic acid complexes (pTP-26mer). Standards shown in kilodaltons. **a** Lanes: *1,* complete reaction mixture as in Fig. 3; *2,* complete reaction mixture plus dATP, dTTP, and ddGTP (20 µ*M* each); *3,* complete reaction mixture plus dATP, dGTP, and dTTP (20 µ*M* each). **b** Lanes: *1,* as in *a,* lane 2; *2,* as in lane 1 plus aphidicolin (100 µ*M*)

HORWITZ and ARIGA 1981). Published sequences of Ad2 terminals indicate that the first 25 nucleotides from the 5′ terminus contain no guanine residues (SHINAGAWA and PADMANABHAN 1979). According to the proposed model of Ad DNA replication, chain termination by ddGTP should result in the formation of an oligonucleotide 26 nucleotides in length linked to an 80K protein (pTP-26mer). When (α^{32}P)-dCTP, dATP, dTTP and ddGTP were incubated with uninfected HeLa nuclear extract, infected cytoplasmic extract, Ad DNA-pro, and other reaction components mentioned above, a band of apparent molecular weight 88K was detected in addition to the 80K band on autoradiograms of SDS-polyacrylamide gels (Fig. 4). No 88K band was detected when ddGTP was omitted and dGTP substituted but a large amount of radioactivity remained near the top of the gel, presumably due to extensive elongation of DNA chains in the absence of the chain terminator. Formation of the 80K and 88K bands was not inhibited by aphidicolin at 100 µ*M*, a concentration that diminished the rate of in vitro Ad DNA synthesis by 90% and reduced the amount of ^{32}P-labeled material migrating near the top of the gel.

Several lines of evidence demonstrate that the 80K protein moiety of the reaction products is the pTP and therefore that the labeled 80K product is pTP-dCMP. These include the following: (a) the size of the protein is the same as that reported for the pTP (CHALLBERG et al. 1981); (b) the requirements for synthesis of the 80K product (other than the deoxynucleotide requirement) are the same as those for synthesis of Ad DNA; (c) the protein-dCMP linkage is acid stable and alkali labile, as is the TP-Ad DNA linkage (CARUSI 1977;

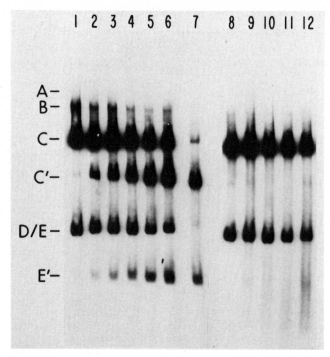

Fig. 5. Origin-specific rounds of Ad DNA synthesis in vitro. Ad DNA-pro (0.15 μg) was digested with *Xba*I and the subsequent synthesis reaction (as in Fig. 2) with (α^{32}P)-dTTP (1.5 μM) was allowed to proceed for 20 min. Then unlabeled dTTP (100 μM) was added to each reaction and the incubation was continued for 0 min (lanes *1* and *8*), 30 min (lanes *2* and *9*), 60 min (lanes *3* and *10*), 90 min (lanes *4* and *11*), 120 min (lanes *5* and *12*), and 180 min (lanes *6* and *7*). The reaction was stopped by the addition of EDTA and cooling to 0° C. In lanes *8–12* the samples were digested with S1 nuclease (0.1 unit/ml) in 30 mM sodium acetate (pH 4.5)/100 mM NaCl/0.3 mM ZnSO$_4$ for 15 min at 37° C. The sample in lane *7* was processed by adding 0.2 M NaOH and holding at 0° C for 10 min before neutralization with HCl. All samples were subsequently deproteinized and processed for electrophoresis and autoradiography. The quantity of sample in lane *7* was 50% of that shown in all other lanes. The terminal restriction fragments were C and E

ROBINSON AND PADMANABHAN 1980; DESIDERIO and KELLY 1981); (d) the same 80K protein is found linked to a 26-base oligonucleotide which probably comprises the 5′-terminal 26 bases of the Ad DNA strand; and (e) in vitro cleavage of the pTP by the viral protease generates fragments similar in size to those produced in the processing of the pTP in vivo.

Specific DNA synthesis on terminal restriction fragments of Ad DNA-pro was studied using a method developed by HORWITZ and ARIGA (1981) for distinguishing replicative from nonreplicative synthesis. The in vitro DNA replication reaction was typically carried out using *Xba*I restriction fragments of Ad DNA-pro (Fig. 5). The ^{32}P-labeled reaction products were separated on an agarose gel and detected by autoradiography. Replicative synthesis resulted in labeling of only the terminal fragments, C and E, while nonreplicative synthesis resulted in labeling of all the fragments in proportion to their size. This assay system permitted the demonstration that at least two rounds of replication occurred in vitro. The strand that was labeled in the first round of replication was displaced in the second round; the displaced single strands were detected on autoradiograms as bands designated C′ and E′, which migrated faster than their corresponding double-stranded fragments C and E (HORWITZ and ARIGA 1981). The decrease of label in double strand during the chase corresponded to the increase of single strand. Both the progeny single- and double-stranded DNA appeared to be linked to protein (Fig. 2).

The availability of the various assay systems which specifically detect the initiation and elongation of nascent Ad DNA has made it possible to identify proteins involved in replication. The goal of developing a reconstituted system for replicating Ad DNA-pro with purified proteins has been achieved. The approaches involved fractionating the crude nuclear and cytosol extracts. The finding that the nuclear extract from uninfected cells and the Ad2-infected cytosol could replace the nuclear extract from infected cells suggested that all the virus-coded proteins required for replication were present in the cytoplasmic extract. Nuclear extracts of uninfected HeLa cells provided a source of two host-coded replication factors which complemented the three proteins derived from Ad-infected cytosol extracts. Extracts of adenovirus mutants which are temperature sensitive for DNA replication have aided in identification of replication factors. Genetic complementation assays were devised in which components deficient in the inactive mutant extracts were added back to restore activity. Such studies, using the adenovirus *ts* mutants H5*ts*125, H5*ts*107, and H5*ts*149, will be described in later sections.

3 Viral Proteins Required for Ad DNA Replication

The synthesis of the pTP-dCMP complex provided a specific assay which was used for the development of a purification procedure for the pTP. A second assay, called the Ad-protein assay, was based on the assumption that fractions containing the adenovirus-coded proteins (Ad proteins) required for replication would complement reaction mixtures containing extracts from uninfected cells in the presence of Ad DNA-pro (IKEDA et al. 1981). Since the Ad DBP was known to be required for viral DNA replication, it was included in reaction mixtures so that only viral proteins other than the Ad DBP would be detected. This reaction was measured by scoring for the incorporation of $(\alpha^{32}P)$-dTTP into an acid-insoluble form. Through each of 4 columns and a glycerol gradient centrifugation step, pTP-dCMP formation and the Ad protein assay identified the same peak of activity. The same peak also contained a DNA polymerase activity detectable on activated calf thymus DNA but not on poly (rA):oligo (dT). On activated DNA, the DNA polymerase was insensitive to aphidicolin. Glycerol gradient centrifugation, the final step in the purification, yielded a single peak of activity sedimenting with an apparent molecular size of 180K

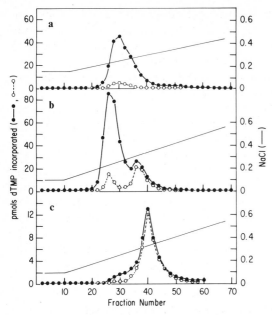

Fig. 6a–c. Purification of DNA polymerases from uninfected and Ad2-infected HeLa cells. DNA polymerases were purified from infected and uninfected extracts, starting with 346 mg protein in each case (LICHY et al. 1982a). DNA polymerase activity was recovered as a single peak on DEAE-cellulose and phosphocellulose columns. The phosphocellulose eluate was chromatographed on denatured DNA-cellulose and fractions were assayed for DNA polymerase activity in the absence (●——●) or presence (o–––o) of 100 μM aphidicolin. **a** DNA-cellulose chromatography of phosphocellulose eluate (9.6 mg protein) derived from the uninfected cell extract. **b** The DNA-cellulose column used in *a* was washed with buffer containing 1.0 M NaCl and reequilibrated with buffer B containing 0.10 M NaCl. The column was then used for chromatography of the phosphocellulose eluate (14.5 mg protein) derived from the infected cell extract. **c** Fractions 34–42 from the column in B were pooled and dialyzed against buffer containing 0.10 M NaCl. The dialyzed fraction was rechromatographed on the same column after washing and reequilibration as described above

relative to marker proteins (ENOMOTO et al. 1981). The most highly purified fraction represented a purification of at least 1000-fold over the crude extract. NaDodSO$_4$-polyacrylamide gel electrophoresis of the glycerol gradient fractions showed major protein bands of 80K and 140K, present in equimolar amounts, which coincided with the peak of Ad-protein activity and pTP-dCMP-forming activity.

The DNA polymerase activity was compared with that of DNA polymerases α, β, and γ in different assay systems. The Ad-protein-associated DNA polymerase (Pol) was different from HeLa cell polymerases β and γ but resembled DNA polymerase α in its template preference. Pol efficiently used activated DNA as a template, but was inactive on poly(rA):oligo(dT). It also resembled polymerase α in its sensitivity to N-ethylmaleimide, NaCl, and cytosine β-D-arabinofuranoside-5′-triphosphate (Ara-CTP). However, Pol was more sensitive to ddTTP than DNA polymerase α and was insensitive to aphidicolin. Aphidicolin (100 μM) inhibited polymerase α activity by approximately 90%, but had no effect on the activity of the Pol. Thus the DNA polymerase activity associated with the purified fraction differed both in its chromatographic and enzymatic properties from HeLa cell DNA polymerases α, β, and γ.

To show that Pol was present only in Ad-infected cells, DNA polymerases were purified in parallel from extracts of infected and uninfected cells (Fig. 6). The peak of Ad-protein and Ad DNA polymerase activities seen on the denatured DNA cellulose column was not detected in the fraction isolated from uninfected cells. Since small amounts of DNA polymerase α contaminated the fractions in the pTP peak, it was possible that the Ad DNA polymerase peak resulted artifactually from stimulation of DNA polymerase α by the pTP rather than from the presence of a chromatographically distinct polymerase. This possibility was ruled out by rechromatography of the pooled fractions containing Ad DNA polymerase activity on denatured DNA cellulose. Only a small portion of the polymerase eluted in the position of DNA polymerase α, whereas almost all of the activity again eluted in the position of the Ad protein (LICHY et al. 1982a).

3.1 Requirements for pTP-dCMP Synthesis with Purified pTP-Pol

Formation of pTP-dCMP was observed with the purified Ad-protein fraction (pTP-Pol) in combination with Ad DNA-pro, MgCl$_2$, and (α^{32}P)-dCTP. No pTP-dCMP was detected when any one of these components was omitted from the reaction mixture or when Ad DNA-pro was replaced by deproteinized Ad DNA. pTP-dCMP synthesis was stimulated by the addition of ATP or nuclear extract from uninfected cells; when both were included, the effect was greater than additive. The addition of 100 μM aphidicolin to the reaction mixture had no effect on pTP-dCMP synthesis.

Since the purified pTP-Pol was free of the Ad DBP, it was possible to examine the effect of the Ad DBP on pTP-dCMP complex formation. In the absence of nuclear extract, addition of the Ad DBP reproducibly inhibited complex formation by a factor of about two. In the presence of nuclear extract, Ad DBP did not stimulate pTP-dCMP synthesis. However, as will be described in a later section, the Ad DBP stimulates complex formation when nuclear extract is replaced by purified nuclear factor I.

The 55K TP was compared (by tryptic peptide mapping) with the 80K protein present in the purified Ad-protein fraction. The peptide map derived from the 80K protein showed extensive homology with that of the 55K TP. In contrast, a map of the Ad DBP showed no such homology (ENOMOTO et al. 1981).

The protein priming model requires that the enzymes involved in Ad DNA replication have the ability to elongate pTP-dCMP. In order to show that pTP-dCMP is an intermediate in the synthesis of pTP-linked nascent DNA chains, a pulse-chase experiment was designed in which the chase was carried out in the presence of dCTP, dATP, dTTP and ddGTP to elongate to the pTP-26mer.

In the presence of the purified pTP-Pol, 30–40% of the pTP-dCMP formed could be chased into the pTP-26mer. The 80K product decreased in intensity concomitant with the appearance of the 88K product (LICHY et al. 1981, 1982). Similar findings were reported by CHALLBERG et al. (1982); at present the reason for the incomplete chase of pTP-dCMP into pTP-26mer is unclear.

3.2 Separation of the pTP from the Ad DNA Polymerase

When the glycerol-gradient-purified pTP-140K complex was treated with 1.7 M urea for 1 h on ice and then sedimented through a 10–30% glycerol gradient

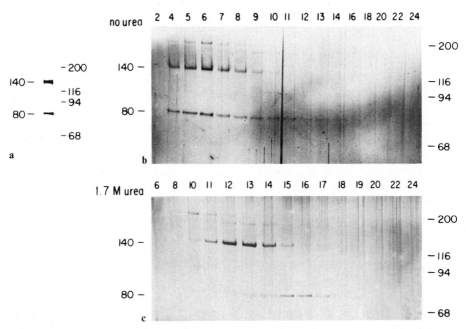

Fig. 7a–c. Glycerol gradient centrifugation of pTP-Pol complex in the presence and absence of urea followed by NaDodSO$_4$-polyacrylamide gel electrophoresis of gradient fractions. The pTP-Pol complex was dialyzed against buffer C (25 mM sodium phosphate, (pH 6.0)/1 mM dithiothreitol/1 mM EDTA/0.5 M NaCl) containing 10% (vol/vol) glycerol. An 80-µl aliquot was adjusted to a final concentration of 1.7 M urea in a volume of 0.2 ml. After 1 h at 0° C, 0.18 ml was applied to a 4.8-ml gradient of 10–30% glycerol in buffer C containing the same concentration of urea. A second aliquot was similarly processed without the addition of urea to the sample gradient. Gradients were centrifuged at 49000 rpm for 24 h in a Beckman SW 50.1 rotor. Fractions were collected from the bottom of the tube. **a** Lane from a Coomassie-blue-strained gel of the pTP-Pol complex (20 µl) used as starting material for the glycerol gradient. **b** NaDodSO$_4$-polacrylamide gel electrophoresis of fractions from the gradient containing no urea. **c** Polyacrylamide gel electrophoresis of fractions from the gradient containing 1.7 M urea. Lanes are labeled by fraction number. Protein bands were visualized by silver staining. Size standards, shown in kilodaltons: myosin (200), β-galactosidase (116), phosphorylase (94), and bovine serum albumin (68)

containing 1.7 M urea, the pTP and 140K proteins no longer cosedimented (Fig. 7). The 140K protein sedimented faster than the pTP; however, each sedimented slower than the pTP-140K complex. DNA polymerase activity on activated DNA coincided with the peak of 140K protein but not with the peak of pTP or either of two minor contaminants of 190K and 205K. The 140K protein does not require pTP for DNA polymerase activity. When glycerol gradient fractions were assayed for synthesis of pTP-dCMP or for Ad-protein activity, a peak was detected only in fractions which contained both the 80K and 140K proteins. pTP-dCMP synthesis was not detected either in fractions containing only the 140K protein or only the 80K protein. These results indicate that both subunits are required for the synthesis of pTP-dCMP complex (LICHY et al. 1982a, b). The requirement for both subunits was observed in the presence or absence of nuclear extract. Purified HeLa DNA polymerases α and β, bacteriophage T4 DNA polymerase, *E. coli* DNA polymerases I, II, and III, calf liver DNA polymerases α and β, and crude extracts containing HeLa DNA polymerase γ failed to substitute for Ad DNA polymerase in this reaction.

3.3 Requirements for Ad DNA-pro Replication with Isolated Subunits

Both the pTP and the Ad DNA polymerase were required for replication of Ad DNA-pro in vitro (Table 1). DNA polymerase α did not substitute for the Ad DNA polymerase. No DNA synthesis was detected in the absence of the Ad DBP, the uninfected nuclear extract, or the Ad DNA polymerase, but in the absence of the pTP, DNA synthesis proceeded at about 10% the rate of the complete system. This residual synthesis probably resulted from the presence of small amounts of the pTP in the Ad DNA polymerase preparations. In contrast to the polymerase activity, pTP-dCMP, and pTP-26mer formation, further elongation of Ad DNA-pro was sensitive to aphidicolin, as previously observed in Ad DNA replication systems reconstituted in vitro with crude extracts (IKEDA et al. 1981; LONGIARU et al. 1979).

3.4 Characterization of the Ad DNA Polymerase

Purified Ad DNA polymerase retained the properties of the pTP-Pol previously described. Polymerase activity was detected with activated calf thymus DNA, but not with the synthetic template-primer poly(rA):oligo(dT). Deoxynucleotide incorporation using the pTP-Pol complex was also detected with the homopolymer template-primers poly(dC):oligo(dG), poly(dA):oligo(dT), poly(dT):oligo(dA), and poly(dT):oligo(rA). With poly(dT) as template and oligo(dA) or oligo(rA) as primers, DNA synthesized by the pTP-Pol complex was stimulated 100-fold by the presence of the Ad DBP (Table 2). No incorporation was observed in the absence of pTP-Pol or Ad DBP. Using the 140K subunit, which

Table 1. Requirements for Ad DNA replication with isolated subunits

Reaction mixture	dTMP incorporation (pmol)
Complete	3.68
Lacking:	
pTP	0.43
Pol	0.06
Ad DBP	0.22
uninfected nuclear extract	0.17
Ad DNA-pro	0.02
Pol but with polymerase α	0.05
Plus:	
polymerase α	3.05
aphidicolin at 10 μM	1.96
aphidicolin at 100 μM	0.64

The complete reaction mixture contained 25 mM Hepes (pH 7.5), 5 mM MgCl$_2$, 2 mM dithiothreitol, 3 mM ATP, 40 μM dATP, 40 μM dCTP, 40 μM dGTP, 4 μM ^{3}H-dTTP (3170 cpm/pmol), 1.5 μg Ad DBP, 0.15 μg Ad DNA-pro, nuclear extract (8.2 μg protein), 0.01 unit of Pol subunit and the pTP subunit. One unit of DNA polymerase incorporated 1 nmol of dTMP into acid-insoluble material in 60 min at 37° C on activated calf thymus DNA (LICHY et al. 1982a)

Table 2. Poly (dT):oligo (dA)-primed DNA synthesis using the Ad DNA polymerase

Additions	dAMP incorporation (pmol)
Experiment I	
pTP-Pol + Ad DBP	18.1
omit pTP-Pol	0.13
omit Ad DBP	0.21
omit pTP-Pol, add Hela pol α	0.14
omit Ad DBP, add E. coli ssb	0.21
Experiment II	
pTP + Pol + Ad DBP	10.2
omit Pol	0.13
omit pTP	28.3
omit Ad DBP	0.10
omit Ad DBP, omit Pol	0.10
omit Ad DBP, omit pTP	0.10

Reaction mixtures (50 μl) contained 50 mM TRIS-HCl (pH 7.9), 10 mM MgCl$_2$, 4.5 mM dithiothreitol, 10 μg bovine serum albumin, 0.4 μg poly (dT), 0.4 μg oligo (dA), 8 μM (^{3}H)-dATP (2500 cpm/pmol), pTP-Pol (experiment I) or isolated pTP and Pol subunits (experiment II), and 0.8 μg Ad DBP or E. coli ssb

had been separated from the 80K subunit, dAMP incorporation was observed only when the 140K Pol and the Ad DBP were combined, suggesting a specific interaction between the Pol and the Ad DBP. *E. coli* single-stranded DNA binding protein (ssb) did not replace Ad DBP and DNA polymerase α did not substitute for the Ad Pol. Addition of the pTP partially inhibited poly(dA) synthesis catalyzed by the Pol. Under optimal conditions, products synthesized in the presence of pTP-Pol, Ad DBP, and poly(dT):oligo(dA) were 30 000 nucleotides in length, suggesting that the Pol is a highly processive enzyme. These experiments were carried out with a large excess of oligo(dA) compared to poly(dT) and Pol.

An exonuclease activity cosedimented with the 140K Pol during glycerol gradient centrifugation, both in the presence and absence of urea (Fig. 8). The nuclease hydrolyzes single-stranded DNA in a $3' \rightarrow 5'$ direction and is at least 10-fold more active on single-stranded than on duplex DNA. No nuclease activity was detected on single-stranded or duplex circular DNA. Addition of the Ad DBP inhibited the exonuclease activity on restriction fragments of single-stranded φX174.

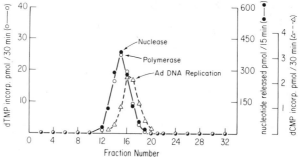

Fig. 8. Cosedimentation of exonuclease activity with the 140K Pol. Glycerol gradient centrifugation of pTP-Pol in the presence of 1.7 M urea was performed as in Fig. 7. Fractions were assayed for DNA polymerase activity on activated calf thymus DNA (o——o); for nuclease activity on ^{3}H-labeled heat-denatured calf thymus DNA (●——●); or for Ad-protein complementing activity in the presence of Ad DNA-pro, Ad DBP, and uninfected nuclear extract (△---△). DNA polymerase activity on activated calf thymus DNA was assayed in reaction mixtures (50 µl) containing 60 mM TRIS-HCl (pH 7.9), 4 mM dithiothreitol, 7.5 mM MgCl$_2$, 10 µg bovine serum albumin, 40 µM each of dATP, dCTP, dGTP, and ^{3}H-dTTP (about 500 cpm/pmol), 10 µg of DNase activated calf thymus DNA, and 2 µl of each fraction. Reaction mixtures were incubated for 30 min at 37° C and stopped by addition of 0.1 ml 50 mM EDTA/0.15 M sodium pyrophosphate. Acid insoluble material was precipitated and radioactivity determined by liquid scintillation counting. To measure nuclease activity, 2-µl aliquots of each fraction were incubated in a 50-µl reaction mixture containing 20 mM TRIS HCl (pH 7.5), 10 mM MgCl$_2$, 4 mM dithiothreitol, 5 µg bovine serum albumin, and 1.2 nmol ^{3}H-labeled heat-denatured calf thymus DNA (100 cpm/pmol). After a 15 min incubation at 37° C, the reaction was stopped by addition of 90 µl 20 mM EDTA (pH 8.2), 200 µg/ml calf thymus DNA, and 60 µl 20% trichloroacetic acid. The mixture was incubated on ice for 5 min, centrifuged at 12000 g for 5 min, and acid-soluble radioactivity was determined

4 Studies with *ts* Mutants

Additional information about the role of the viral-coded proteins in Ad DNA replication was obtained from the study of several Ad DNA negative *ts* mutants. Two complementation groups of Ad *ts* mutants defective in DNA replication have been described. One group includes the Ad DBP mutants H5*ts*125 and H5*ts*107, which map in early region E2A (62–68 map units) (GRODZICKER et al. 1977). Mutants in a second group, the N complementation group, including H5*ts*149 and H5*ts*36, map between coordinates 18 and 22 from the left end of the Ad genome, within an open reading frame extending from 22.9 leftward to 14.2 in the early region E2B (GALOS et al. 1979; ALESTROM et al. 1982; GINGERAS et al. 1982). This region is adjacent to the coding region for pTP, which has recently been localized between 28.9 and 23.5 map units. Based on the following studies, it appears likely that mutants in the N group code for the Pol gene.

4.1 Ad5*ts*149 and Ad5*ts*36 (N-Group) Mutants

In vitro complementation assays using extracts made from these viral mutants have been developed. Restoration of replication activity to these deficient extracts was accomplished by the addition of appropriate fractions purified from cells infected with wild-type virus, or from cells infected with mutant virus from a different complementation group. To characterize the replication defect in an N-group mutant, extracts were prepared from Ad5ts149 or Ad5ts36 viral-infected cells grown at the nonpermissive temperature. These extracts were unable to synthesize viral DNA. The defect in these extracts could be reversed by the addition of a fraction containing pTP-Pol purified from wild-type cells (LICHY et al. 1982b; STILLMAN et al. 1982; FRIEFELD et al. 1983b; OSTROVE et al. 1983). To further define the nature of the N-group mutation, cytosol extracts prepared from H5ts149-infected cells were mixed with isolated wild-type pTP (80K) or Pol (140K) subunits. H5ts149 extracts were assayed for their ability to support synthesis of pTP-dCMP in the presence and absence of added pTP or Pol subunit (LICHY et al. 1982b; FRIEFELD et al. 1983b). The addition of the 80K subunit to the H5ts149 extract had little effect on the amount of product formed. However, the addition of the 140K subunit greatly stimulated the reaction, indicating that the mutant extract was deficient in a functional 140K protein. The lack of stimulation by the 80K subunit could not be attributed to the presence of an inhibitor, because the addition of both subunits to the reaction mixture did not block the stimulation due to the 140K subunit, but rather resulted in further enhancement of the reaction. As controls, extracts prepared both from cells infected with wild-type virus and from cells infected with H5ts149 at permissive temperatures were incubated with isolated subunits. Such extracts supported DNA synthesis and the addition of either pTP or Pol subunits had little effect; stimulation was only observed upon the addition of both subunits.

Cytosol extracts prepared from cells infected with H5ts149 at both permissive (33° C) and nonpermissive (39° C) temperatures in vivo were also assayed for their replicative activity using XbaI restriction fragments of Ad DNA-pro (Fig. 9). This assay was totally dependent on the presence of uninfected HeLa nuclear extract and infected cytosol fractions containing the Ad DBP, 80K pTP, and 140K Pol. Cytosol extracts prepared from cells infected with H5ts149 at permissive temperatures and wild-type extracts prepared at both permissive and nonpermissive temperatures showed specific incorporation of radioactivity into terminal restriction fragments containing the origins of Ad DNA replication. Extracts prepared from H5ts149-infected cells which were grown at 39° C and contained functional Ad DBP were inactive. However, addition of the 140K Pol subunit to the extract restored activity to normal levels, further indicating that mutant extracts were deficient in active 140K Pol protein.

Furthermore, glycerol gradient sedimentation of extracts showed that a replicative activity representing the pTP-Pol complex was greatly reduced in H5ts149 extracts as compared with wild-type extracts, suggesting some alteration in the mutant. Both initiation and elongation of DNA by H5ts149 extracts isolated from cells grown at permissive temperature were more sensitive to urea inactivation than were wild-type Ad2 extracts. These results, along with the mapping data of ALESTROM et al. (1982) and GINGERAS et al. (1982), the absence of the Pol from uninfected extracts, and the differing properties of the Pol from the known host DNA polymerases α, β, and γ, strongly suggest that the Pol is a viral-encoded protein, as is the pTP.

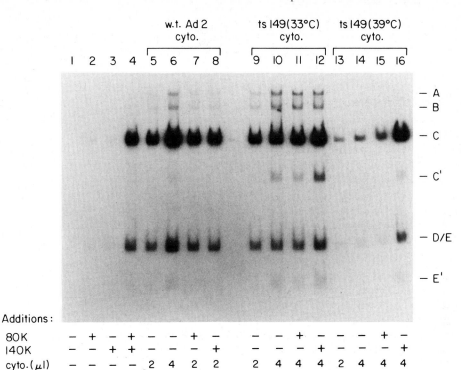

Fig. 9. Complementation of H5*ts*149 cytosol extracts with isolated wild-type subunits (pTP or Pol) in the elongation reaction. Replication of *Xba*I restriction fragments was carried out using cytosol extracts (*cyto*) of wild-type Ad2-infected cells grown at 33° C (lanes *5–8*) and H5*ts*149 infected cells grown at either the permissive temperature (33° C; lanes *9–12*) or the nonpermissive (39° C; lanes *13–16*) temperature. All reaction mixtures contained uninfected nuclear extract (8.2 µg protein); cytosol extracts and the purified 80K and 140K subunits were added as indicated. In lanes *1–4*, in which no cytoplasmic extract was present, 1.0 µg Ad DBP was added to the reaction mixtures. Ad2, H5*ts*149 (33° C), and H5*ts*149 (39° C) extracts were used at protein concentrations of 10.4, 10.2, and 8.9 mg/ml respectively; the 80K and 140K subunits were used at 10 ng. Reaction mixtures contained 25 mM Hepes (pH 7.5), 5 mM MgCl$_2$, 0.5 mM dithiothreitol, 50 µM dATP/dGTP/dCTP, 1.5 µM (α^{32}P)dTTP (20000–40000 cpm/pmol), 3.75 mM ATP, uninfected nuclear extract (4–8 µg of protein), 0.5 µg of Ad DBP, 0.07 µg of Ad DNA-pro that had been cleaved at 37° C with 2.5 units *Xba*I, and various cytosol extracts or isolated subunits. Reactions were terminated after 120 min at 30° C by the addition of 0.2% SDS

4.2 Ad5*ts*125 and Ad5*ts*107 DBP Mutants

Similar complementation studies using in vitro extracts from the mutants H5*ts*125 and H5*ts*107 have been used to explore the role of another viral gene product, the Ad DBP. From the nucleotide sequence of the Ad DBP gene, KRUIJER et al. (1981) determined that the Ad DBP contained 529 amino acid residues and had an actual molecular weight of 59K. Previous determinations from mobilities of the protein in SDS-polyacrylamide gels placed the molecular weight of the Ad DBP at 72K. For historical reasons, the Ad DBP will be referred to as 72K for the remainder of this review.

Recent DNA sequencing data has shown that both the H5*ts*125 and H5*ts*107 mutations consist of a single-base change in amino acid 413 near the C-terminus of the Ad DBP coding region (KRUIJER et al. 1983). The role of the Ad DBP in initiation has been studied by the formation of the 80K-dCMP complex. Extracts made from cells infected with H5*ts*125 or H5*ts*107 can form nearly identical amounts of 80K-dCMP complex at both permissive and nonpermissive temperatures (CHALLBERG et al. 1982; FRIEFELD et al. 1983a). The addition of purified Ad DBP does not enhance 80K-dCMP complex formation in either wild-type or mutant infected extracts. The 80K-dCMP complex can also be formed in a purified system consisting of protein factors isolated from uninfected HeLa nuclei and pTP-Pol purified free of Ad DBP (ENOMOTO et al. 1981; IKEDA et al. 1981). These data indicate that the Ad DBP is not essential for the initiation of Ad DNA synthesis under the conditions used. However, the role of Ad DBP in initiation using purified proteins is more complicated and is discussed in a later section.

The role of the Ad DBP has also been studied during the early elongation of the 80K-dCMP to the 26th deoxynucleotide, the first dG in the viral nucleotide sequence. The addition of Ad DBP to this reaction enhanced pTP-26mer production two- to fourfold in H5*ts*125 and H5*ts*107 extracts incubated at nonpermissive temperatures, but had little effect on wild-type or mutant extracts incubated at permissive temperature. Dependence of this reaction on Ad DBP is not complete, as a residual amount of the pTP-26mer is formed in the *ts* extracts at nonpermissive temperatures. Similar residual amounts of the pTP-26mer are formed in the presence of HeLa nuclear extract and wild-type pTP-Pol purified free of Ad DBP. Early elongation may be facilitated by a component in HeLa nuclear extract, such as a host DBP, which may partially substitute for the Ad DBP.

Specific DNA synthesis, measured in an assay using *Xba*I cleaved Ad DNA-pro, required the presence of a functional Ad DBP. The effects of purified *ts* Ad DBPs were assayed in the presence of purified pTP-Pol and uninfected HeLa nuclear extract (Fig. 10). At permissive temperatures, Ad DBP isolated from H5*ts*125 or H5*ts*107 infected cells by chromatography on DEAE-cellulose and single-strand DNA agarose columns complemented purified pTP-Pol and HeLa nuclear extract to allow specific replication; however, at nonpermissive temperatures, the Ad DBPs isolated from H5*ts*125 and H5*ts*107 were inactive. Controls using Ad2 DBP were active at both temperatures, indicating no inhibition by the elevated temperatures alone (FRIEFELD et al. 1983a).

Ad DBP is phosphorylated asymmetrically; the phosphate residues are concentrated at the amino end of the protein (KLEIN et al. 1979; LINNE and PHILIPSON 1980). Proteolytic fragments of the Ad DBP were prepared and purified in order to define the active site on the 72K DBP. Chymotryptic digestion of the 72K Ad DBP produced a 27K, heavily phosphorylated, N-terminal fragment and a 44K C-terminal fragment which contained one or a few phosphorylation sites (KLEIN et al. 1979). The 44K C-terminus complemented in vitro Ad DNA replication in an elongation system using crude nuclear extracts prepared from H5*ts*125-infected cells (ARIGA et al. 1980). These extracts contained endogenous *ts* Ad DBP, but became dependent on exogenous wild-type Ad DBP

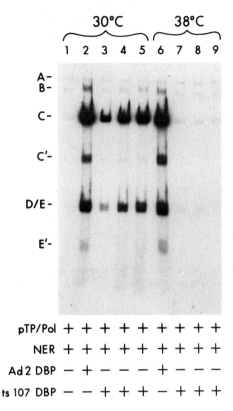

Fig. 10. Requirements for elongation with purified H5ts107 Ad DBP. Elongation on *Xba*I terminal restriction fragments was analyzed as in Fig. 9. All lanes contained Ad2 DNA-pro, pTP-Pol, uninfected HeLa nuclear extract (*NER*), and the additions of DBP as indicated. The reactions were incubated at 120 min at the temperatures indicated. *Ad2 DBP,* 1.5 µg in lanes 2 and 6. ts*107Ad DBP,* 0.5 µg in lanes 3 and 7; 1 µg in lanes 4 and 8; 1.5 µg in lanes 5 and 9

at nonpermissive temperatures. Subsequently, a more purified system devoid of endogenous Ad DBP and dependent only upon the pTP-Pol and an uninfected nuclear extract has been used to show that all the Ad DBP activity necessary for DNA replication resides in a 34K fragment derived from the 44K C-terminal (FRIEFELD et al. (1983a). This 34K fragment, which was approximately as active as intact 72K DBP, contained no detectable ^{32}P when cleaved from Ad DBP which was heavily labeled in vivo with ^{32}P-orthophosphate; thus it appears that the phosphorylated region at the N-terminus of the intact Ad DBP is unnecessary for DNA synthesis in vitro under the conditions used (Fig. 11).

Nitrocellulose filter binding studies were performed to compare Ad DBP binding to Ad single-strand DNA and elongation on terminal restriction fragments of Ad DNA-pro under the conditions of the in vitro synthesis reaction (Krevolin and Horwitz, manuscript in preparation). Both the 72K Ad DBP and the 34K C-terminus from wild-type-infected cells bound to DNA and supported DNA elongation in vitro. A 34K chymotryptic C-terminal fragment prepared from Ad DBP isolated from H5ts107-infected cells was shown to be *ts* both for in vitro DNA elongation and for DNA binding. However, the 72K Ad DBP prepared from H5ts107-infected cells was shown to be *ts* for elongation, but still bound to DNA as well as wild-type Ad DBP. It was con-

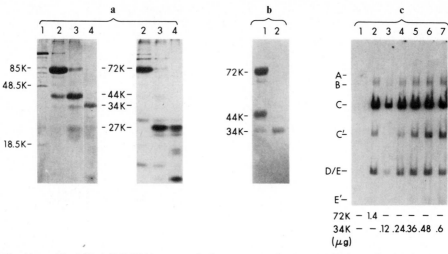

Fig. 11 a–c. The 34K Ad2 DBP chymotryptic fragment complements Ad DNA replication in vitro.
a ^{32}P-labeled Ad2 DBP was digested for 30 min with chymotrypsin (0.34 μg/ml, lane *2;* 0.91 μg/ml,
lane *3;* 9.1 μg/ml, lane *4*) and electrophoresed on a 15% NaDodSO$_4$-polyacrylamide gel. The gel
was stained with Coomassie blue (*left*) and autoradiographed for 48 h (*right*). The numbers to the
left represent the molecular weight of virion markers (lane 1). The numbers in the *center* represent
the calculated molecular weight of Ad2 DBP and its fragments. **b** The 34K fragment of Ad2 DBP
was purified through single-stranded DNA agarose; a Coomassie blue stain of an acrylamide gel
electropherogram of 2 μg of the fragment is shown in lane 2. Markers of a partial digest of the
purified 72K Ad DBP are shown in lane 1. **c** The purified 34K fragment of Ad2 DBP shown
in *b* was used to complement the replication of Ad2 terminal restriction fragments in vitro. All
reactions contained Ad2 DNA-pro, uninfected nuclear extract, and pTP-Pol freed of endogenous
DBP. Lane *1* contained no 72K or 34K DBP. Lane 2 contained 72K DBP and lanes *3–7* contained
increasing concentrations of the 34K fragment as indicated in the figure. The reactions were incubated
at 30° C for 120 min

cluded from this data that DNA binding was necessary but not sufficient to
ensure DNA replication. The C-terminus of the Ad DBP appears to be involved
in DNA binding as well as the in vitro elongation reaction; the phosphorylated
amino end of the Ad DBP is not directly needed for these two reactions but
may play a role in helping to stabilize a conformation needed for DNA binding.

5 Host Factors

The separation of the in vitro system into an infected cytoplasmic component
and an uninfected nuclear component has permitted the characterization of
host-coded factors involved in Ad DNA replication. The uninfected nuclear
extract, which is required for both pTP-dCMP complex formation and chain
elongation, has been fractionated and two host-derived proteins have been identified. Nuclear factor I, a 47K protein that stimulates pTP-dCMP complex
formation and dNMP incorporation in the Ad DNA elongation system, and

Table 3. Requirements for Ad DNA-pro replication with purified proteins

Conditions	DNA synthesis (%)	
	A	B
Complete	100	
− pTP-Pol fraction or − Ad DBP or − Ad DNA-pro	<1	
− nuclear factor I and nuclear factor II	6	
− nuclear factor II	30	
− nuclear factor I	9	
Complete		100
+ aphidicolin (10 μM)		45
+ aphidicolin (100 μM)		10
− ATP		31

100% synthesis in A and B was 6.13 and 5.90 pmol respectively of dTMP incorporation in 60 min at 30° C. Reaction mixtures were as in Table 1

nuclear factor II, which stimulates dNMP incorporation only in the presence of nuclear factor I, have been purified (NAGATA et al. 1982, 1983a). In the presence of both nuclear factors and the three viral proteins (described above), full-length 36-kb Ad DNA is synthesized with Ad DNA-pro as the template.

DNA synthesis using the completely purified system containing the pTP-Pol, Ad DBP, nuclear factors I and II, and Ad DNA-pro was totally dependent on the presence of Ad DNA-pro, pTP-Pol, and Ad DBP (Table 3). In the presence of both the pTP-Pol and Ad DBP, synthesis was stimulated fivefold by the addition of nuclear factor I, but not by the addition of nuclear factor II. The simultaneous addition of nuclear factors I and II stimulated DNA synthesis 15-fold. Stimulation of DNA synthesis by nuclear factor II was completely dependent on the presence of nuclear factor I. Maximal replication of Ad DNA-pro with purified proteins required ATP and was inhibited by aphidicolin to the same extent found with crude extracts which supported in vitro Ad DNA replication.

5.1 Nuclear Factor I

Nuclear factor I has been purified free of detectable DNA polymerase α, β, and γ activities to yield a single peak of activity sedimenting with an apparent molecular mass of 47K after glycerol gradient centrifugation. In the presence of pTP-Pol and Ad DNA-pro as template, low levels of pTP-dCMP complex can be formed in the absence of nuclear fractions. This reaction is stimulated by nuclear factor I and by ATP. The addition of Ad DBP (in the absence of nuclear fractions) inhibits pTP-dCMP complex formation markedly. This inhibition can be overcome by the addition of nuclear factor I. Under these

Table 4. Requirements for pTP-dCMP complex formation with purified components

pTP-Pol	Nuclear factor I	Ad DBP	ATP	pTP-dCMP formed (fmol)
+	+	+	+	0.93
+	+	+	−	0.43
+	−	+	−	0.05
−	+	+	+	0.05
+	+	−	+	0.33
+	−	−	+	0.15
+	+	−	−	0.13
+	−	−	−	0.07

Reaction mixtures contained 25 mM Hepes (pH 7.5), 5 mM MgCl$_2$, 4 mM dithiothreitol, 3 mM ATP, 0.5 µM (α^{32}P)-dCTP (specific activity 400–410 Ci/mmol), 10 µg bovine serum albumin, 0.1 µg Ad DNA-pro, and, where indicated, glycerol-gradient-purified pTP-Pol, 1 µg Ad DBP, and 10 ng nuclear factor I. No detectable pTP-dCMP complex was observed in the absence of Ad DNA-pro, the Ad protein fraction, or MgCl$_2$. Incubation was for 60 min at 30° C

conditions, complex formation is completely dependent on nuclear factor I, and ATP further stimulates this reaction (Table 4).

The formation of the pTP-dCMP complex (80K) and its elongation to the pTP-26mer (88K) have been studied using the purified nuclear factors (NAGATA et al. 1983a). In the presence of pTP-Pol and Ad DNA-pro as template, the formation of both 80K and 88K complexes were stimulated by the addition of nuclear factor I; however, the 80K product predominated. When Ad DBP was added to the reaction, the 88K product predominated, in agreement with previous data using crude nuclear extracts which showed that Ad DBP stimulated formation of pTP-26mer by two- to fourfold. Nuclear factor I both stimulates pTP-dCMP complex formation and appears to act in the early stages of the elongation reaction in concert with the pTP, Pol, and Ad DBP. Products synthesized by these proteins are elongated to approximately 30% of the length of full-sized Ad DNA-pro (Fig. 12).

The nuclear factor I stimulatory activity for pTP-dCMP complex formation and the complementing activity in the Ad DNA-pro elongation assay were both sensitive to N-ethylmaleimide treatment. Both activities were unaffected by heat treatment at 55° C for 15 min but were totally inactivated at 90° C for 2 min. Nuclear factor I contained no detectable nuclease, topoisomerase I, DNA-dependent and independent ATPase, RNA polymerase, or DNA polymerase activities. The presence of nuclear factor I did not alter the nucleotide specificity of complex formation. Maximal stimulation of pTP-dCMP complex formation by nuclear factor I required the presence of ATP in both the presence and the absence of Ad DBP. pTP-dCMP complex formation can occur on single-stranded DNA in the presence of pTP-Pol (IKEDA et al. 1982). This reaction, which is inhibited by Ad DBP, is unaffected by nuclear factor I and thus differs from the reaction on double-stranded DNA template.

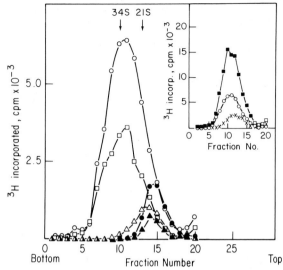

Fig. 12. Alkaline sucrose gradient sedimentation of Ad DNA synthesized in vitro. Products were formed with pTP-Pol fraction, Ad DBP, and nuclear factor I in the absence (Δ) or presence of nuclear factor II (o) or 2 units HeLa type I DNA topoisomerase (□). Similar reactions were carried out in the presence of 100 μM aphidicolin and are represented by the filled-in symbols (•, ▲). Reaction mixtures (50 µl) contained 25 mM Hepes (pH 7.5), 5 mM MgCl$_2$, 4 mM dithiothreitol, 3 mM ATP, 40 µM each of dATP, dGTP and dCTP, 4 µM ^{3}H-dTTP (6600 cpm/pmol), 10 µg bovine serum albumin, and 0.5 µg Ad DNA-pro. Reactions were carried out at 30° C for 120 min. Products were processed and centrifuged at 45000 rpm in a Beckman SW 50.1 rotor for 2.5 h at 4° C in 5–20% alkaline sucrose gradients (0.3 N NaOH/1 M NaCl/10 mM EDTA/0.1% sarkosyl). *Arrows* indicate the positions of the 34S ^{14}C-Ad-DNA single strands as an internal marker and of a 21S ^{32}P-labeled pBR322 recombinant DNA single strand as an external marker in a parallel gradient. Sedimentation was from right to left. The *insert* shows profiles of products formed after incubation of pTP-Pol, Ad DBP, nuclear factor I, and nuclear factor II at 30° C for 30 min (x), 120 min (o), or 360 min (■)

Nuclear factor I, Ad DBP, and ATP may stimulate initiation of Ad DNA-pro by exposing a single-stranded region near the terminal which contains a specific DNA sequence or structure needed for pTP-dCMP synthesis. Studies using cloned Ad DNA fragments lacking the 55K parental TP have provided evidence for such a sequence or structure. These experiments utilized plasmid pLA1 DNA, which contains a 3290-bp fragment derived from the left-hand terminal (0–9.4 map units) of Ad5 DNA (TAMANOI and STILLMAN 1982). It has recently been shown that nuclear factor I binds selectively to a 451-bp DNA fragment containing the adenoviral terminal sequence from 0 to 3 map units, but lacking the 55K TP (NAGATA et al. 1983b) (Fig. 13). Retention of the labeled DNA fragment on nitrocellulose filters by nuclear factor I did not require Mg^{2+} or ATP. Selective binding of nuclear factor I to the 451-bp sequence did not require the sequence to be at the termini of the DNA fragment in which it was located, nor was binding affected by the distance of the sequence from the termini. The binding of nuclear factor I may facilitate strand separation of the template Ad DNA-pro, exposing single-stranded regions that could interact with pTP and Pol.

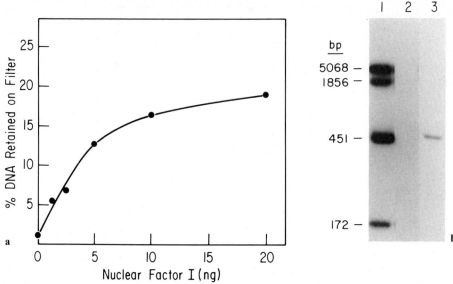

Fig. 13a, b. DNA-binding property of nuclear factor I. **a** Nitrocellulose filter binding assay. DNA-binding activity of nuclear factor I (glycerol gradient fraction) was assayed as a function of the amount of protein added. pLA1 DNA was digested with *Eco*RI and *Pvu*II and treated with *E. coli* alkaline phosphatase. The 5′ ends of DNA fragments were labeled with (γ^{32}P)-ATP and T4 polynucleotide kinase. Nuclear factor I was incubated in a reaction mixture (50 μl) containing 25 mM Hepes/NaOH (pH 7.5), 5 mM MgCl$_2$, 4 mM dithiothreitol, 3 mM ATP, 10 μg bovine serum albumin, 150 mM NaCl, and 40 ng 5′-^{32}P-labeled DNA (1.6×10^2 cpm/ng). After 20 min at 30° C the mixture was filtered through a nitrocellulose membrane (Millipore HAWP). The filter was washed five times with 0.5 ml of a buffer containing 25 mM Hepes/NaOH (pH 7.5), 5 mM MgCl$_2$, 4 mM dithiothreitol, and 150 mM NaCl, dried, and the radioactivity retained was counted by Cerenkov radiation. **b** Analysis of DNA retained on nitrocellulose filters. DNA fragments retained on the filter under the above condition were eluted with 10 mM TRIS-HCl (pH 7.5) 5 mM EDTA/0.2% NaDodSO$_4$. *E. coli* tRNA (30 μg) was added to each eluate and the DNA was precipitated with ethanol. DNA fragments in each sample were analyzed by polyacrylamide slab gel electrophoresis (3.5%; 10 cm × 15 cm × 0.1 cm) with TRIS-borate buffer (89 mM TRIS base/89 mM boric acid/2 mM EDTA) and autoradiographed. Lane *1*, control sample; lane *2*, no protein added; lane *3*, nuclear factor 1 (10 ng)

Footprinting experiments using pancreatic DNase I have revealed that nuclear factor I specifically protected a 32-bp sequence located between nucleotides 17 and 48 of the Ad DNA region cloned onto plasmid pLA1; the sequence on the complementing strand was also protected (Fig. 14) (NAGATA et al. 1983b). The 32-bp sequence has the potential to form a hairpin structure, and remarkably it contains the four "consensus" sequences found at the DNA terminus of many Ad serotypes (Fig. 15).

The binding of Ad DBP, pTP-Pol complex, and nuclear factor I to DNA containing the 451-bp sequence noted in Fig. 14 has been examined (Table 5). At low ionic strength (0.05 M NaCl), nuclear factor I binds to duplex DNA containing this sequence. Ad DBP can also bind to duplex DNA at low ionic strength. In the presence of 0.15 M NaCl, only nuclear factor I binds significantly to this DNA. The same sequence contained within heat-denatured DNA supports the binding of Ad DBP, pTP-Pol, and nuclear factor I at low ionic

SEQUENCES PROTECTED BY FACTOR I; HIGHER ORDER STRUCTURE

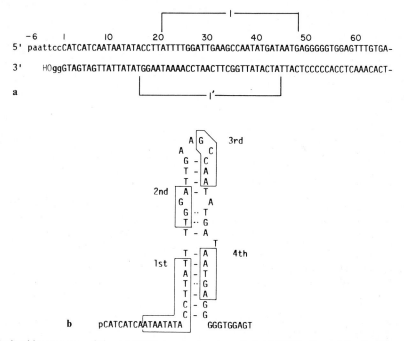

Fig. 14. a Nucleotide sequence of the Ad DNA terminal region of pLA1 DNA digested by *Eco*RI. Small letters *aattcc* represent the *Eco*RI linker sequence which was added in the construction of pLA1 DNA. Capital letters represent the left-hand terminal nucleotide sequence derived from Ad5 DNA. Brackets 1 and 1′ indicate regions protected against DNase 1 attack by nuclear factor 1. **b** Possible secondary structure of the DNA region at the nuclear factor I binding site. The boxed sequences represent four consensus sequences found in several serotypes of Ad DNA as shown in Fig. 15

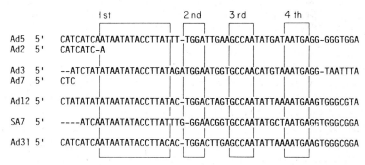

Fig. 15. Comparison of the terminal nucleotide sequence from different adenoviruses. Sequences which are shared between different adenoviruses are boxed (1st, 2nd, 3rd and 4th consensus sequences). The Ad5 sequence is taken from STEENBERGH et al. (1977), the Ad2 sequence from ARRAND and ROBERTS (1979) and SHINAGAWA and PADMANABHAN (1979), the Ad3, Ad12, and SA7 sequences from TOLUN et al. (1979), the Ad7 sequence from DIJKEMA and DEKKER (1979), the Ad31 from STILLMAN et al. (1982), and the Ad12 from SUGISAKI et al. (1980). Human adenoviruses are categorized into five serological subgroups (A to E). The 1st consensus sequence is common to all of the human adenoviruses. Ad12 and Ad31 (group A), Ad3 and Ad7 (group B), and Ad2 and Ad5 (group C) contain the other three consensus sequences. Ad9 and Ad10 (group D) do not contain the 2nd and 3rd consensus sequences but do contain the 4th (STILLMAN et al. 1982b)

Table 5. Influence of salt and DNA secondary structure on protein-DNA interaction

Protein added	% DNA retained on filter			
	Native		Heat-denatured	
	0.05 M NaCl	0.15 M NaCl	0.05 M NaCl	0.15 M NaCl
None	1.8	1.5	3.7	1.4
Ad DBP	28.5	1.8	84.5	90.2
pTP-Ad Pol	1.7	0.8	78.5	2.0
Nuclear factor I	81.9	40.7	36.0	3.2

The nitrocellulose filter binding assay was done in a 50-μl reaction mixture containing ^{32}P-end-labeled DNA, 25 mM Hepes (pH 7.5), 5 mM MgCl$_2$, 4 mM dithiothreitol, 10 μg bovine serum albumin, various protein fractions, and NaCl concentrations as indicated. Reactions were incubated at 0° C for 20 min and filtered through a nitrocellulose filter (Millipore Corp. HA 0.45 μm). Filters were washed five times with 0.5 ml of a buffer containing 25 mM Hepes (pH 7.5), 5 mM MgCl$_2$, 4 mM dithiothreitol, and the same concentration of NaCl as added to the reaction mixture. After drying, filters were counted by Cerenkov radiation. Assays for filter binding studies contained 7.5 ng of either the native or heat-denatured 451-bp *Eco*RI-*Pvu*II DNA fragment as in Fig. 13 in the presence of Ad DBP (0.9 μg), pTP-Pol (8 ng), nuclear factor I (10 ng), or with no protein

strength. However, at high ionic strength, only Ad DBP retains the ability to bind to single-strand DNA.

Footprinting experiments have been carried out in the presence of both Ad DBP and pTP-Pol. Under the conditions used (high ionic strength), Ad DBP alone protected the entire 451-nucleotide region, indicating its lack of binding specificity. Interestingly, in the presence of both nuclear factor I and Ad DBP, significant nuclease attack was detected between nucleotides 10 and 20; no cleavage was detected within the region between positions 21 and 48 protected by nuclear factor I alone (Fig. 14a). VAN BERGEN et al. (1983) have reported that the first consensus sequence may be essential for the formation of the pTP-dCMP initiation complex. It is possible that the first consensus sequence is exposed in the presence of nuclear factor I and Ad DBP and that this exposed region is utilized by the pTP-Pol complex as a site for binding. Such a model suggests a complex involving five proteins essential for the initiation of DNA replication. These proteins, the pTP-Pol, Ad DBP, nuclear factor I, and the 55K TP must interact in a specific manner occupying the first 50 bp of the Ad DNA. In addition, we know that ATP stimulates initiation and elongation reactions; however, it is not clear whether ATP plays any role in the generation of the proposed protein complexes.

5.2 Nuclear Factor II

Nuclear factor II complementing activity was separated from nuclear factor I by chromatography on DEAE-cellulose and on carboxymethylcellulose. DNA

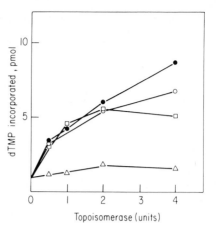

Fig. 16. Substitution of nuclear factor II by DNA topoisomerases. Reaction mixtures, as described in Fig. 12, contained nuclear factor II (●), type I topoisomerase purified from HeLa cells (o), type I topoisomerase purified from calf thymus (□), or *E. coli* type I topoisomerase (△). One unit of topoisomerase activity was the amount required for complete conversion of 0.3 µg ΦX174 from I DNA to topoisomers in 60 min at 30° C

polymerases α and γ were removed by adsorption to DEAE-cellulose, while DNA polymerase β was removed by chromatography on denatured DNA cellulose (NAGATA et al. 1983a).

Nuclear factor II had no effect on the formation of the pTP-dCMP complex, the synthesis of the 88K pTP-26mer, or the replication of *Xba*I-generated terminal restriction fragments of Ad DNA-pro. In the presence of pTP-Pol and Ad DBP, elongation on Ad DNA-pro template was stimulated by the addition of nuclear factor I alone, but not by the addition of nuclear factor II alone. However, the addition of both nuclear factors stimulated DNA synthesis 15-fold, a value higher than that expected from the additive effect of each alone. Omission of nuclear factor II resulted in the synthesis of DNA which was approximately 25–30% of full-length 34S Ad DNA.

Gel filtration indicated that nuclear factor II complementing activity eluted as a protein with native molecular weight varying between 25K and 45K with a Stokes radius of 26Å. NaDodSO$_4$-polyacrylamide gel electrophoresis of fractions obtained by gel filtration showed the presence of two major bands at 14.5 and 15.5K and a minor band at 30.5K. Nuclear factor II contained no detectable DNA or RNA polymerase, DNA-dependent or -independent ATPase activities, or ribo- or deoxyribonuclease. The most purified fractions of nuclear factor II contained a DNA topoisomerase activity. Both the nuclear factor II DNA-complementing activity and topoisomerase activities were sensitive to *N*-ethylmaleimide and were inactivated by heat. The topoisomerase activity did not require Mg^{2+} or ATP and remained unaffected by 0.2 *M* NaCl or KCl; the enzyme changed the linking number of a unique topoisomer of plasmid pAO3 in steps of one, characteristic of a type I DNA topoisomerase. Aphidicolin and nuclear factor I had no effect on the topoisomerase.

Eukaryotic topoisomerases substituted for nuclear factor II in the presence of pTP-Pol, Ad DBP, Ad DNA-pro, and nuclear factor I, while *E. coli* type I topoisomerase was inactive in the complementation assay (Fig. 16). Purified type I topoisomerase from HeLa cells and calf thymus replaced nuclear factor II in the formation of full-length Ad DNA in vitro. These results indicate that topoisomerase I may play an important role in altering higher-order DNA structures near the replication fork only after extensive DNA synthesis. The topoisomerase may act to untangle complicated DNA structures which inhibit the orderly translocation of the replication complex generated by strand displacement and fork movement.

6 DNA Requirements

DNA replication using either crude extracts or purified proteins required Ad DNA-pro as template. No DNA synthesis or initiation (pTP-dCMP complex formation) was observed with protease-treated Ad DNA. These results suggest that initiation of replication may involve recognition of the 55K TP bound to the template, or possibly some structure near the terminal that is maintained by the covalently bound protein. However, it remains unclear whether the protein bound to the template DNA is required for replicative DNA synthesis.

The observation that single-stranded ϕX174 DNA supported the synthesis of protein-linked DNA chains by the action of the purified pTP-Pol (IKEDA et al. (1982) indicated that protein bound to the template was not required for initiation under certain conditions. Products of the elongation of pTP-dCMP complex formed with ϕX174 single-stranded circular DNA as template were predominantly derived from the sequences between nucleotides 2363 and 2977 and nucleotides 3760 and 4206. Computer search showed that the heptanucleotide T-A-T-T-T-T-G, present between nucleotides 19 and 25 from the 5' ends of Ad2 DNA, was present in both sites of ϕX174 DNA that supported protein-primed DNA chain elongation. However, the reaction observed with ϕX174 DNA differed from that observed with Ad DNA-pro in two fundamental characteristics (IKEDA et al. 1982). First, the Ad DBP strongly inhibited pTP-dCMP complex formation with ϕX174 DNA. In the presence of uninfected nuclear extract and Ad-infected cytosol, the Ad DBP had no effect on complex formation using Ad DNA-pro as template. The addition of nuclear extract abolished the reaction with single-stranded DNA. Second, ATP, which stimulated pTP-dCMP synthesis two- to fivefold and DNA synthesis by more than tenfold when Ad DNA-pro was the template, inhibited pTP-dCMP synthesis with ϕX174 DNA. Thus the reaction on ϕX174 DNA seemed to be a type of nonreplicative initiation of DNA synthesis, leaving open the possibility that the TP bound to the template was required for replicative synthesis. Furthermore, restriction fragments isolated from double-stranded ϕXRFI using *HaeIII* were totally inactive in supporting pTP-dCMP complex formation. However, heat denaturation of the fragments rendered all sequences active.

TAMANOI and STILLMAN (1982) have argued that the inactivity of deproteinized Ad DNA in the in vitro system is an artifact due to the method used to remove the TP. They found that treatment of Ad DNA-pro with proteases, which leaves a short peptide at the 5'-terminals of the DNA strands, rendered the DNA inactive. In contrast, removal of the protein with piperidine, which cleaves the alkali-labile phosphodiester bond between the protein and the DNA terminus, leaving no residual peptide, yielded a protein-free DNA template which supported pTP-dCMP synthesis and elongation to lengths of about 100 bases. However, the piperidine-treated DNA did not support these reactions in crude extracts (which did replicate Ad DNA-pro), but only with extracts which had been adsorbed to and eluted from DNA-cellulose columns.

TAMANOI and STILLMAN (1982) and VAN BERGEN et al. (1983) studied DNA synthesis on plasmids containing cloned origins of Ad DNA replication. When these protein-free DNAs are used as templates, pTP-dCMP complex can be formed only when the plasmid is linearized so that the origin of Ad DNA replication is located at the end of the molecule. Neither linearized plasmid DNA with an internal origin nor supercoiled plasmid DNA supported complex formation. After heat denaturation, the linear plasmid DNA supported complex formation; no specific origin is required under these conditions. These results suggest that a specific duplex DNA sequence, and not the presence of the parental TP, is required for the initiation reaction. This sequence must be located at the termini of duplex DNA. However, initiation and elongation on the double-stranded Ad sequence devoid of TP is only about 3–5% of that observed with Ad DNA-pro (Guggenheimer et al., manuscript in preparation).

Recent studies by Guggenheimer et al. (manuscript in preparation) indicate that the replication of pLA1 RFIII DNA containing the cloned origin of Ad DNA at an end requires another host protein in addition to nuclear factors I and II. This host protein has been isolated from nuclear extracts of uninfected HeLa cells. In the presence of this newly identified protein, pTP-Pol, Ad DBP, and nuclear factor I, both pTP-dCMP complex formation and DNA synthesis occur. All nucleotide incorporation on nascent chains occurred covalently linked to protein; full-length duplex DNA products were formed, their size dependent upon the length of the RFIII pLA1 derivative used in the reaction. The nature and mechanism of action of the new host protein which is specific for pLA1 DNA should help to define the role played by the Ad DNA terminal protein.

7 Inhibition of Ad DNA Synthesis by SLE Sera

It has been found that some patients with systemic lupus erythematosus (SLE) have a serum inhibitor that interferes with in vitro Ad DNA replication (HORWITZ et al. 1982). The inhibitor, which was present in sera containing antibody to *ds* DNA, copurified with IgG by sodium sulfate precipitation, DEAE-cellulose chromatography, polyacrylamide gel electrophoresis, immunoelectrophoresis, and sucrose density gradient sedimentation, and was presumably *ds* DNA antibody. The site of action of the *ds* DNA antibody appeared to be after the polymerization of the 26th deoxynucleotide in the elongation reaction.

8 Summary and Prospects

Analysis of eukaryotic replication mechanisms depends on the use of model systems which can be readily manipulated in vitro. Of the available systems, adenovirus is the only one for which the entire process of replication can be carried out in vitro. For this reason, the adenovirus system has proved uniquely suitable to biochemical analysis of the type described in this review. The results obtained have helped define some of the mechanisms used and proteins required in adenovirus DNA replication. These findings can be used to construct a working model. The observations governing this model include the following:

1. Progeny DNA synthesis begins with the covalent linkage of the first nucleotide to protein.
2. The specific initiation reaction with Ad DNA-pro most likely involves the pTP, Pol, TP covalently linked to Ad DNA, the Ad DBP, and nuclear factor I. These purified proteins may form a specific complex governed by the four consensus sequences found in many Ad serotypes.
3. The only DNA polymerase which functions in Ad DNA replication is the 140K viral-coded polymerase (Pol). This enzyme can elongate synthetic polynucleotides [such as oligo (dA):poly (dT)] in the presence of the Ad DBP. Poly (dA) chains as large as 30kb can be formed, and chains are synthesized at a rate of 20 nucleotides/s at 30° C. In vitro, Ad DNA-pro supports nucleotide incorporation at a rate of about 25 nucleotides/s at 30° C, a rate close to the in vivo rate of Ad DNA replication (NAGATA et al. 1983a).
4. In the absence of nuclear factor II, elongation of Ad DNA proceeds until chains of 10kb are formed. Full-length 35-kb Ad DNA can be formed in the presence of this factor or eukaryotic topoisomerase I.
5. To date, none of the proteins isolated possesses a helicase type activity; none of the fractions contains a DNA-dependent ATPase activity. We assume that by virtue of its ability to displace oligo(dA) hydrogen bonded to the poly(dT) template strand, the complex of Pol and Ad DBP can displace the nontemplate strand, eventually leading to the complete displacement of this strand.

9 Model of Ad DNA-pro Replication

The initiation reaction results in the formation of pTP-dCMP. Maximal synthesis with the Ad DNA-pro requires the pTP, Pol, nuclear factor I, Ad DBP, and ATP. In the absence of pTP, Pol, Ad DNA-pro, or Mg^{2+}, no initiation is detected. In the presence of Ad DBP, the reaction is markedly dependent on nuclear factor I and the reaction is stimulated by ATP. The small but detectable formation of the pTP-dCMP complex that occurs in the presence of pTP and Pol alone is inhibited by *E. coli* ssb, as well as Ad DBP. We suspect that this reflects nonspecific initiation events occurring on single-stranded regions, presumably at the end of DNA chains which may be frayed.

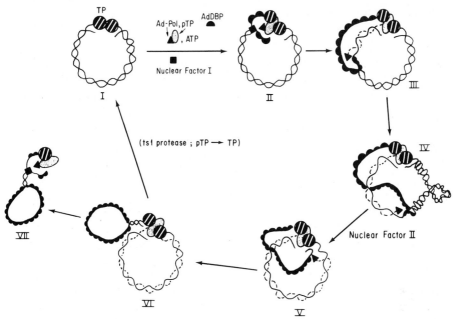

Fig. 17. Proposed model of Ad DNA-pro replication (see text for details)

Thus we envisage an initial reaction in which Ad DBP and nuclear factor I play an important role. The pTP-Pol complex (which is held together by noncovalent linkage) is probably capable of binding to the Ad DNA-pro through interaction between the TP and the pTP. We hypothesize that the specific binding of nuclear factor I to the duplex region between nucleotides 17 and 49 unwinds the duplex at the 5′ end, which aids in the binding of the pTP-Pol complex and Ad DBP. Ad DBP binds to single strands generated by the unwinding or fraying at the 5′ ends accompanying the binding of the 80K pTP.

The incorporation catalyzed by the Pol probably leads to the dissociation of the Pol from the pTP-Pol complex. We know that the further elongation reaction is absolutely dependent on the Ad DBP. This reaction, studied with synthetic polynucleotides, indicates a specific interaction between the Ad Pol and the Ad DBP. We have also found that ATP stimulates the elongation reaction, but this role has yet to be defined.

Electron micrographs of Ad DNA-pro suggest that its structure is circular (ROBINSON et al. 1973; ROBINSON and BELLETT 1975). Removal of the protein results in the formation of linear duplex structures. With this in mind, we suggest that the overall pathway can be summarized as described in Fig. 17. In this model, initiation and elongation result in the displacement reaction leading to the formation of structure II. With continued elongation, a replication intermediate (III) is formed. In the absence of topoisomerase I activity, structure IV accumulates. It is interesting to note that aphidicolin, which has no effect on the Ad polymerase in the usual activated calf thymus DNA assay (which is carried out in the presence of a large excess of primer 3'-OH ends), does inhibit extensive Ad DNA replication and leads to DNA chains similar in size to those found in reactions lacking topoisomerase. Several explanations for the aphidicolin sensitivity of Ad DNA replication remain plausible. First, aphidicolin may act at some target other than DNA polymerase, such as the Ad DBP, one of the host-coded factors provided by the nuclear extract, or the replication complex at the branch of the replicating fork (FOSTER et al. 1982). The possibility of aphidicolin action at multiple sites might explain, in part, the greater aphidicolin sensitivity of host DNA replication in comparison to the effect on activity of the purified DNA polymerase α. Second, DNA polymerase α may itself play a role in Ad DNA replication, but be required in such minute quantities that the amount present in the components of the purified system cannot be detected by conventional DNA polymerase assays. A third possibility is that aphidicolin acts directly on the Ad DNA polymerase, but inhibition of DNA synthesis only becomes apparent with the synthesis of long DNA chains, which do not occur in the polymerase assay containing activated DNA. However, aphidicolin does not inhibit the extensive Pol-Ad DBP-dependent translocation of the replication fork that occurs on poly dT:oligo dA.

The addition of topoisomerase I permits the chains to be further elongated, resulting in the displacement of an intact single strand (VI) which can form the panhandle structure shown as structure VII. The complementary regions (the 102 bases at each end) which generate structure VII result in the formation of an end identical to that present in structure I (without circularity). This product contains the duplex nucleotide sequence essential for the binding of nuclear factor I which supports the specific initiation reaction. We suspect that the topoisomerase removes knotted DNA complexes which alter the fork movement. Why it should occur only with chains elongated more than 25% of the length of the genome remains to be elucidated.

The model proposed for the replication of Ad DNA is a modified rolling circle model in which a single-strand displacement occurs concomitant with synthesis. What happens to the proteins upon termination of one round of DNA synthesis remains to be determined, but we have shown that the formation of a replication complex facilitates the use of the replicating molecule for repeated multiple rounds of initiations. We have detected reinitiation in this reaction after as little as 2% net synthesis.

References

Abboud M, Horwitz MS (1979) The DNA polymerase associated with the adenovirus type 2 replication complex: effect of 2'-3'-dideoxythymidine-5'-triphosphate on viral DNA synthesis. Nucleic Acids Res 6:1025

Alestrom P, Akusjarvi G, Pettersson M, Pettersson U (1982) DNA sequence analysis of the region encoding the terminal protein and the hypothetical N-gene product of adenovirus type 2. J Biol Chem 257:13492

Arens M, Yamashita T (1978) In vitro termination of adenovirus DNA synthesis by a soluble replication complex. J Virol 25:698

Ariga H, Klein H, Levine AJ, Horwitz MS (1980) A cleavage product of the adenovirus DNA binding protein is active in DNA replication in vitro. Virology 101:307

Arrand J, Roberts RJ (1979) The nucleotide sequences at the termini of adenovirus 2 DNA. J Mol Biol 128:577

Brison O, Kedinger C, Wilhelm J (1977) Enzymatic properties of viral replication complexes isolated from adenovirus type 2-infected HeLa cell nuclei. J Virol 24:423

Carusi EA (1977) Evidence for blocked 5'-termini in human adenovirus. Virology 76:380

Challberg MD, Kelly TJ Jr (1979a) Adenovirus DNA replication in vitro. Proc Natl Acad Sci USA 76:655

Challberg MD, Kelly TJ Jr (1979b) Adenovirus DNA replication in vitro: Origin and direction of daughter strand synthesis. J Mol Biol 135:999

Challberg MD, Kelly TJ Jr (1981) Processing of the adenovirus terminal protein. J Virol 38:272

Challberg MD, Ostrove JM, Kelly TJ (1982) Initiation of adenovirus DNA replication: Detection of covalent complexes between nucleotide and the 80-kilodalton terminal protein. J Virol 41:265

Challberg MD, Desiderio SV, Kelly TJ Jr (1980) Adenovirus DNA replication in vitro: Characterization of a protein covalently linked to nascent DNA strands. Proc Natl Acad Sci USA 77:5105

Daubert SD, Bruening G, Najarian RC (1978) Protein bound to the genome RNAs of cowpea mosaic virus. Eur J Biochem 92:45

Desiderio SV, Kelly TJ Jr (1981) Structure of the linkage between adenovirus DNA and the 55,000 molecular weight terminal protein. J Mol Biol 145:319

Dijkema R, Dekker BMM (1979) The inverted terminal repetition of the DNA of weakly oncogenic adenovirus type 7. Gene 8:7

Enomoto T, Lichy JH, Ikeda J-E, Hurwitz J (1981) Adenovirus DNA replication in vitro: Purification of the terminal protein in a functional form. Proc Natl Acad Sci USA 78:6779

Foster DA, Hontzopoulos P, Zubay G (1982) Resistance of adenoviral DNA replication to aphidicolin is dependent on the 72-kilodalton DNA-binding protein. J Virol 43:679

Friefeld BR, Krevolin MD, Horwitz MS (1983a) Effects of the adenovirus H5ts125 and H5ts107 DNA binding proteins on DNA replication in vitro. Virology 124:380

Friefeld BR, Lichy JH, Hurwitz J, Horwitz MS (1983b) Evidence for an altered adenovirus DNA polymerase in cells infected with the mutant H5ts149. Proc Natl Acad Sci USA 80:1589

Galos R, Williams J, Binger MH, Flint SJ (1979) Location of additional early gene sequences in the adenoviral chromosome. Cell 17:945

Garon CF, Berry KW, Rose JA (1972) A unique form of terminal redundancy in adenovirus DNA molecules. Proc Natl Acad Sci USA 69:2391

Garon CF, Berry KW, Rose JA (1975) Arrangement of sequences in the inverted terminal repetition of adenovirus 18 DNA. Proc Natl Acad Sci USA 72:3039

Gerlich WH, Robinson WS (1980) Hepatitis B virus contains protein attached to the 5' terminus of its complete DNA strand. Cell 21:801

Gingeras TR, Sciaki D, Gelinas RE, Bing-Dong J, Yen CE, Kelly MM, Bullock PA, Parsons BL, O'Neill KE, Roberts RJ (1982) Nucleotide sequences from the adenovirus 2 genome. J Biol Chem 257:13475

Golini F, Nomoto A, Wimmer E (1978) The genome-linked protein of picornaviruses. IV. Difference in the VPg's of encephalomyocarditis virus and poliovirus as evidence that genome-linked protein are virus-coded. Virology 89:112

Grodzicker TC, Anderson CW, Sambrook J, Mathews MB (1977) The physical locations of structural genes in adenovirus DNA. Virology 80:111

Guggenheimer RA, Nagata K, Field J, Lindenbaum J, Gronostajski RM, Horwitz MS, Hurwitz J (1983) In vitro synthesis of full length adenoviral DNA. Mechanisms of DNA Replication and Recombination Vol X 395

Horwitz MS (1978) Temperature sensitive replication of H5ts125 adenovirus DNA in vitro. Proc Natl Acad Sci USA 75:4291

Horwitz MS, Ariga H (1981) Multiple rounds of adenovirus DNA synthesis in vitro. Proc Natl Acad Sci USA 78:1476

Horwitz MS, Friefeld BR, Keiser HD (1982) Inhibition of adenovirus DNA synthesis in vitro by sera from patients with systemic lupus erythematosus. Mol Cel Biol 2:1492

Ikeda J-E, Enomoto T, Hurwitz J (1981) Replication of the adenovirus DNA protein complex with purified proteins. Proc Natl Acad Sci USA 78:884

Ikeda J-E, Enomoto T, Hurwitz J (1982) Adenoviral protein-primed initiation of DNA chains in vitro. Proc Natl Acad Sci USA 79:2442

Kaplan LM, Kleinman RE, Horwitz MS (1977) Replication of adenovirus type 2 DNA in vitro. Proc Natl Acad Sci USA 74:4425

Kaplan LM, Ariga H, Horwitz MS, Hurwitz J (1979) Complementation of the temperature-sensitive defect in H5ts125 adenovirus DNA replication in vitro. Proc Natl Acad Sci USA 76:5534

Klein H, Maltzman W, Levine AJ (1979) Structure-function relationships of the adenovirus DNA-binding protein. J Biol Chem 254:11051

Kruijer W, van Schaik FMA, Sussenbach JS (1981) Structure and organization of the gene coding for the DNA binding protein of adenovirus type 5. Nucleic Acid Res 9:4439

Kruijer W, Nicolas JC, van Schaik FMA, Sussenbach JS (1983) Structure and function of DNA binding proteins from revertants of adenovirus type 5 mutants with a temperature sensitive DNA replication. Virology 124:425

Lechner RL, Kelly TJ Jr (1977) The structure of replicating adenovirus 2 DNA molecules. Cell 12:1007

Lichy JH, Horwitz MS, Hurwitz J (1981) Formation of a covalent complex between the 80,000 dalton adenovirus terminal protein and 5'-dCMP in vitro. Proc Natl Acad Sci USA 78:2678

Lichy JH, Field J, Horwitz MS, Hurwitz J (1982a) Separation of the adenovirus terminal protein precursor from its associated DNA polymerase: role of both proteins in the initiation of adenovirus DNA replication. Proc Natl Acad Sci USA 79:5225

Lichy JH, Nagata K, Friefeld BR, Enomoto T, Field J, Guggenheimer RA, Ikeda J-E, Horwitz MS, Hurwitz J (1982b) Isolation of proteins involved in the replication of adenoviral DNA in vitro. Cold Spring Harbor Symp Quant Biol 47:731

Linne T, Philipson L (1980) Further characterization of the phosphate moiety of the adenovirus type 2 DNA-binding protein. Eur J Biochem 103:259

Longiaru M, Ikeda J-E, Jarkovsky Z, Horwitz SB, Horwitz MS (1979) Effect of aphidicolin on adenovirus DNA synthesis. Nuc Acid Res 6:3369

Mellado RP, Penalva MA, Inciarte MR, Salas M (1980) The protein covalently linked to the 5' termini of the DNA of *Bacillus subtilis* phage φ29 is involved in the initiation of DNA replication. Virology 104:84

Nagata K, Guggenheimer R, Enomoto T, Lichy JH, Hurwitz J (1982) Adenovirus DNA replication in vitro: Identification of a host factor that stimulates the synthesis of the preterminal protein dCMP-complex. Proc Natl Acad Sci USA 79:6438

Nagata K, Guggenheimer RA, Hurwitz J (1983a) Adenovirus DNA replication in vitro: synthesis of full-length DNA with purified proteins. Proc Natl Acad Sci USA 80:4266

Nagata K, Guggenheimer RA, Hurwitz J (1983b) Specific binding of a cellular DNA replication protein to the origin of replication of adenovirus DNA. Proc Natl Acad Sci USA 80:6177

Ostove JM, Rosenfeld P, Williams J, Kelly TJ (1983) In vitro complementation as an assay for purification of adenovirus DNA replication proteins. Proc Natl Acad Sci USA 80:935

Pénalva MA, Salas M (1982) Initiation of phage φ29 DNA replication in vitro: Formation of a covalent complex between the terminal protein, p3, and 5'-dAMP. Proc Natl Acad Sci USA 79:5522

Pincus S, Robertson W, Rekosh D (1981) Characterization of the effect of aphidicolin on adenovirus DNA replication: evidence in support of a protein primer model of initiation. Nucleic Acid Res 9:4919

Rekosh DMK, Russell WC, Bellett AJD, Robinson AJ (1977) Identification of a protein linked to the ends of adenovirus DNA. Cell 11:283

Revie D, Tseng BY, Grafstrom RH, Goulian M (1979) Covalent association of protein with replicative form DNA of parvovirus H-1. Proc Natl Acad Sci USA 76:5539

Robinson AJ, Younghusband HB, Bellett AJD (1973) A circular DNA protein complex from adenoviruses. Virology 56:54

Robinson AJ, Bellett AJD (1975) Complementary strands of CELO virus DNA. J Virol 15:458

Robinson I, Padmanabhan R (1980) Studies on the nature of the linkage between the terminal protein and the adenovirus DNA. Biochem Biophys Res Commun 94:398

Shinagawa M, Padmanabhan R (1979) Nucleotide sequence at the inverted terminal repetition of adenovirus type 2 DNA. Biochem Biophys Res Commun 87:671

Shinagawa M, Padmanabhan R (1980) Comparative sequence analysis of the inverted terminal repetitions from different adenoviruses. Proc Natl Acad Sci USA 77:3831

Smart J, Stillman BW (1982) Adenovirus terminal protein precursor (Partial amino acid sequence and the site of covalent linkage to virus DNA). J Biol Chem 257:13499

Steenbergh PH, Maat J, van Ormondt H, Sussenbach JS (1977) The nucleotide sequence at the termini of adenovirus type 5 DNA. Nucleic Acids Res 4:4371

Stillman BW (1981) Adenovirus DNA replication in vitro: a protein linked to the 5' end of nascent DNA strands. J Virol 37:139

Stillman BW, Lewis JB, Chow LT, Mathews MB, Smart JE (1981) Identification of the gene and mRNA for the adenovirus terminal protein precursor. Cell 23:497

Stillman BW, Tamanoi F, Mathews MB (1982a) Purification of an adenovirus coded DNA polymerase that is required for initiation of DNA replication. Cell 31:613

Stillman BW, Topp WC, Engler JA (1982b) Conserved sequences at the origin of adenovirus DNA replication. J Virol 44:530

Sugiasaki H, Sugimoto K, Takanami M, Shiroki K, Saito I, Shimojo H, Sawada Y, Yemizu Y, Uesugi S, Fujinage K (1980) Structure and gene organization in the transforming Hind III-G fragment of Ad12. Cell 20:777

Tamanoi F, Stillman BW (1982) Function of adenovirus terminal protein in the initiation of DNA replication. Proc Natl Acad Sci USA 79:2221

Tolun A, Alestrom P, Pettersson U (1979) Sequence of inverted terminal repetitions from different adenoviruses: demonstration of conserved sequences and homology between SA7 termini and SV40 DNA. Cell 17:705

Van Bergen BGM, van der Ley PA, van Driel W, van Mansfeld ADM, van der Vliet PC (1983) Replication of origin containing adenovirus DNA fragments that do not carry the terminal protein. Nucleic Acids Res 11:1975

Van der Werf S, Bouche JP, Mechali M, Girard M (1980) Involvement of both DNA polymerase and in the replication of adenovirus deoxyribonucleic acid in vitro. Virology 104:56

Wolfson J, Dressler D (1972) Adenovirus 2 DNA contains an inverted terminal repetition. Proc Natl Acad Sci USA 69:3054

Note Added in Proof

Deletion mutant derivatives of the Adenovirus DNA replication origin contained within the 6.6 kb plasmid, pLAI, have been used to analyze the nucleotide sequences required for the formation and subsequent elongation of the pTP-dCMP initiation complex[1]. The existence of two domains within the first fifty base-pairs of the Ad genome has been demonstrated. Both of these are required for the efficient use of recombinant DNA molecules as templates in crude as well as in purified in vitro DNA replication systems. The first domain, consisting of a ten base pair "core" sequence located at nucleotide position 9–18 has been tentatively identified as a binding site for the pTP (RIJINDERS et al. 1983). The second required domain, consisting of a 32 base pair region spanning nucleotides 17–48, has been shown to be essential for the binding of nuclear factor I (NAGATA et al. 1983).

---

1 Guggenheimer RA, Stillman BW, Nagata K, Tamanoi F, Hurwitz J (1984). DNA Sequence Required for the in vitro Replication of Adenovirus DNA. Proc. Natl. Acad. Sci. USA (in press)

Erratum

to Current Topics in Microbiology and Immunology, Vol. 109
DOERFLER et al.: On the Mechanism of Recombination Between Adenoviral
and Cellular DNAs: The Structure of Junction Sites

On page 218, lines 10/11 the sentence should read:
"..., in that in some of the clones specific alterations were introduced..."

Subject Index

The Molecular Biology of Adenoviruses 1

30 Years of Adenovirus Research 1953–1983

Editor: **W. Doerfler**

1983. 69 figures. XII, 232 pages
(Current Topics in Microbiology and Immunology,
Volume 109)
ISBN 3-540-13034-9

Contents:
L. Philipson: Structure and Assembly of Adenoviruses. – *J.S. Sussenbach, P.C. van der Vliet:* The Mechanism of Adenovirus DNA Replication and the Characterization of Replication Proteins. – *F. Tamanoi, B.W. Stillman:* The Origin of Adenovirus DNA Replication. – *M. Salas:* A New Mechanism for the Initiation of Replication of $\phi 29$ and Adenovirus DNA: Priming by the Terminal Protein. – *U. Pettersson, A. Virtanen, M. Perricaudet, G. Akusjärvi:* The Messenger RNAs from the Transforming Region of Human Adenoviruses. – *R. Weinmann, S. Ackerman, D. Bunick, M. Concino, R. Zandomeni:* In Vitro Transcription of Adenovirus Genes. – *W.D. Richardson, H. Westphal:* Adenovirus Early Gene Regulation and the Adeno-associated Virus Helper Effect. – *M. Green, K.H. Brackmann, L.A. Lucher, J.S. Symington:* Antibodies to Synthetic Peptides Targeted to the Transforming Genes of Human Adenoviruses – An Approach to Understanding Early Viral Gene Function. – *W. Doerfler, R. Gahlmann, S. Stabel, R. Deuring, U. Lichtenberg, M. Schulz, D. Eick, R. Leisten:* On the Mechanism of Recombination Between Adenoviral and Cellular DNAs: The Structure of Junction Sites. – Subject Index.

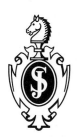

Springer-Verlag
Berlin
Heidelberg
New York
Tokyo

The Molecular Biology of Adenoviruses 3

30 Years of Adenovirus Research 1953-1983

Editor: **Walter Doerfler**

1984.
(Current Topics in Microbiology and
Immunology, Volume 111)
ISBN 3-540-13138-8
In preparation

Contents:

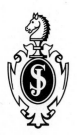

Springer-Verlag
Berlin
Heidelberg
NewYork
Tokyo